Mental and Behavioral Health of Immigrants in the United States

Mental and Behavioral Health of Immigrants in the United States

Cultural, Environmental, and Structural Factors

Edited by

Gordon C. Nagayama Hall

ELSEVIER

ACADEMIC PRESS

An imprint of Elsevier

Academic Press
125 London Wall, London EC2Y 5AS, United Kingdom
525 B Street, Suite 1650, San Diego, CA 92101, United States
50 Hampshire Street, 5th Floor, Cambridge, MA 02139, United States
The Boulevard, Langford Lane, Kidlington, Oxford OX5 1GB, United Kingdom

Notices

Knowledge and best practice in this field are constantly changing. As new research and experience broaden our understanding, changes in research methods, professional practices, or medical treatment may become necessary.

Practitioners and researchers must always rely on their own experience and knowledge in evaluating and using any information, methods, compounds, or experiments described herein. In using such information or methods they should be mindful of their own safety and the safety of others, including parties for whom they have a professional responsibility.

To the fullest extent of the law, neither the Publisher nor the authors, contributors, or editors, assume any liability for any injury and/or damage to persons or property as a matter of products liability, negligence or otherwise, or from any use or operation of any methods, products, instructions, or ideas contained in the material herein.

Library of Congress Cataloging-in-Publication Data
A catalog record for this book is available from the Library of Congress

British Library Cataloguing-in-Publication Data
A catalogue record for this book is available from the British Library

ISBN 978-0-12-816117-3

Publisher: Nikki Levy
Editorial Project Manager: Barbara Makinster
Production Project Manager: Swapna Srinivasan
Cover Designer: Mark Rogers

Typeset by SPi Global, India

Contents

Contributors

Numbers in paraentheses indicate the pages on which the authors' contributions begin.

Carmela Alcántara (279), School of Social Work, Columbia University, New York, NY, United States

Francheska Alers-Rojas (135), University of Michigan, Ann Arbor, MI, United States

Miriam J. Alvarez (71), University of Texas at El Paso, El Paso, TX, United States

Angel D. Armenta (71), University of Texas at El Paso, El Paso, TX, United States

Germine H. Awad (201), The University of Texas at Austin, Austin, TX, United States

R. Gabriela Barajas-Gonzalez (253), Department of Population Health, New York University School of Medicine, New York, NY, United States

David M. Barnes (219), Department of Epidemiology, School of Global Public Health, New York University, New York, NY, United States

Esther J. Calzada (253), Steve Hicks School of Social Work, University of Texas at Austin, Austin, TX, United States

Flor Castellanos (201), The University of Texas at Austin, Austin, TX, United States

Rosario Ceballo (135), University of Michigan, Ann Arbor, MI, United States

Tania Chowdhury (179), New York University, New York, NY, United States

Cory L. Cobb (3), College of Education, University of Texas at Austin, Austin, TX, United States

Luciana Giorgio Cosenzo (279), School of Social Work, Columbia University, New York, NY, United States

Sarah Valentina Diaz (279), School of Social Work, Columbia University, New York, NY, United States

J. Mark Eddy (3), Family Translational Research Group, New York University, New York, NY, United States

Evan L. Eschliman (219), Department of Sociomedical Sciences, Mailman School of Public Health, Columbia University, New York, NY, United States

Hanan Hashem (201), The University of Texas at Austin, Austin, TX, United States

Yang Hou (25), University of Kentucky, Lexington, KY, United States

Keng-Yen Huang (253), Department of Population Health, New York University School of Medicine, New York, NY, United States

Alejandra Garcia Isaza (3), College of Education, Center for Equity Promotion, University of Oregon, Eugene, OR, United States

Su Yeong Kim (25), University of Texas at Austin, Austin, TX, United States

Hee Yun Lee (157), School of Social Work, University of Alabama, Tuscaloosa, AL, United States

YiPing Li (219), Clinical Psychology (Psychology in Education), Teachers College, Columbia University, New York, NY, United States

Sarah A. Lieff (219), Department of Social and Behavioral Sciences, School of Global Public Health, New York University, New York, NY, United States

Cristal Lopez (95), Texas A&M University, College Station, TX, United States

Elma I. Lorenzo-Blanco (113), Department of Human Development and Family Sciences, University of Texas at Austin, Austin, TX; Department of Public Health Sciences, University of Miami, Miami, FL, United States

P. Priscilla Lui (45), Southern Methodist University, Dallas, TX, United States

Charles R. Martinez. Jr (3), College of Education, University of Texas at Austin, Austin, TX, United States

Heather H. McClure (3), College of Education, Center for Equity Promotion, University of Oregon, Eugene, OR, United States

Jessica P. Montoro (135), University of Michigan, Ann Arbor, MI, United States

Andrea S. Mora (135), University of Michigan, Ann Arbor, MI, United States

Melanie Morris (279), School of Social Work, Columbia University, New York, NY, United States

Jessica A. Neese (157), School of Social Work, University of Alabama, Tuscaloosa, AL, United States

Hien Nguyen (201), The University of Texas at Austin, Austin, TX, United States

Lizette Ojeda (95), Texas A&M University, College Station, TX, United States

Sumie Okazaki (179), New York University, New York, NY, United States

Taylor Payne (201), The University of Texas at Austin, Austin, TX, United States

Savannah Pham (45), Southern Methodist University, Dallas, TX, United States

Seth J. Schwartz (113), Department of Human Development and Family Sciences, University of Texas at Austin, Austin, TX; Department of Public Health Sciences, University of Miami, Miami, FL, United States

Abigail Sharer (95), Texas A&M University, College Station, TX, United States

Yishan Shen (25), Texas State University, San Marcos, TX, United States

Lawrence H. Yang (219), Department of Social and Behavioral Sciences, School of Global Public Health, New York University; Department of Epidemiology, Mailman School of Public Health, Columbia University, New York, NY, United States

Byron L. Zamboanga (45), Smith College, Northampton, MA, United States

Michael A. Zárate (71), University of Texas at El Paso, El Paso, TX, United States

Minyu Zhang (25), University of Texas at Austin, Austin, TX, United States

Preface

The goal of this book is to address the complexities of immigration and their effects on mental health. Immigration often does not involve a smooth and linear transition from one culture to another. Cultural and sociocultural factors influence the transition. The cultural distance between the immigrant's home culture and the host culture influences adjustment. Optimal adjustment may involve retaining one's home culture as well as acculturation to the host culture. In addition to cultural adjustment, immigrants undergo sociocultural adjustment. After immigration, many experience minority status and group-based discrimination for the first time in their lives. Such sociocultural stressors complicate the process of moving from one culture to another. Successful coping with both cultural and sociocultural stressors is the challenge immigrants face in achieving and maintaining mental health.

This book is particularly timely, given the recent efforts of the United States to restrict immigration. Immigrants are wrongly scapegoated for problems such as scarcity of jobs and crime. Whereas refugee status was once a source of sympathy for immigrants, such sympathy now seems to be in short supply. Nonrefugee immigrants are also not welcomed. Legal immigration status does not protect immigrants from scapegoating. Documented immigrants are often lumped together with undocumented immigrants in public perceptions. These political pressures create fear among immigrants that has deleterious effects on their mental health.

Most immigration to the United States historically has been from Latin America and Latinx Americans have become the largest population of color in the United States. However, immigration laws have changed immigration patterns. The largest group of new immigrants is now from Asia. In the past, Asian immigration to the United States generally has been from East Asia (China, Japan, and Korea). Recent immigration has been from Southeast and South Asia. Another wave of recent immigrants has come from Arab and Middle Eastern countries.

This book includes contributions of leading researchers from psychology, education, and social work. The three sections of the book are: (a) Acculturation; (b) Mental Health; and (c) Psychopathology. The section on Acculturation addresses geographic and social contexts of immigration, how parents and children navigate the acculturation process, how different cultural orientations affect behavior, and research methods on acculturation. The Mental Health section covers specific mental health issues among Latinx, Asian, and Arab/Middle Eastern immigrants. The third section on Psychopathology addresses epidemiology, internalizing symptoms, and sleep disorders among immigrants.

In the Acculturation section, Chapter 1 by Cobb and colleagues addresses the complexity of reasons for immigration and the diversity of receiving contexts for immigrants. What is known from traditional receiving contexts where there are large immigrant populations is not necessarily applicable in emerging contexts. Kim and colleagues in Chapter 2 focus on Chinese and Mexican immigrant families, the two largest immigrant groups to the United States. They discuss how acculturation influences parenting behaviors, focusing on how the acculturation gap between parents and children, and language brokering influence adolescent mental health. In Chapter 3, Zamboanga and Lui review conceptual models of acculturation that can help identify mechanisms of alcohol use. The authors discuss the promise of bicultural orientation approaches to acculturation for research and practice. Zarate and colleagues in Chapter 4 review and critique historical and contemporary theories and measures of acculturation. Their cultural inertia theory addresses many of the limitations of other approaches and offers guidance for future research.

The Mental Health section begins with Chapter 5 by Ojeda and colleagues on the challenges immigrants face in work contexts. They highlight the diversity within immigrant groups and the demands of navigating between work and family. Lorenzo-Blanco and Schwartz in Chapter 6 review the current status of the Latinx population in the United States. They emphasize the systems in which stressors and barriers are embedded. Chapter 7 by Ceballo and colleagues dovetails Chapter 6 with a focus on Latinx immigration issues and their psychological effects. The unique contribution of Chapter 7 is the discussion of the mental health effects of religion and spirituality. Lee and Neese in Chapter 8 offer a social work perspective on the mental and behavioral health of immigrants from multiple global regions. The need for culturally sensitive assessment and intervention methods is emphasized. In Chapter 9, Chowdhury and Okazaki consider the impact of the events of September 11, 2001 on South Asian Muslim Americans' mental health. The authors review specific challenges within South Asian Muslim American communities and challenges found within subgroups of those communities such as women, individuals who identify as LGBTQ+, youth, and older adults. Awad and colleagues in Chapter 10 focus on immigrants of Arab and Middle Eastern/North African descent, examining within-group diversity, misconceptions, and migration history. They contextualize these issues with conceptual frameworks and explain pre- and postmigration stressors that affect mental health.

In the final section on Psychopathology, Yang and colleagues in Chapter 11 review proposed mechanisms of the immigrant health paradox that immigrants tend to be healthier than subsequent generations born in the United States. They illustrate with Black immigrants how the proposed mechanisms operate.

In Chapter 12, Calzada and colleagues review internalizing disorders in Latinx children. Included are new longitudinal data on Dominican and Mexican American children's developmental trajectories of depression, anxiety, and somatization. Cosenzo and colleagues have provided a systematic review of insomnia among multiple immigrant groups in Chapter 13. Their review underscores the need to expand traditional treatment models to include contextual factors beyond the individual level.

I thank Ellen Huang for her help in editing the book. I also thank Dennis McGonagle for his initial encouragement to take on this project, and Barbara Makinster and Sandra Harron for seeing this book through with their helpful editorial work. I hope that this book will help advance research, education, practice, and policy on immigration during a time when such guidance is desperately needed.

Gordon C. Nagayama Hall
University of Oregon, Eugene, OR, United States

Section A

Acculturation

Chapter 1

Linking acculturation factors, family environments, and mental health outcomes among Latino families in traditional, emerging, and crisis immigrant receiving contexts in the United States

Cory L. Cobb[a], Charles R. Martinez. Jr[a], Alejandra Garcia Isaza[b], Heather H. McClure[b] and J. Mark Eddy[c]

[a]*College of Education, University of Texas at Austin, Austin, TX, United States,* [b]*College of Education, Center for Equity Promotion, University of Oregon, Eugene, OR, United States,* [c]*Family Translational Research Group, New York University, New York, NY, United States*

Introduction

The literature on recent Latino[a] immigrants to the United States is replete with evidence linking acculturation processes to the psychological and behavioral health of immigrant individuals and families. *Acculturation* broadly refers to the continuous exchange of cultural information (i.e., values, beliefs, behavioral norms) between groups of people, and the subsequent changes in culture that occur as part of that exchange (Berry, 2017). Acculturation is a multidimensional construct, incorporating several interacting variables such as language use/proficiency, nativity status, and cultural identity processes. Such definitional complexity has led to a lack of consensus among researchers on how to measure acculturation (Schwartz & Unger, 2017). In turn, findings related to acculturation effects are often inconsistent, with some studies showing negative effects of acculturation on mental and behavioral health outcomes, and other studies showing neutral or positive effects (Schwartz & Unger, 2017). Nevertheless, the

a. The US Office of Management and Budget uses the word "Latino" to refer to peoples of Cuban, Mexican, Puerto Rican, Central or South American, or of other Spanish cultures or origins, regardless of race.

Mental and Behavioral Health of Immigrants in the United States
https://doi.org/10.1016/B978-0-12-816117-3.00001-4

process of acculturation and the stressors that accompany it have been linked to a host of deleterious outcomes for immigrant families (Bekteshi & Kang, 2018). Such outcomes include decreased well-being, internalizing symptoms, externalizing symptoms, disease biomarkers, and health-risk behaviors (Fuligni et al., 2009; Martinez, 2006; Schwartz et al., 2015).

One critical factor influencing immigrant acculturation and adjustment to a new homeland is the context of reception of the receiving society. *Context of reception* for immigrants broadly refers to the "the opportunity structure, degree of openness versus hostility, and acceptance in the local community" (Schwartz et al., 2014, p. 2). An emerging body of research demonstrates how the context of reception matters in understanding acculturation and mental health among Latino immigrants, where a wide variation in receiving contexts can drastically change the adaptation experiences of immigrants once they have arrived in the United States (Salas-Wright & Schwartz, 2019). Although many immigrants experience common, reception-related challenges during acculturation process (e.g., discrimination, learning a new language, adjusting to school), such experiences can play out quite differently depending on the factors related to the context of reception.

Throughout the 20th century, Latino population tended to be concentrated primarily in *traditional receiving contexts* where local communities and states have a long history of receiving and accommodating Latino immigrants, most notably California, Florida, Illinois, New Jersey, New York, and Texas (Radford & Noe-Bustamante, 2019). These states have been classified as the "Big 6," the top geographic locations where the majority of the foreign-born Latino population has been concentrated throughout various immigration waves in the past century (Camarota, 2012). However, beginning in the 1990s and continuing today, Latino immigrants have increasingly settled in *emerging receiving contexts*, 22 other states, such as Georgia, Minnesota, Washington, and Wisconsin, which in prior decades had little presence of Latino immigrant population but are now receiving a rapid influx (Pew Research Center, 2016). In contrast to traditional receiving contexts, Latino immigrants in emerging receiving contexts face more language barriers, restricted access to culturally responsive social services, more fragmented social networks, and education and health systems that are ill-prepared to support Latino newcomers, especially those who are non-English speakers and economically disadvantaged (Kiang, Grzywacz, Marín, Arcury, & Quandt, 2010; Martinez, McClure, & Eddy, 2016). Thus, traditional receiving contexts and emerging receiving contexts differ for immigrants in terms of opportunities, resources, and acceptance, and these differences have important implications for the mental and behavioral health outcomes of Latino immigrant population.

Unfortunately, much of what is known about the effects of acculturation on health-related outcomes stems from research conducted in traditional immigrant settlement states as opposed to emerging receiving contexts. This raises concerns regarding the generalizability of epidemiological research linking acculturation to health outcomes for Latino immigrants, and it points to potential limitations in existing prevention and clinical treatment approaches designed to support and sustain immigrant health. For example, although prior research—largely conducted in traditional receiving contexts—documented positive effects of adolescent language brokering (i.e., acting as linguistic and cultural intermediaries in support of immigrant families navigating the host society) on outcomes such as adolescent confidence, maturity, academic self-efficacy, and pride in being able to help their families (Tilghman-Osborne, Bámaca-Colbert, Witherspoon, Wadsworth, & Hecht, 2016; Weisskirch, 2017), findings from a study in Oregon, an emerging context, found negative effects of language brokering not only on parental depression, stress, and anxiety, parenting practices, but also on youth academic adjustment, internalizing symptoms, externalizing symptoms, and substance use among youth (Martinez, McClure, & Eddy, 2009).

These findings underscore how receiving contexts can profoundly matter to health and well-being. Thus, the objective of this chapter is to review salient factors associated with traditional and emerging receiving contexts, as well as the role that such factors can play in understanding the links between acculturation processes and mental and behavioral health outcomes among Latino immigrant families. We also consider a currently active third context, crisis migration, and how the ecology of this context can impact health. We conclude with a discussion of ways in which contexts of reception might be considered in creating policy, as well as designing and adapting interventions to support and sustain the mental and behavioral health of Latino immigrant families.

Traditional contexts of reception and immigrant mental health

In a little over 50 years, the Latino population in the United States experienced a ninefold increase, from 6.3 million in 1960 to 56.5 million by 2015 (Flores, 2017). This was driven by the 1965 amendment to the Immigration and Nationality Act that lifted restrictive immigration quotas favoring European immigration and marked the beginning of the Contemporary Immigration Era (Pew Research Center, 2016). Of the over 59 million immigrants that have arrived during this era, half came from Latin America. These new arrivals are projected to drive US population growth through 2065 (Pew Research Center, 2016).

Prior to 2000, 78% of Latino immigrants to the United States from Latin American and Spanish-speaking Caribbean nations settled in the Big 6 states (Vásquez, Seales, & Marquardt, 2008). For many immigrants in these states, and particularly those settling in ethnically dense enclaves, the acculturation process has become easier due to well-established immigrant communities and the availability of more linguistically and culturally responsive services at both the local and state levels (Schwartz & Unger, 2017). Indeed, one consequence of having an ethnically dense concentration of foreign-born people that share a language, traditions, and needs is that the social infrastructure within the immediate context is shaped to better serve the communities that have settled there. As noted by Portes and Manning (1986), "Once an enclave economy has fully developed, it is possible for a newcomer to live his life entirely within the confines of the community. Work, education, and access to health care, recreation, and a variety of other services can be found without leaving the bounds of the ethnic economy" (pp. 63–64). Thus, in areas where significant Latino social, cultural, political, and business enclaves already exist, maintenance of one's cultural heritage is not only possible but also functional.

Research has documented that residing in ethnic enclaves can preserve cognitive schemata within Latino immigrants because they reproduce the sounds, sights, smells, tastes, and feelings of the homelands of immigrants (Falicov, 2013). Furthermore, residing in states with ethnically dense communities provides immigrants with a sense of cultural continuity by allowing them to navigate their daily lives in ways that make them feel more "at home" in their new country of settlement. Such cultural continuity not only helps to reduce the painful feelings of loss associated with migrating to a new country, but also permits Latino immigrants to further transform their local communities into more familiar places and to maintain salient group identities (Falicov, 2007, 2013). Thus, residing in ethnic enclaves can yield both sociocultural and psychological benefits for Latino immigrants.

Residing in ethnic enclaves also permits new Latino immigrants to more easily develop community networks and social support systems. During migration, immigrants typically experience the loss of social ties around which they have built their lives (Hull, Kilbourne, Reece, & Husaini, 2008). Community networks, comprising neighborhoods, churches, and schools, become key sources of new personal relationships. Strong identification with community networks has been found to protect immigrants' self-esteem against discrimination (Jetten et al., 2015) and provide immigrants with stronger feelings of personal control of their lives (Greenaway et al., 2015). The availability of community networks in established immigrant communities assists in helping immigrants to reduce stress and locate important health-care information (Bender & Castro, 2000), buffers cultural stress (Jasinskaja-Lahti, Liebkind, Jaakkola, & Reuter, 2006), and provides religious support important for well-being and academic achievement (Thompson & Gurney, 2003). Thus, migrating to traditional receiving contexts, where community networks are well-established, facilitates positive adjustment because immigrants are able to quickly forge new social relationships and reap the benefits of such relationships to health.

Researchers have also documented differing outcomes of Latino immigrants *between* ethnic enclaves in traditional contexts of reception. Specifically, Schwartz et al. (2014) compared depressive symptoms associated with the perceived context of reception between samples of Latino residents from Miami, Florida and from Los Angeles, California. Results showed that individuals in Los Angeles reported experiencing more discrimination and a more negative context of reception compared to individuals in Miami; in addition, the perceived negative context of reception significantly predicted depressive symptoms at 6-month follow-up only for residents in Los Angeles. Interestingly, Schwartz et al. (2014) also noted the advantage of wealth and power held by many Cubans relative to other Latino ethnic groups in Miami. The authors also noted that several contextual factors, such as reasons for migrating, resources available to immigrants, and legal status that might result in differing levels of empowerment and political power, which may help explain why Miami residents perceived a more positive context of reception than those residing in Los Angeles, where Latinos hold less wealth and power and where there tends to be a greater concentration of undocumented immigrants relative to Miami (Schwartz et al., 2014). These findings highlight that, although ethnic enclaves generally provide similar sets of experiences for many Latino immigrants, not all enclaves are created equal—some may yield some deleterious effects for immigrant health.

For instance, ethnic density does not necessarily result in a fully developed enclave economy that facilitates positive immigrant adjustment. A dense concentration of immigrant ethnic minorities can spark reactionary policymaking that can severely impact Latino immigrant population. Indeed, research examining the relationship between state-level immigration policies and Latino mental health across 31 states showed that, compared to non-Latinos, Latino individuals residing in states with more exclusionary immigration policies had higher rates of poor mental health than those residing in states with less exclusionary immigration policies (Hatzenbuehler et al., 2017). Even among the states considered to be traditional receiving contexts, differences regarding the policy climate were evident: California and New Jersey were found to be the most inclusionary, followed by New York and Illinois that were modestly inclusionary; Texas was neither inclusionary nor exclusionary; and Florida was found to be modestly exclusionary. Thus, ethnic enclaves, even in traditional receiving contexts, may differ in the psychosocial experiences they confer to Latino immigrants due to differences in inclusionary versus exclusionary state-level policies.

Other possibilities as to why some ethnic enclaves with traditional receiving contexts yield negative effects on residents are structural factors such as poverty and limited access to quality education. Recently, Arévalo, Tucker, and Falcón (2015) examined the relationship between self-reported depressive symptoms of middle and older-aged Puerto Ricans and ethnic population density within the city of Boston. Although results showed a protective effect of neighborhood ethnic density on depressive symptoms, this relation was only present after controlling for neighborhood poverty (Arévalo et al., 2015). This finding provides a partial account of the disparate results reported in the literature that have produced evidence both in favor of (Mair et al., 2010; Ostir, Eschbach, Markides, & Goodwin, 2003) and against (Dinwiddie, Gaskin, Chan, Norrington, & McCleary, 2013; Lee, 2009) the protective effect of ethnic density for mental health. Essentially, Arévalo et al. (2015) demonstrated that ethnic enclaves usually have high levels of poverty, and such poverty may exert an undue influence on the relationship between ethnic density and mental health. They also showed that although individuals in neighborhoods with high ethnic density may report fewer depressive symptoms, they were also more likely to be less educated, older, and poor, as well as have lower language proficiency and engage in less recreational activities. This set of findings highlights the complex interplay of factors that can potentially affect the mental health of Latino immigrants, even in traditional receiving contexts—illustrating the need to consider the specific immigrant context and the multiple levels of influence that may impact the health of Latino immigrants.

Emerging contexts of reception and immigrant mental health

In contrast to traditional contexts of reception, since 2000, 22 US states have been recognized as "emerging" contexts due to recent and rapid immigrant population growth (Vásquez et al., 2008). Most Latino immigrants settling in emerging immigrant states have been from Mexico. Between 1990 and 2000, the Mexican immigrant population increased more than 1800% in Alabama, North Carolina, and Tennessee, more than 1000% in Arkansas and Minnesota, over 800% in Georgia, and between 500% and 700% in Indiana, Iowa, Nebraska, and Utah (Zúñiga & Hernández-León, 2005). By 2000, the overall proportion of Mexicans settling in new destination states grew from 13% to 35% (Durand, Massey, & Capoferro, 2005). Despite the predominance of Mexican immigrants in the United States, by 2000, diversity was increasing, with Latinos from countries other than Cuba, Mexico, and Puerto Rico accounting for 63% of all Latinos in Virginia, 55% in Louisiana, 34% in Mississippi, 31% in Kentucky, and 24% in Nebraska (Zúñiga & Hernández-León, 2005).

In emerging immigrant contexts, demands on Latino newcomers can be high due to limited Spanish language support and barriers to accessing social services, and may increase the likelihood that encounters with native English speakers and their US-born counterparts, when they do occur, will be stressful (Martinez et al., 2009). Moreover, Latino immigrants in emerging states may encounter several social-structural challenges, most notably few established ethnic enclaves and weak infrastructure to support newly arrived immigrants. The social-structural characteristics of many Latino communities influence the nature, complexity, and magnitude of potential contextual stressors related to cultural adaptation and residential integration (Hall & Stringfield, 2014). In turn, these stressors can have significant impacts on mental health.

Community and neighborhood characteristics in emerging immigrant contexts may also increase the frequency of stressful life events (Latkin, Curry, Hua, & Davey, 2007), as well as the degree of psychological distress experienced by community members (Galea et al., 2007). For instance, Ornelas and

Perreira (2011) documented that immigrants living in North Carolina who reported experiencing ethnic or racial discrimination in their neighborhoods were more likely to experience depressive symptoms. Acculturative stress, when combined with neighborhood and other stressors, can diminish individuals' coping resources, making mental health disorders and maladaptive coping behaviors more likely (Bekteshi & Kang, 2018). Further, coping in response to acculturative stressors may also influence mental health, with one study of Puerto Rican adults in Central Florida indicating that participants who coped with acculturative stress through self-blame were more likely to experience depressive symptoms (Capielo, Delgado-Romero, & Stewart, 2015).

In addition to fewer developed infrastructure services in new growth states (e.g., bilingual education, medical interpreters in health settings, immigrant organizations), formal and informal policies and practices may limit immigrants' access to the social safety net in ways that Big 6 states historically have not (Capps et al., 2002). The sociodemographic characteristics and premigration experiences of new immigrants also may interact in important ways with US-based social and economic contexts to increase risk or protective factors for families and youth. When new immigrants have lower educational levels, limited English language proficiency, and lower incomes—sociodemographic characteristics that are more common among immigrants in emerging versus traditional settlement states (Capps et al., 2002)—they may establish lives in neighborhoods, schools, and jobs that contain more psychosocial stressors.

Stressors related to social-structural characteristics also impact key elements of the early family environment such as parent-child relationships, parental affection, and family conflict (Schwartz et al., 2015). These, in turn, can influence the development of emotional and cognitive responses to environmental challenges in youth (e.g., psychosocial stressors), which are predictive of concurrent and subsequent emotional adjustment (Schwartz et al., 2015). Poor adjustment in childhood or early adolescence, including the display of aggression and other antisocial behaviors, is predictive of poor mental and behavioral health later in life, including adolescent and adult substance use (Doom, Vanzomeren-Dohm, & Simpson, 2016). While these are common "malleable" issues often discussed by prevention researchers, a variety of other issues, including socioeconomic and cultural protective factors, are considered of great importance for Latino immigrants in emerging states.

Immigrants in emerging contexts of reception, especially recent arrivals, may experience acute and intense psychosocial stress (Kiang et al., 2010). Such stress may contribute to several poor outcomes for Latino parents and youth, including depression, anxiety, and substance use (Kiang et al., 2010; Martinez et al., 2009; Martinez, 2006). For example, findings from one study with foreign-born Mexican origin youth in Oregon showed that recent immigrant youth and parents (i.e., living in the United States for 2–4 years) may experience higher levels of internalizing and emotional distress that diminish in intensity over time, echoing findings from other emerging immigrant sites

(Martinez, McClure, Eddy, & Wilson, 2011). In addition, discrimination and other social-contextual stressors have been linked to depression and anxiety among children and youth in Latino migrant farmworker families in Indiana (Taylor & Ruiz, 2017). In this study, children and youth were above established norms for self-reported anxiety and depression, and were more likely to experience loneliness, economic hassles, and discrimination.

It is not surprising that during immigrant families' first few years in the United States, when it is expected that they would experience the steepest adjustment and most intense stress, Mexican immigrant parents reported the highest levels of both stress and frequency of past year binge drinking (Martinez et al., 2011). This finding runs counter to previous findings that recently arrived immigrant adults have lower levels of alcohol use compared with immigrants who had lived in the United States longer and with US-born Latinos (Vega, Sribney, Aguilar-Gaxiola, & Kolody, 2004). Such a finding also raises questions as to whether recently immigrated parents in Oregon and similar emerging contexts experience higher levels of stress compared with those in traditional contexts where most prior research has been conducted. The scant evidence suggests that epidemiological studies focusing on Latinos in states with established immigrant communities—and the interventions that have been developed based on the data from these studies—may fail to reflect unique vulnerabilities for immigrants in emerging states (Martinez, 2006; Prado et al., 2009).

Other factors that may impact Latino mental health in emerging contexts of reception are legal status and the presence of community organizations. For example, in Oklahoma, Latina adults reported fewer depressive symptoms than Latinas in traditional contexts (Zapata Roblyer, Carlos, Merten, Gallus, & Grzywacz, 2017), and undocumented women reported significantly higher stress than documented women. Although the authors noted that even the moderate levels of depressive symptoms reported are concerning given the barriers to depression treatment experienced by many Latinos (Alegría et al., 2008)—barriers that are exacerbated for immigrants who are undocumented (Vargas Bustamante et al., 2012)—vigorous efforts by Oklahoma community organizations to reach out to Latino immigrants and provide services across the lifespan may be credited, at least in part, with the relatively positive findings regarding Latinas' depressive symptoms. This finding highlights the importance of available, proactive, community-level resources in emerging contexts and how such resources can positively impact the psychological health of immigrants.

Finally, gender and occupation status may intersect with risk for depressive symptoms in emerging contexts of reception. Specifically, one study found that Latina farmworkers in North Carolina reported experiencing greater stress and anxiety than both employed and unemployed non-farmworker Latinas (Arcury et al., 2018). Furthermore, employed Latinas, whether farmworkers or in other occupations, reported greater stress and anxiety than unemployed Latinas. Although preliminary, these findings provide an impetus to further examine the intersection between various social identities and their relationship to mental health among Latino immigrants residing in emerging versus traditional contexts of reception.

In sum, research on Latino immigrants in emerging contexts of reception remains in its early stages. It is clear that immigrants in emerging contexts undergo a very different experience than immigrants in more traditional contexts of reception, and such differing experiences can be attributed largely to the specific histories, resources, social structure, and other features available in the receiving context. Whereas traditional contexts of reception tend to possess several protective features, such as the presence of ethnic enclaves and established social services, many emerging contexts do not possess these features. Further research is needed to explore the context-specific factors that promote and protect—as well as exacerbate and harm—the psychological and behavioral health of Latino immigrants in new growth states.

Crisis migrant contexts of reception and mental health

There is a third context of reception for Latinos that has been gaining much attention: the context of *crisis migration*. Crisis migration broadly refers to (often large) movements of people(s) that occur because of anticipated or real threats—whether acute or chronic, natural or man-made—to one's life, safety, health, and/or basic subsistence (Martin, Weerasinghe, & Taylor, 2014). These threats may be social, political, economic, and/or environmental, and often result in abrupt, unexpected, relocation of families from their home countries. Recent examples of crisis migration for Latinos include the exodus of immigrants from the Northern Triangle countries (Honduras, Guatemala, and El Salvador) due to extreme violence and crime; the fleeing of millions of Venezuelans in the wake of their country's political turmoil and economic collapse; and the resettlement of many Puerto Ricans due to the aftermath of Hurricane Maria. Thus, crisis migrants can entail those who are displaced and compelled to migrate by current situations beyond their control; who migrate because they anticipate future threats to their lives; and/or who migrate because they may otherwise be trapped in place due to financial, security, safety, health, or other logistical reasons (Blizzard & Batalova, 2019; McAdam, 2014).

Given the abrupt and adverse nature of crisis migration, it is not surprising that meta-analytic and large-scale narrative research reviews have consistently linked it with significant acute stress (anxiety, depression, substance use) and trauma (PTSD; e.g., Porter & Haslam, 2005; Scaramutti, Salas-Wright, Vos, & Schwartz, 2019; Schwartz et al., 2018). In fact, research has shown that refugees settling in Western countries are 10 times more likely to report PTSD, depression, and anxiety symptoms compared with the general population and other comparable immigrant groups (e.g., Fazel, Wheeler, & Danesh, 2005; Lindert, von Ehrenstein, Priebe, Mielck, & Brähler, 2009). Not only can the adverse effects of crisis migration remain for years after resettlement (Bogic, Njoku, & Priebe, 2015), but can also be exacerbated if destination contexts are ill-equipped to receive crisis migrants due to limited resources or unwelcoming contexts of reception (Kim, 2016; Schwartz et al., 2014, 2018). These patterns of psychopathology in refugees and asylum seekers have been found in a variety of studies (cf. Fazel et al., 2005; Porter & Haslam, 2005). Taken together, these studies suggest that refugees and asylum seekers experience significant psychological distress as they attempt to resettle in new homelands.

To understand the stressful effects of crisis migration, it is important to understand its social dimensions and to situate such migration within an ecological context. Whether a hazardous event becomes a crisis that spurs people to flee their countries and experience symptoms of mental health problems depends largely on the resources and capacities of those who migrate to cope with the event, as well as the availability (or accessibility) of resources in the country, state, and locality where they resettle (McAdam, 2014). Of course, whether an event per se leads to crisis migration may depend on how that event interacts with other existing psychosocial stressors such as poverty, weak political institutions, poor economic infrastructure, overcrowding, limited access to resources, and the destination country's context of reception. Therefore, crisis migration and its stressful psychological effects are best understood as a complex interaction between political, social, environmental, and economic factors triggered (but not necessarily caused) by an event. In this sense, crisis migration is more rooted in systemic inequities that place certain groups more vulnerable to displacement because they lack sufficient resources to cope with an adverse event. Such vulnerability to stress may be compounded when migrants are displaced to receiving contexts that are ill-equipped to provide them with the resources they need. Thus, like for other immigrant groups, the ecology of specific contexts of reception is critical when predicting the degree of stress crisis migrants might experience (Marks, McKenna, & Coll, 2018; Schwartz et al., 2014).

For instance, socioeconomic factors in postmigration contexts, such as housing and financial security, have been linked with refugee mental health. Research findings suggest that unemployment and financial instability are strong risk factors for depression and anxiety among refugees (Kim, 2016), and refugees with less access to economic resources report poorer mental health outcomes than refugees with more access to these financial resources (Porter & Haslam, 2005). Financial resource limitations in receiving contexts may mean that refugees will have limited access to stable housing, which has been linked to psychological distress and impairment in global functioning among refugees (Kim, 2016; Porter & Haslam, 2005). Given the relatively decentralized refugee resettlement system in the United States, placement into a specific state or local community context can have ramifications for refugees' level of access to public services and financial assistance programs. For example, a refugee family of three might receive a monthly *Temporary Assistance for Needy Families* payment of $789 in New York but only $281 in Texas; to qualify for Medicaid, the same refugee family must have an income significantly below the federal poverty level in Florida and Texas but could earn more in New York and California (Fix, Hooper, & Zong, 2017).

Furthermore, growing reliance on state and local resources has resulted in backlash and discrimination against refugees in various parts of the country, as concerns from politicians and some of their constituents have been expressed about strain on public assistance programs and scarcity of additional resources such as safety nets (e.g., food pantries) and legally mandated interpretation and translation services (Migration Policy Institute, 2015). Also, the political climate and receptivity of voters and politicians vary significantly from state to state. For example, governors of Texas and Florida have recently openly opposed the resettlement of Syrian refugees in their states, while governors in other states, such as California and New York, have not opposed such resettlement (Fix et al., 2017). Discrimination within resettlement environments has been negatively linked with quality of life and positively linked with depression for refugees after controlling for other pre- and postmigration factors (Li, Liddell, & Nickerson, 2016).

In contrast, research shows more positive mental health among refugees in environments they perceive to be more welcoming. In a study of recently migrated Venezuelan refugees, results show that migrants resettling in South Florida reported less depression, a more positive context of reception, and less anxiety than migrants resettling in the country of Colombia (Schwartz et al., 2018). This was explained by the fact that South Florida represents a receiving context with a long and welcoming history of resettling refugees whereas refugee resettlement in Colombia began only recently. Moreover, Venezuela and Colombia have a long rivalry in politics, sports, trade, and other domains, which may have increased the likelihood of discrimination against Venezuelans resettling in Colombia (Schwartz et al., 2018). Thus, refugee mental health depends, in part, on the receiving context's history and experience with resettling refugees, the historical relationship between the specific refugee group resettling and receiving society, and the availability and accessibility of resources within new receiving contexts.

Another important factor in refugee resettlement and mental health is the growing trend toward more limited and restrictive asylum policies in nations that experience large, acute influxes of crisis migrants. In 2014, the United States experienced a surge of refugees and asylum seekers from the Northern Triangle countries to the US-Mexico border. In response, and particularly within the past few years, the United States sharply increased its capacity and tendency to detain families, including the separation of children from their parents, for indefinite periods of time, and has consistently messaged a strong "zero-tolerance" stance regarding most forms of immigration from southern countries (Martin, 2012; Society for Research in Child Development, 2018).

Crisis migrants who are detained, especially for extended periods of time, may manifest a variety of mental health problems. A systematic review found that detainees reported high levels of depression, anxiety, and PTSD, and symptom severity increased with time in detention (Robjant, Hassan, & Katona, 2009). In a recent study, Keller, Joscelyne, Granski, and Rosenfeld (2017) found that 32% of asylum seekers from Central America who arrived at the US-Mexico border met diagnostic criteria for PTSD, 24% for depression, and 7% for both disorders. The severity of symptoms was correlated with the length of the time spent in detention. Two-month follow-up interviews revealed that individuals who were released from detention reported marked decreases in stress, whereas those who remained in detention reported an increase in symptoms. In the broader literature, factors contributing to psychological distress among detainees include little to no access to legal services, extended separation from family (including children), proximity to others experiencing severe psychological distress, lack of personal agency, and uncertainty regarding duration of detention (Li et al., 2016; von Werthern et al., 2018). These findings suggest that prolonged detention while waiting asylum outcomes is associated with several deleterious outcomes on refugees' psychological health.

Taken together, crisis migration is a stressful process that poses significant psychological and behavioral health risks for refugees and asylum seekers. Such risks are best understood within an ecological context as several pre- and post-migration factors interact in complex ways to impact crisis migrants' health. Such factors include, but are not limited to, the abrupt nature of crisis migration, trauma accrued during the migration journey, availability and accessibility of resources in destination societies, receiving contexts' attitudes and policies toward crisis migrants, destination countries' experience with resettling crisis migrants, and indefinite amounts of time spent in detention centers.

Conclusions and implications for policy, prevention, and treatment

Today, new Latino immigrants to the United States are likely to experience at least one of three contexts of reception: traditional, emerging, and/or crisis. Each of these contexts possesses unique ecologies that confer very different experiences to Latino immigrants depending on where they settle. In general, traditional contexts have well developed, formal, and informal support systems for receiving and assisting immigrants, which tend to ease their transition into the United States. Emerging contexts typically do not have these support systems and thus tend to present more challenging circumstances compared to traditional receiving contexts. Crisis contexts have few supports and may present extreme challenges to immigrants' psychological and behavioral health. Research within traditional and emerging contexts indicates that the psychological and behavioral health of immigrants can vary widely, and such variation is a function of social-contextual factors such as the characteristics of the specific context where immigrants arrive, what life was like for immigrants before leaving their countries of origin, the experiences of immigrants in transit, and what happened after arrival. In contrast, within current crisis contexts, and particularly for newly arrived immigrants residing in border settlements in Mexico or in US-based detention centers, both mental and physical health may suffer. Thus, the specific context of reception should be considered when developing policy, as well as interventions to support and sustain the psychological and behavioral health of Latino immigrants.

Regarding policy, there is considerable evidence that local, state, and/or national policies reflect anti-immigrant sentiments that can negatively impact Latino communities (e.g., Hatzenbuehler et al., 2017; Philbin, Flake, Hatzenbuehler, & Hirsch, 2018). For example, one of the most notorious anti-immigrant policies, Arizona's State Bill 1070 (SB 1070), required all local and state law enforcement officials to investigate the immigration status of anyone suspected of being undocumented—making it a state crime for noncitizen immigrants to fail to carry proper immigrant documentation (Lam & Morse, 2012). Following SB 1070, several other states implemented similar bills, the majority of which were framed as protecting communities from undocumented immigrants (Morse, 2011). The passage of anti-immigrant bills not only creates a discriminatory context that legalizes racial profiling among anyone presumed to be a foreigner (Viruell-Fuentes, Miranda, & Abdulrahim, 2012), but it also results in reduced access to important social services and poorer psychological health for Latino immigrants residing in such contexts (Almeida, Biello, Pedraza, Wintner, & Viruell-Fuentes, 2016; Roche, Vaquera, White, & Rivera, 2018; Szkupinski Quiroga, Medina, & Glick, 2014). Although anti-immigrant policies generally target undocumented immigrants, ethnicity and immigrant status tend to be conflated such that most Latinos are assumed to be recent immigrants, and most immigrants are assumed to be undocumented—resulting in the marginalization of an entire group of people with great diversity on the issue of both immigration status and recency of arrival (Almeida et al., 2016; Viruell-Fuentes et al., 2012). In actuality, in parts of some regions of the United States (e.g., the southeast, the southwest), Latinos were residents long before non-Hispanic White immigrants arrived.

Other policy issues that continue to impact some Latino communities regard differential access to quality health care. For instance, the passage of the Affordable Care Act (ACA) in 2010 promised to be a defining moment for Latino health care, particularly the expansion of Medicaid. However, a 2012 Supreme Court decision made the expansion of Medicaid optional for states (Supreme Court of the United States, 2012), resulting in a decrease in Latino uninsured rates in states that expanded Medicaid but stagnation in Latino uninsured rates in states that have not expanded Medicaid. This policy hurts many Latino communities because nearly 75% (10.2 million) of the nation's eligible but uninsured Latinos live in states without Medicaid expansion (Doty, Beutel, Rasmussen, & Collins, 2015). Thus, Latino families may experience disparate health-related outcomes depending on the specific state and community in which they live.

Similar to health care, policies surrounding education for Latinos has resulted in disparate educational outcomes. Intersecting with social-structural issues that impact Latino educational achievement (e.g., poverty, racism, parents' low educational attainment, low-resource schools), a lack of uniform federal policy has resulted in state policies that differentially impact Latino communities depending on the state in which they live (Flores, 2010; Flores & Chapa, 2009).

For instance, although there are no laws in most states preventing undocumented Latinos from attending college, they are generally prohibited from competing for state financial aid. The problem of no financial aid intensifies for undocumented Latinos who live in poverty and are charged tuition rates three to seven times higher than that for legal residents or US citizens. Such policies not only contribute to negative educational trajectories of undocumented families in these states, but they also significantly limit their upward social and economic mobility (Abrego & Gonzales, 2010). Only a handful of states have passed laws allowing undocumented Latinos to qualify for in-state tuition (Philbin et al., 2018). Clearly, Latinos may experience differing educational opportunities depending on the specific context in which they reside.

A lack of policy regarding the humane treatment of Latino immigrant families in detention centers also greatly impacts Latino families. As noted by Guttentag and Driscoll (2019), the issue at the border is less about the number of Latino individuals arriving and more about system policies that fail to respond in a humane, efficient, and orderly way among those seeking asylum. Indeed. Latino crisis migrants are often separated from their families and detained for indefinite periods of time. Such treatment often results in symptoms of anxiety, depression, and PTSD (Robjant et al., 2009). Latino crisis migrants who are detained at the border also face little or no access to legal representation, extended isolation from their children, proximity to others experiencing severe psychological distress, and feelings of uncertainty regarding duration of detention (Li et al., 2016; von Werthern et al., 2018). Due to the lack of policy surrounding humane treatment of crisis migrants seeking asylum in the United States, they will continue to experience significant psychological issues associated with residing in ill-prepared detention centers while waiting an indefinite amount of time regarding the outcome of their case.

In light of the evidence regarding the impact of policy (or lack thereof) on Latino families, there are several recommendations that policymakers may consider when developing legislation surrounding Latino communities. Broadly, there is no "one size fits all," approach and policymakers should pay careful attention to the specific state and community context in which Latinos reside. For example, policymakers may consider settling Latino immigrants either in a traditional ethnic enclave or in an emerging immigrant context. This is important because immigration entails a loss of social ties around which immigrants have built their lives, and ethnic enclaves provide a sense of cultural continuity for Latino immigrants as they reproduce the sights, sounds, smells, and feelings of their heritage culture. Such enclaves also provide Latino immigrants with significant community networks that can provide social support as well as assistance in locating and accessing important social resources and in obtaining gainful employment. However, there is often significant poverty and segregation in many ethnic enclaves. Thus, for second- and third-generation Latino youth, who tend to be more bicultural, such enclaves may be less beneficial for individuals who remain there as they may stifle educational and career advancement. In short, upwardly mobile opportunities may simply be unavailable within the local community. Policymakers may wish to communicate more directly with other local communities and states where immigration policies/programs have been successful, and tailor such programs to the specific community where policy is being considered.

On a more specific note, policymakers should ensure that Latino families have access to quality health care through expanding Medicaid and other health-insurance programs, especially in states where there are a significant number of Latino communities but Medicaid has not been expanded. Furthermore, legislators should consider educational policies that center on lowering tuition rates or providing access to quality education, particularly among undocumented youth who complete high school but cannot attend college due to restrictive immigration policies. Such a policy would not only result in a more educated Latino community, but also contribute to upward social mobility that could impact future generations of Latino families. Finally, policymakers should seriously consider the psychological and behavioral impact that current immigration policy at the border has on immigrant families and communities. This does not mean ignoring federal law, but it does mean taking a second look on ensuring that policies in place provide humane treatment to crisis migrants and that keep Latino migrant families together as they wait to hear about their residency status.

With respect to prevention and intervention, interventionists should consider conducting a multilevel assessment of both the target Latino population and the characteristics of the setting where an intervention will be attempted. Indeed, the specific receiving context influences the experiences of immigrants within any setting and may include scaffolding upon which an intervention can be built. Such scaffolding may include financial resources, immigrant-serving institutions, social services, and community-based networks. Intervention developers should also make efforts to clearly understand the target population in terms of their countries of origin, cultural backgrounds, life histories in the country of origin, postmigration experiences, current psychological and behavioral problems they are experiencing, and the specific resources they bring to bear while adapting to a new homeland. In other words, merely knowing who the members of a target population are—for example, newly arrived Latino immigrants living in a traditional receiving context—provides insufficient information for the development of culturally specific prevention and intervention programs.

It is also important to search the scientific literature for promising approaches to assist with the problems at hand in the population of interest. Unfortunately, the literature on clinical or preventive interventions designed and tested specifically for various Latino population in the United States remains small. This means that a program developer will likely be in the position of having, as a starting place, an intervention that was not developed for the target population but has been successful for the targeted issue within another population. Thus, systematic program adaptation is likely to be the primary task of the developer in order to ensure cultural responsiveness and fit of the intervention to the target population. It seems to us that the program adaption process should include, at minimum, elements of a community-based participatory approach, an approach that our team has used successfully in developing culturally informed interventions addressing behavioral and psychological health in Latino population (e.g., Martinez & Eddy, 2005).

Considering the challenges faced by Latino immigrants within each of the contexts of reception, fundamental elements to any intervention include the provision of knowledge, skills training, and individualized supports. In terms of knowledge, interventions need to provide immigrants with crucial information regarding available legal options, community networks, social services, employment opportunities, public schools, and access to housing. In terms of skills training, interventions need to provide immigrants with instruction and practice to cope with stressors associated with migrating to and residing within their new social context(s). Such training should start with individual-focused strategies aimed at providing immigrants with the necessary psychological resources to buffer against acculturative stress, and continue on to issues, if appropriate, such as parenting skills aimed at assisting families to effectively navigate life within their reception context. Finally, in terms of individualized supports, it is clear that there is a great variation within the immigrant population in terms of needs and available resources, and it is important to tailor interventions to the needs of the individual or community.

Both prevention and clinical treatment efforts to support Latino immigrant families should include a careful consideration of the contextual challenges and assets of the receiving context. For example, preventive interventions in emerging receiving contexts must respond to parental disempowerment that often accompanies immigration in an environment with limited social support networks and community resources. Enhancing parent self-efficacy is essential to any intervention effort to disrupt this dynamic (Martinez & Eddy, 2005). Likewise, recent immigrants bring many strengths that can serve as positive supports during the adaptation process. For example, students in Latino immigrant and non-English speaking families have long been shown to do their homework outside of school than their White or English-speaking peers, and their parents have been shown to be more involved in supporting homework completion than their White peers (Martinez, DeGarmo, & Eddy, 2004; Noel, Stark, & Redford, 2016). Given the challenges that often accompany immigrants' adaptation to the United States, such cultural strengths might be easier to overlook in well-meaning efforts to support children and families.

In conclusion, research findings across multiple studies and contexts consistently link contexts of reception with the psychological and behavioral health of Latino immigrant population. Differences in the receiving contexts experienced by immigrants may partially explain why research linking acculturation to mental health outcomes produces inconsistent findings to the extent that many studies fail to directly measure or compare aspects of the receiving contexts in such studies. Understanding the pathways toward healthy adaption to life in the United States for Latino immigrant families requires a more nuanced understanding about how place and context matter in promoting and sustaining healthy adjustment. Future research should pay special attention to understanding the social-contextual mechanisms that drive variance in outcomes based on receiving contexts. Moreover, policies, as well as prevention and treatment approaches, should be developed that respond directly to the characteristics of each of the unique receiving contexts in which Latino immigrants must cope as they attempt to thrive in the United States.

References

Abrego, L. J., & Gonzales, R. G. (2010). Blocked paths, uncertain futures: The postsecondary education and labor market prospects of undocumented Latino youth. *Journal of Education for Students Placed at Risk*, *15*, 144–157.

Alegría, M., Canino, G., Shrout, P. E., Woo, M., Duan, N., Vila, D., et al. (2008). Prevalence of mental illness in immigrant and non-immigrant US Latino groups. *American Journal of Psychiatry*, *165*, 359–369.

Almeida, J., Biello, K. B., Pedraza, F., Wintner, S., & Viruell-Fuentes, E. (2016). The association between anti-immigrant policies and perceived discrimination among Latinos in the US: A multilevel analysis. *SSM-Population Health*, *2*, 897–903.

Arcury, T. A., Sandberg, J. C., Talton, J. W., Laurienti, P. J., Daniel, S. S., & Quandt, S. A. (2018). Mental health among Latina farmworkers and other employed Latinas in North Carolina. *Journal of Rural Mental Health*, *42*, 89–101.

Arévalo, S. P., Tucker, K. L., & Falcón, L. M. (2015). Beyond cultural factors to understand immigrant mental health: Neighborhood ethnic density and the moderating role of pre-migration and post-migration factors. *Social Science & Medicine*, *138*, 91–100.

Bekteshi, V., & Kang, S. W. (2018). Contextualizing acculturative stress among Latino immigrants in the United States: A systematic review. *Ethnicity & Health*, *23*, 1–18.

Bender, D. E., & Castro, D. (2000). Explaining the birth weight paradox: Latina immigrants' perceptions of resilience and risk. *Journal of Immigrant Health*, *2*, 155–173.

Berry, J. W. (2017). Theories and models of acculturation. In S. J. Schwartz & J. B. Unger (Eds.), *Oxford handbook of acculturation and health* (pp. 15–27). New York, NY: Oxford University Press.

Blizzard, B., & Batalova, J. (2019). *Refugees and asylees in the United States*. Washington, DC: Migration Policy Institute.

Bogic, M., Njoku, A., & Priebe, S. (2015). Long-term mental health of war-refugees: A systematic literature review. *BMC International Health and Human Rights*, *15*, 29–70.

Camarota, S. A. (2012). *Immigrants in the United States. A profile of America's foreign-born population*. Retrieved from https://cis.org/sites/cis.org/files/articles/2012/immigrants-in-the-united-states-2012.pdf.

Capielo, C., Delgado-Romero, E. A., & Stewart, A. E. (2015). A focus on an emerging Latina/o population: The role of psychological acculturation, acculturative stress, and coping on depression symptoms among Central Florida Puerto Ricans. *Journal of Latina/o Psychology*, *3*, 209–223.

Capps, R., Ku, L., Fix, M. E., Furgiuele, C., Passel, J. S., Ramchand, R., et al. (2002). *How are immigrants faring after welfare reform? Preliminary evidence from Los Angeles and New York City?: Final report*. Washington, DC: The Urban Institute.

Dinwiddie, G. Y., Gaskin, D. J., Chan, K. S., Norrington, J., & McCleary, R. (2013). Residential segregation, geographic proximity and type of services used: Evidence for racial/ethnic disparities in mental health. *Social Science & Medicine*, *80*, 67–75.

Doom, J. R., Vanzomeren-Dohm, A. A., & Simpson, J. A. (2016). Early unpredictability predicts increased adolescent externalizing behaviors and substance use: A life history perspective. *Development and Psychopathology*, *28*, 1505–1516.

Doty, M. M., Beutel, S., Rasmussen, P. W., & Collins, S. R. (2015, April 27). *Latinos have made coverage gains but millions are still uninsured [Blog post]*. Retrieved from http://www.commonwealthfund.org/publications/blog/2015/apr/latinos-have-made-coverage-gains.

Durand, J., Massey, D. S., & Capoferro, C. (2005). The new geography of Mexican migration. In V. Zúñiga & R. Hernández-León (Eds.), *New destinations: Mexican immigration in the United States* (pp. 1–20). New York, NY: Russell Sage Foundation.

Falicov, C. J. (2007). Working with transnational immigrants: Expanding meanings of family, community, and culture. *Family Process*, *46*, 157–171.

Falicov, C. J. (2013). *Latino families in therapy*. New York, NY: Guilford Press.

Fazel, M., Wheeler, J., & Danesh, J. (2005). Prevalence of serious mental disorder in 7000 refugees resettled in western countries: A systematic review. *The Lancet*, *365*, 1309–1314.

Fix, M., Hooper, K., & Zong, J. (2017). *How are refugees faring? Integration at U.S. state levels*. Washington, DC: Migration Policy Institute.

Flores, S. M. (2010). State dream acts: The effect of in-state resident tuition policies on the college enrollment of undocumented Latino students in the United States. *The Review of Higher Education*, *33*, 239–283.

Flores, A. (2017). *Facts on U.S. Latinos, 2015: Statistical portrait of Hispanics in the United States*. Retrieved from https://www.pewhispanic.org/2017/09/18/facts-on-u-s-latinos/#growth-sources.

Flores, S. M., & Chapa, J. (2009). Latino immigrant access to higher education in a bipolar context of reception. *Journal of Hispanic Higher Education*, *8*, 90–109.

Fuligni, A. J., Telzer, E. H., Bower, J., Cole, S. W., Kiang, L., & Bowen, M. R. (2009). A preliminary study of daily interpersonal stress and C-reactive protein levels among adolescents from Latin American and European backgrounds. *Psychosomatic Medicine*, *71*, 329–333.

Galea, S., Ahern, J., Nandi, A., Tracy, M., Beard, J., & Vlahov, D. (2007). Urban neighborhood poverty and the incidence of depression in a population-based cohort study. *Annals of Epidemiology*, *17*, 171–179.

Greenaway, K. H., Haslam, S. A., Cruwys, T., Branscombe, N. R., Ysseldyk, R., & Heldreth, C. (2015). From "we" to "me": Group identification enhances perceived personal control with consequences for health and well-being. *Journal of Personality and Social Psychology*, *109*, 53–74.

Guttentag, L., & Driscoll, S. (2019). *Crisis at the border? An update on immigration policy with Stanford's Lucas Guttentag*. Stanford Law School. Retrieved from https://law.stanford.edu/2019/04/22/crisis-at-the-border-an-update-on-immigration-policy-with-stanfords-lucas-guttentag/.

Hall, M., & Stringfield, J. (2014). Undocumented migration and the residential segregation of Mexicans in new destinations. *Social Science Research*, *47*, 61–78.

Hatzenbuehler, M. L., Prins, S. J., Flake, M., Philbin, M., Frazer, M. S., Hagen, D., et al. (2017). Immigration policies and mental health morbidity among Latinos: A state-level analysis. *Social Science & Medicine*, *174*, 169–178.

Hull, P., Kilbourne, B., Reece, M., & Husaini, B. (2008). Community involvement and adolescent mental health: Moderating effects of race/ethnicity and neighborhood disadvantage. *Journal of Community Psychology*, *36*, 534–551.

Jasinskaja-Lahti, I., Liebkind, K., Jaakkola, M., & Reuter, A. (2006). Perceived discrimination, social support networks, and psychological well-being among three immigrant groups. *Journal of Cross-Cultural Psychology*, *37*, 293–311.

Jetten, J., Branscombe, N. R., Haslam, S. A., Haslam, C., Cruwys, T., Jones, J. M., et al. (2015). Having a lot of a good thing: Multiple important group memberships as a source of self-esteem. *PLoS One*, *10*, e0124609.

Keller, A., Joscelyne, A., Granski, M., & Rosenfeld, B. (2017). Pre-migration trauma exposure and mental health functioning among Central American migrants arriving at the US border. *PLoS One*, *12*(1), e0168692.

Kiang, L., Grzywacz, J. G., Marín, A. J., Arcury, T. A., & Quandt, S. A. (2010). Mental health in immigrants from nontraditional receiving sites. *Cultural Diversity and Ethnic Minority Psychology*, *16*, 386.

Kim, I. (2016). Beyond trauma: Post-resettlement factors and mental health outcomes among Latino and Asian refugees in the United States. *Journal of Immigrant and Minority Health*, *18*, 740–748.

Lam, C., & Morse, A. (2012). *U.S. supreme court rules on Arizona's immigration enforcement law*. Washington, DC: National Conference of State Legislatures.

Latkin, C. A., Curry, A. D., Hua, W., & Davey, M. A. (2007). Direct and indirect associations of neighborhood disorder with drug use and high-risk sexual partners. *American Journal of Preventive Medicine*, *32*, 234–241.

Lee, M. A. (2009). Neighborhood residential segregation and mental health: A multilevel analysis on Hispanic Americans in Chicago. *Social Science & Medicine*, *68*, 1975–1984.

Li, S. S., Liddell, B. J., & Nickerson, A. (2016). The relationship between post-migration stress and psychological disorders in refugees and asylum seekers. *Current Psychiatry Reports*, *18*, 82.

Lindert, J., von Ehrenstein, O. S., Priebe, S., Mielck, A., & Brähler, E. (2009). Depression and anxiety in labor migrants and refugees—A systematic review and meta-analysis. *Social Science & Medicine*, *69*, 246–257.

Mair, C., Roux, A. V. D., Osypuk, T. L., Rapp, S. R., Seeman, T., & Watson, K. E. (2010). Is neighborhood racial/ethnic composition associated with depressive symptoms? The multi-ethnic study of atherosclerosis. *Social Science & Medicine*, *71*, 541–550.

Marks, A. K., McKenna, J. L., & Coll, C. G. (2018). National immigration receiving contexts. *European Psychologist*, *23*, 6–20.

Martin, L. L. (2012). "Catch and remove": Detention, deterrence, and discipline in US noncitizen family detention practice. *Geopolitics*, *17*, 312–334.

Martin, S. F., Weerasinghe, S., & Taylor, A. (Eds.), (2014). *Humanitarian crises and migration: Causes, consequences and responses*. New York, NY: Routledge.

Martinez, C. R., Jr. (2006). Effects of differential family acculturation on Latino adolescent substance use. *Family Relations*, *55*, 306–317.

Martinez, C. R., Jr., DeGarmo, D. S., & Eddy, J. M. (2004). Promoting academic success among Latino youths. *Hispanic Journal of Behavioral Sciences*, *26*, 128–151.

Martinez, C. R., Jr., & Eddy, J. M. (2005). Effects of culturally adapted parent management training on Latino youth behavioral health outcomes. *Journal of Consulting and Clinical Psychology*, *73*, 841–851.

Martinez, C. R., Jr., McClure, H. H., & Eddy, J. M. (2009). Language brokering contexts and behavioral and emotional adjustment among Latino parents and adolescents. *Journal of Early Adolescence*, *20*(1), 71–98.

Martinez, C. R., Jr., McClure, H. H., & Eddy, J. M. (2016). Latino youth substance use in states with emerging immigrant communities. In Y. F. Thomas, L. N. Price, & A. V. Lybrand (Eds.), *Drug use trajectories among minority youth* (pp. 305–330). New York, NY: Springer Publishing.

Martinez, C. R., Jr., McClure, H. H., Eddy, J. M., & Wilson, D. M. (2011). Time in US residency and the social, behavioral, and emotional adjustment of Latino immigrant families. *Hispanic Journal of Behavioral Sciences*, *33*, 323–349.

McAdam, J. (2014). Conceptualizing "crisis migration": A theoretical perspective. In S. F. Martin, S. Weerasinghe, & A. Taylor (Eds.), *Humanitarian crises and migration: Causes, consequences and responses* (pp. 28–50). New York, NY: Routledge.

Migration Policy Institute. (2015). *Economic, social, and health effects of discrimination on Latino immigrant families*. Retrieved from https://www.migrationpolicy.org/research/economic-social-and-health-effects-discrimination-latino-immigrant-families.

Morse, A. (2011). *Arizona's immigration enforcement laws*. Washington, DC: National Conference of State Legislatures.

Noel, A., Stark, P., & Redford, J. (2016). *National parent and family involvement in education, from the National Household Education Surveys 2012 (NCES 2013–028.REV2)*. Washington, DC: National Center for Education Statistics, Institute of Education Sciences, U.S. Department of Education. Retrieved from http://nces.ed.gov/pubsearch.

Ornelas, I. J., & Perreira, K. M. (2011). The role of migration in the development of depressive symptoms among Latino immigrant parents in the USA. *Social Science & Medicine*, *73*, 1169–1177.

Ostir, G. V., Eschbach, K., Markides, K. S., & Goodwin, J. S. (2003). Neighbourhood composition and depressive symptoms among older Mexican Americans. *Journal of Epidemiology & Community Health*, *57*, 987–992.

Pew Research Center. (2016). *Modern immigration wave brings 59 million to US, driving population growth and change through 2065. Views of immigration's impact on U.S. Society mixed*. Retrieved from https://www.pewresearch.org/hispanic/wp-content/uploads/sites/5/2015/09/2015-09-28_modern-immigration-wave_REPORT.pdf.

Philbin, M. M., Flake, M., Hatzenbuehler, M. L., & Hirsch, J. S. (2018). State-level immigration and immigrant-focused policies as drivers of Latino health disparities in the United States. *Social Science & Medicine*, *199*, 29–38.

Porter, M., & Haslam, N. (2005). Predisplacement and postdisplacement factors associated with mental health of refugees and internally displaced persons: A meta-analysis. *JAMA*, *294*, 602–612.

Portes, A., & Manning, R. D. (1986). The immigrant enclave: Theory and empirical examples. In O. Olzac & J. Nagel (Eds.), *Competitive ethnic relations*. Orlando, FL: Academic Press.

Prado, G., Huang, S., Schwartz, S. J., Maldonado-Molina, M. M., Bandiera, F. C., de la Rosa, M., et al. (2009). What accounts for differences in substance use among U.S.-born and immigrant Hispanic adolescents?: Results from a longitudinal prospective cohort study. *Journal of Adolescent Health*, *45*, 118–125.

Radford, J., & Noe-Bustamante, L. (2019). *Facts on U.S. immigrants, 2017: Statistical portrait of the foreign-born population in the United States*. Pew Hispanic Research Center. Retrieved from https://www.pewresearch.org/hispanic/2019/06/03/facts-on-u-s-immigrants-trend-data/.

Robjant, K., Hassan, R., & Katona, C. (2009). Mental health implications of detaining asylum seekers: Systematic review. *The British Journal of Psychiatry*, *194*, 306–312.

Roche, K. M., Vaquera, E., White, R. M., & Rivera, M. I. (2018). Impacts of immigration actions and news and the psychological distress of US Latino parents raising adolescents. *Journal of Adolescent Health*, *62*, 525–531.

Salas-Wright, C. P., & Schwartz, S. J. (2019). The study and prevention of alcohol and other drug misuse among migrants: Toward a transnational theory of cultural stress. *International Journal of Mental Health and Addiction*, *17*, 346–369.

Scaramutti, C., Salas-Wright, C. P., Vos, S. R., & Schwartz, S. J. (2019). The mental health impact of Hurricane Maria on Puerto Ricans in Puerto Rico and Florida. *Disaster Medicine and Public Health Preparedness*, *13*(1), 24–27.

Schwartz, S. J., Salas-Wright, C. P., Pérez-Gómez, A., Mejía-Trujillo, J., Brown, E. C., Montero-Zamora, P., et al. (2018). Cultural stress and psychological symptoms in recent Venezuelan immigrants to the United States and Colombia. *International Journal of Intercultural Relations*, *67*, 25–34.

Schwartz, S. J., & Unger, J. B. (2017). Acculturation and health: State of the field and recommended directions. In S. J. Schwartz & J. B. Unger (Eds.), *Oxford handbook of acculturation and health* (pp. 1–14). New York, NY: Oxford University Press.

Schwartz, S. J., Unger, J. B., Baezconde-Garbanati, L., Zamboanga, B. L., Lorenzo-Blanco, E. I., Des Rosiers, S. E., et al. (2015). Trajectories of cultural stressors and effects on mental health and substance use among Hispanic immigrant adolescents. *Journal of Adolescent Health*, *56*, 433–439.

Schwartz, S. J., Unger, J. B., Lorenzo-Blanco, E. I., Des Rosiers, S. E., Villamar, J. A., Soto, D. W., et al. (2014). Perceived context of reception among recent Hispanic immigrants: Conceptualization, instrument development, and preliminary validation. *Cultural Diversity and Ethnic Minority Psychology*, *20*(1), 1–15.

Society for Research in Child Development. (2018). *The science is clear: Separating families has long-term damaging psychological and health consequences for children, families, and communities*. Retrieved from http://www.srcd.org/policy-media/statements-evidence.

Supreme Court of the United States. (2012). *National Federation of Independent Business v. Sebelius. Patient Protection and Affordable Care Act Litigation. Paper 333*. Retrieved from http://digitalcommons.law.scu.edu/aca/333.

Szkupinski Quiroga, S., Medina, D. M., & Glick, J. (2014). In the belly of the beast: Effects of anti-immigration policy on Latino community members. *American Behavioral Scientist*, *58*, 1723–1742.

Taylor, Z. E., & Ruiz, Y. (2017). Contextual stressors and the mental health outcomes of Latino children in rural migrant-farmworker families in the Midwest. *Journal of Rural Mental Health*, *41*, 284–298.

Thompson, N. E., & Gurney, A. G. (2003). "He is everything": Religion's role in the lives of immigrant youth. *New Directions for Youth Development*, *2003*, 75–90.

Tilghman-Osborne, E. M., Bámaca-Colbert, M., Witherspoon, D., Wadsworth, M. E., & Hecht, M. L. (2016). Longitudinal associations of language brokering and parent-adolescent closeness in immigrant Latino families. *The Journal of Early Adolescence*, *36*, 319–347.

Vargas Bustamante, A., Fang, H., Garza, J., Carter-Pokras, O., Wallace, S. P., Rizzo, J. A., et al. (2012). Variations in healthcare access and utilization among Mexican immigrants: The role of documentation status. *Journal of Immigrant and Minority Health*, *14*, 146–155.

Vásquez, M. A., Seales, C. E., & Marquardt, M. F. (2008). *New Latino destinations*. In *Latinas/os in the United States: Changing the face of América*. (pp. 19–35). Boston, MA: Springer.

Vega, W. A., Sribney, W. M., Aguilar-Gaxiola, S., & Kolody, B. (2004). 12-Month prevalence of DSM-III-R psychiatric disorders among Mexican Americans: Nativity, social assimilation, and age determinants. *The Journal of Nervous and Mental Disease*, *192*, 532–541.

Viruell-Fuentes, E. A., Miranda, P. Y., & Abdulrahim, S. (2012). More than culture: Structural racism, intersectionality theory, and immigrant health. *Social Science & Medicine*, *75*, 2099–2106.

von Werthern, M., Robjant, K., Chui, Z., Schon, R., Ottisova, L., Mason, C., & Katona, C. (2018). The impact of immigration detention on mental health: A systematic review. *BMC Psychiatry*, *18*(1), 1–19.

Weisskirch, R. S. (2017). *Language brokering in immigrant families: Theories and contexts*. New York, NY: Routledge/Taylor & Francis Group.

Zapata Roblyer, M. I., Carlos, F. L., Merten, M. J., Gallus, K., & Grzywacz, J. G. (2017). Psychosocial factors associated with depressive symptoms among Latina immigrants living in a new arrival community. *Journal of Latina/o Psychology*, *5*, 103–117.

Zúñiga, V. & Hernández-León, R. (Eds.), (2005). *New destinations: Mexican immigration in the United States*. New York, NY: Russell Sage Foundation.

Further reading

Castañeda, H., Holmes, S. M., Madrigal, D. S., Young, M. E. D., Beyeler, N., & Quesada, J. (2015). Immigration as a social determinant of health. *Annual Review of Public Health*, *36*, 375–392.

Chapter 2

Acculturation, parent-child relationships, and mental health of adolescents in Chinese and Mexican immigrant families

Su Yeong Kim[a], Minyu Zhang[a], Yang Hou[b] and Yishan Shen[c]
[a]*University of Texas at Austin, Austin, TX, United States,* [b]*University of Kentucky, Lexington, KY, United States,* [c]*Texas State University, San Marcos, TX, United States*

Acculturation can profoundly influence the way parent-child relationships are expressed in immigrant families. Acculturation refers to the culture change that occurs when immigrants settle in a host culture (Schwartz, Unger, Zamboanga, & Szapocznik, 2010). Within immigrant families, parents' acculturation levels can influence their parenting behaviors. A difference in the acculturation levels of parents and children, which is described as acculturation gap, often results in children performing language translation tasks (language brokering) for parents who are less proficient in the language of the host culture. At present, Asian and Latinx immigrants represent 26% and 51%, respectively, of the immigrant population in the United States (Lopez, Passel, & Rohal, 2015). This review draws on the literature on adolescents in Chinese and Mexican immigrant families whenever possible, as these two ethnic groups are the largest among US Asians and Latinxs, respectively (Lopez et al., 2015). We present consistencies as well as divergences among studies on acculturation and parent-child relationships in Chinese (Asian) and Mexican (Latinx) immigrant families as a means to understand the development of children of immigrants in the United States more broadly.

Garcia Coll et al.'s (1996) integrative model of minority children's development provides a useful framework for our conceptual review. This model describes *adaptive culture* as a coping mechanism in which aspects of culture are modified in recognition of the contextual demands of the environment. Our review highlights the *adaptive culture* and *family* components of Garcia Coll et al.'s model, placing them at the core of our understanding of minority children's developmental outcomes in immigrant families. We do so by examining

Mental and Behavioral Health of Immigrants in the United States
https://doi.org/10.1016/B978-0-12-816117-3.00002-6

how acculturation, as one aspect of adaptive culture, can inform parent-child relationships in immigrant families. Our review extends Garcia Coll et al.'s model, which is relevant to minorities more generally, by addressing the demographic shifts in the United States that have made it important to study minority children with immigrant backgrounds.

Garcia Coll et al.'s (1996) notion of *adaptive culture* in immigrant communities has been shown to promote positive adjustment (Perez-Brena, Rivas-Drake, Toomey, & Umaña-Taylor, 2018). *Adaptive culture* in immigrant communities can also function as a risk enhancer that can be associated with poor adjustment (Perez-Brena et al., 2018). We provide examples of the conditions where promotive or risk enhancing effects may occur in the context of acculturation, parent-child relationship, and mental health among adolescents in Chinese and Mexican immigrant families.

Our review focuses on the developmental period of adolescence because it is characterized by a search for autonomy and independence that potentially puts the children of Chinese and Mexican immigrants into conflict with their collectivistic cultural background (Bámaca-Colbert, Umaña-Taylor, Espinosa-Hernández, & Brown, 2012). This period of heightened tension in the parent-child relationship represents an opportune time for preventive interventions to improve the health and well-being of children of immigrants.

Parenting

Parenting is at the core of understanding parent-child relationships, and acculturation is at the core of understanding parenting in immigrant families. Acculturation has been conceptualized along multiple dimensions and encompasses both the heritage culture and receiving culture orientations (Schwartz et al., 2010). Immigrant parents' acculturation can influence their expression of parenting behaviors in at least two ways: first, the degree to which they espouse cultural values in their parenting behaviors; and second, the ways in which they express ethnic or bicultural socialization beliefs in their parenting behaviors.

Before we understand how acculturation may alter Chinese and Mexican immigrant parents' expression of cultural values in their parenting behaviors, it is important to review how parenting in these groups has been studied. Parental warmth and control are the two parenting dimensions used to derive classic parenting styles—for example, authoritarian (low warmth and high control) and authoritative (high warmth and high control), which are described in the literature on European American children (Maccoby & Martin, 1983). The extant literature on Chinese American and Mexican American parenting practices has focused on each group separately; however, there are striking similarities in the findings of these two groups. For example, earlier studies on Chinese American and Mexican American parenting characterized their parenting as more negative, or authoritarian, relative to European American parenting (e.g., Dornbusch, Ritter, Leiderman, Roberts, & Fraleigh, 1987). More recent studies examining within-group variation in Chinese American or Mexican American parenting have found that parents are more likely to be authoritative than authoritarian (Domenech Rodríguez, Donovick, & Crowley, 2009; Kim, Wang, Orozco-Lapray, Shen, & Murtuza, 2013; White, Zeiders, Gonzales, Tein, & Roosa, 2013). Although the classic parenting styles are still widely used to describe parenting in ethnic and racial groups, when studies have focused on within-group variability, another similarity between the two groups is the emergence of culturally unique parenting styles. Characterized by high levels of warmth, high levels of control, and also a particular cultural value or cultural adaptation in response to the environment, these culturally unique styles include *training* parenting (Chao, 1994) and *tiger* parenting (Kim, Wang, et al., 2013) among Chinese Americans, and *no-nonsense* parenting (White et al., 2013) and *always aware* parenting (Ceballo, Kennedy, Bregman, & Epstein-Ngo, 2012) among Mexican Americans.

One of the first studies on the role of culture in parenting to gain wide attention was by Chao (1994), who described a culturally unique parenting style among Chinese Americans that shared similarities with the classic definition of authoritarian parenting but was different in motivation and meaning. According to Chao (1994), "training" is accomplished through parental involvement, especially through parental devotion and sacrifice (Chao, 1994). More recently, another form of culturally specific parenting in Chinese American families gained popular attention in the press, *tiger* parenting (Chua, 2011). Kim, Wang, et al. (2013) defined *tiger* parenting as a style characterized by high levels of shaming (a culturally relevant parenting dimension), along with more traditional parenting dimensions that are positive (e.g., warmth, monitoring) and negative (e.g., hostility, punitive parenting). They found that even *supportive* parenting, which is akin to authoritative parenting, involves low to moderate levels of shaming in Chinese Americans.

According to Sue and Okazaki (1990), Asian Americans see academic achievement as a form of *relative functionalism*. They argue that achieving academically is seen as an important avenue for achieving upward mobility. For this reason, Chinese American parents may adopt a strategy, such as *tiger* parenting, that results in high academic adjustment for their adolescents (Kim, Wang, et al., 2013). Such a strategy, however, often results in adolescents who are *paradoxically adjusted* (high levels of academic adjustment, low levels of socio-emotional adjustment) (Kim, Wang, Shen, & Hou, 2015). Therefore, while *tiger* parenting can result in a high academic adjustment for adolescents, it comes at the cost of their socio-emotional adjustment (Kim et al., 2015). It appears that *supportive* parenting relates to more positive academic and socio-emotional adjustment of adolescents relative to *tiger* parenting in Chinese American adolescents (Kim et al., 2015).

Studies on culture and parenting in Latinxs have focused on cultural values of *familismo* (reciprocity among family members) and *respeto* (respect for authority) (Halgunseth, Ispa, & Rudy, 2006). These cultural values are positively related to authoritative parenting in Mexican American families (White et al., 2013). Cultural values such as *familismo* can also mitigate the negative effects of economic stressors on Mexican American parenting. For example, White, Liu, Nair, and Tein (2015) found that among mothers endorsing low levels of *familismo*, economic pressure can undermine the mothers' ability to be warm toward their children. However, among mothers endorsing high *familismo*, their ability to prioritize their children's needs in fulfilling their maternal role means that despite facing economic pressure, they are still able to be warm toward their children. Culturally informed parenting of adolescents in Mexican American families is often described in the context of neighborhood adversity, as in the case of *no-nonsense* parenting (White et al., 2013) and *always aware* (*siempre pendiente*) parenting (Ceballo et al., 2012). *No-nonsense* parenting combines moderate levels of harshness with elements of authoritative parenting (high levels of warmth and control). Similarly, *always aware* parenting involves physical and emotional awareness of children through effective communication and monitoring in high risk neighborhoods (Ceballo et al., 2012). These types of parenting are described as adaptations parents make to meet the demands of their high-risk neighborhood environment. Just as authoritative parenting relates to more advantageous outcomes in adolescents, adaptation in parenting, such as *no-nonsense* parenting in fathers, relates to declines in internalizing problems across the course of adolescence in Mexican Americans (White, Liu, Gonzales, Knight, & Tein, 2016).

The scholarship on parenting in both Chinese American (Kim et al., 2015; Kim, Wang, et al., 2013) and Mexican American (White et al., 2013, 2016) families together highlight the importance of going beyond the classic parenting dimensions of warmth and control (Maccoby & Martin, 1983) to consider culture-specific dimensions (such as shaming in Chinese Americans), and culture-specific contexts (such as high-adversity neighborhoods), as a way to capture adaptive parenting in immigrant families.

Parenting and acculturation

Given that immigrant families are likely to express their parenting through their cultural values and/or the contextual demands of their environment (White, Roosa, Weaver, & Nair, 2009), do parents' acculturation levels play a role in how their parenting behaviors are expressed? Studies examining parental acculturation in Chinese and Mexican immigrant families generally find that parental acculturation can relate to parenting behaviors directly, or indirectly through stressors that parents experience as minorities and immigrants. For example, Chinese American parents' higher levels of orientation toward Chinese culture relate to more bicultural difficulty (difficulty managing two cultures) and subsequently parental depressive symptoms, which in turn relate to lower levels of reasoning in parenting; in contrast, parents' higher levels of American orientation relate to lower levels of bicultural difficulty and subsequently parental depressive symptoms, which in turn relate to less punitive parenting and more reasoning in parenting (Kim, Shen, Huang, Wang, & Orozco-Lapray, 2014). Acculturative stressors experienced by parents also influence parenting behaviors directly or indirectly. For example, among Chinese Canadian parents, acculturation stress, such as language stress and discrimination, relates to less positive parenting (lower levels of warmth, lower levels of monitoring, lower levels of reasoning, and higher levels of rigid psychological control) toward their adolescent children (Miao, Costigan, & MacDonald, 2018). Another salient acculturative stressor facing Chinese immigrant parents is being perceived as a foreigner, which indirectly influences adolescents' adjustment through interparental and parent-child relationships (Hou, Kim, & Wang, 2016).

Similar to findings on Chinese immigrant parents, in studies with Mexican American parents, acculturative stressors, such as pressure to learn English, relate to more parental depressed mood, which in turn relates to less parental warmth (White et al., 2009). White and colleagues also found that among Mexican immigrant mothers espousing a high level of *familismo*, neighborhood danger relates to mothers' use of harsh parenting strategies (White, Pasco, Gonzales, Knight, & Burleson, 2019). White and colleagues also contend that the use of harsh parenting among immigrant mothers espousing *familismo* represents an adaptive response to their dangerous host culture environment by giving them the means to ensure their children's safety (White et al., 2019).

Studies show a direct association between the acculturation level of Mexican immigrant parents and their parenting, in which higher levels of parental Mexican orientation relate to more positive parenting, such as more parental involvement and effective discipline (Santisteban, Coatsworth, Briones, Kurtines, & Szapocznik, 2012). Bicultural orientation, or a high level of acculturation toward both the American culture and the heritage culture, also appears to be adaptive. Specifically, when Mexican immigrant mothers and fathers feel a connection to both Latinxs and Americans, they demonstrate more warmth in their parenting and show lower levels of aversive and withdrawn parenting behaviors toward their children (Gassman-Pines & Skinner, 2018).

Parental acculturation's influence on parenting behaviors can also inform immigrant parents' socialization strategies, such as which aspects of the heritage culture they retain and which aspects of the host culture they promote in their children. *Ethnic or cultural socialization* refers to the process by which parents teach their children about their heritage, history and customs, and promote ethnic pride in their children (Umaña-Taylor, Zeiders, & Updegraff, 2013). In Chinese American families, more frequent experiences of interpersonal discrimination in the mother's workplace is a stressor that relates to lower levels of cultural socialization practices (Hagelskamp & Hughes, 2014). According to these authors, Chinese immigrant mothers are likely to attribute workplace discrimination to their foreigner status and limited English proficiency. Parents respond to such workplace discrimination by encouraging their children to assimilate to

US culture while downplaying the distinctiveness of being Chinese. In Mexican American adolescents, ethnic socialization can relate to a stronger sense of ethnic identity, ultimately influencing positive developmental outcomes in multiple domains (Umaña-Taylor et al., 2014). In both Chinese and Mexican immigrant families, ethnic socialization also involves *bicultural socialization*, or transmitting ethnic cultural values to children while also socializing them to become American. This includes teaching children to be aware of discrimination and pointing out the realities of being an ethnic minority (Halgunseth et al., 2006; Juang, Shen, Kim, & Wang, 2016).

Scholarship on parenting in immigrant families is increasingly recognizing the need to consider classic parenting practices together with cultural socialization practices. Calzada and colleagues conceptualize cultural socialization dimensions as representing Mexican cultural values of *respeto,* and *sense of independence* as representing American cultural values in immigrant parents (Calzada, Huang, Anicama, Fernandez, & Brotman, 2012). Mexican immigrant parents' cultural value of *respeto* relates to authoritarian parenting, whereas the American cultural value of independence relates to authoritative parenting (Calzada, Barajas-Gonzalez, Huang, & Brotman, 2017). When the cultural socialization dimensions of *respeto* and sense of independence were combined with general parenting measures such as warmth and parental control, various parenting profiles emerged in a sample of Mexican immigrant parents (Kim, Chen, Hou, Zeiders, & Calzada, 2019). Specifically, six profiles emerged for adolescent report of mothers, including *integrated-authoritative* (high on socialization toward *respeto* and high on socialization toward independence; high on warmth, monitoring, and reasoning; and relatively low on hostility), *moderately integrated-indulgent* (moderate on both socialization toward *respeto* and independence; moderate on positive parenting aspects; and relatively low on hostility), *moderately integrated-no-nonsense* (moderate on both socialization toward *respeto* and independence; moderate on positive parenting aspects; and high on hostility), *moderately integrated-authoritative* (moderate on both socialization toward *respeto* and independence; relatively high on monitoring, reasoning, and warmth; and low on hostility), *separated-no-nonsense* (high on socialization toward *respeto*, low on socialization toward independence; moderate on warmth, monitoring, and reasoning; high on hostility) and *marginalized-harsh* (low on socialization toward *respeto*, low on socialization toward independence; moderate on positive parenting aspects; and relatively high on hostility). In addition, two more profiles for an adolescent report of fathers were found, including *moderately integrated-harsh* (moderate on both socialization toward *respeto* and independence; relatively low on positive parenting aspects; and relatively high on hostility), and *marginalized-neglectful* (very low on all indicators). Of the eight parenting profiles that emerged, parents who espoused the *integrated-authoritative* parenting profile showed the most optimal adolescent outcomes (i.e., better grades, higher sense of life meaning, and fewer delinquent behaviors) (Kim et al., 2019).

In summary, in both Chinese and Mexican Americans, parenting is influenced by their cultural values. Parental acculturation can directly and indirectly alter their parenting behaviors through stressors that arise from their minority and immigrant status. Through bicultural socialization, parents play an active role in socializing their children about their heritage and also about how to become American. Culturally sensitive parenting interventions that reflect the reality of immigration-related challenges show more success when compared to parenting interventions that focus on improving skills related to general parenting practices alone (López-Zerón, Parra-Cardona, & Yeh, 2019). For this reason, there is added value in recognizing contextual stressors and cultural aspects of parenting when developing evidence-based parenting interventions for immigrant families. In the next section, we examine how the acculturation levels of both parents and children in immigrant families influence parent-child relationships.

Parent-child acculturation gap

In immigrant families, members can vary in their orientation (comprised of language, values, behaviors, and practices) toward both heritage and host cultures. A cultural orientation mismatch between parents and children is referred to as generational dissonance by sociologists, and as cultural dissonance, acculturation gap, or acculturation discrepancy by psychologists (Kim, Chen, Li, Huang, & Moon, 2009; Lau et al., 2005). The generational/cultural dissonance literature contains four conflicting propositions: (1) expected acculturation gap (where children acculturate faster and are more oriented toward the host culture than their parents are) creates tensions in the parent-child relationship that relate to negative adolescent outcomes; (2) acculturation gap is normative and does not have negative consequences on adolescent outcomes; (3) reverse or unexpected acculturation gap (where children are more oriented to the heritage culture than their parents are) is what drives negative developmental outcomes in adolescents; and (4) adolescents' adjustment drives the acculturation gap.

The first proposition is the most long-held, dominant view in the literature, and is known as the acculturation gap-distress model, which proposes that high levels of parent-child acculturation discrepancy is a risk factor for child development (Kim, Chen, Wang, Shen, & Orozco-Lapray, 2013; Lui, 2015; Schofield, Parke, Kim, & Coltrane, 2008). In this view, parent-child acculturation discrepancy relates to child maladjustment (e.g., lower academic performance, more depressive symptoms, and more delinquent behaviors) either directly, or indirectly through family processes such as parenting. For example, in a Chinese American sample, higher levels of parent-child acculturation discrepancy in American orientation related to lower levels of parental warmth, monitoring, and reasoning, and consequently to adolescent maladjustment (Kim, Chen, et al., 2013). Similarly, in a Mexican American sample, it was found that higher levels of parent-child acculturation discrepancy were related to more family conflict, and consequently to adolescent maladjustment (Schofield et al., 2008).

From the *adaptive culture* perspective of Garcia Coll et al. (1996), the amplification of risk from the acculturation gap is the dominant view, as acculturation gap is expected to relate to distress. Despite its intuitive appeal, the acculturation gap-distress model has also been critiqued. Using a sample of Mexican Americans, other researchers found that acculturation gap does not relate to maladjustment in adolescents (Telzer, Yuen, Gonzales, & Fuligni, 2016). These authors explain their findings by suggesting that the expected acculturation gap (where children are more oriented to the host culture than their parents are) is normative for children in immigrant families, as it allows children to facilitate familial adjustment to the cultural values and customs of the host society. From Garcia Coll et al.' (1996) *adaptive culture* perspective, then, Telzer et al.' (2016) findings demonstrate how acculturation gap can also be promotive without having negative consequences on the mental health of children of immigrants. Others have critiqued the acculturation gap-distress model by suggesting that reverse acculturation gap, or acculturation gap in the unexpected direction, is what relates to child maladjustment. Using a sample of Mexican Americans, Lau et al. (2005) found that unexpected acculturation gap, where adolescents were more oriented toward the heritage culture than their parents were, was associated with more conduct problems, while acculturation gap in the expected direction did not relate to negative child outcomes.

Although studies have generally tested the relationship from the acculturation gap to adolescent outcomes, the reverse direction of effects has also been proposed and empirically supported (Lui, 2018). Specifically, adolescents' own adjustment appears to be the driving force in predicting acculturation gap: Asian American adolescents' reports of internalizing and externalizing symptoms were found to relate indirectly to acculturation gap through intergenerational cultural conflict (Lui, 2018).

We contend that the inconsistent support for the acculturation gap-distress model found in these studies may be related to differences in methodology. Such differences include variation in the way the acculturation gap is conceptualized and operationalized in empirical studies. Some of these studies used a single informant design and took a difference score approach to assess acculturation gap. The more favored approaches are to assess acculturation from the parent and child directly, and to leverage the following: (1) an interaction approach to assess acculturation gap; (2) multilevel modeling to account for the multilevel structure of parent-child dyads in modeling acculturation gap; (3) the actor-partner interdependence model to account for the dyadic data structure in modeling parent-child acculturation gap; (4) a person-centered latent profile analysis to capture the variation in acculturation dimensions of parents and children; or (5) acculturation gap conceptualized as acculturative family distancing.

Although acculturation gap between parents and children is conceptualized as a dyadic process, studies often use a single informant design to assess parent and child acculturation from the child's perspective (e.g., Céspedes & Huey, 2008). Specifically, an acculturation measure was completed twice by children, once from the child's perspective and a second time where the child reported on the parent's acculturation level (Céspedes & Huey, 2008). This may result in informant bias, such that the acculturation gap may be perceived by the child as larger than it would have been had it been assessed by the parent and child separately. The most intuitive method of assessing acculturation gap is using a difference score approach, in which the difference in acculturation scores between a parent and child is calculated (Birman, 2006). The difference score is then used to represent the acculturation gap and determine its role in child mental health. The difference score approach has been heavily critiqued as invalid (De Los Reyes & Kazdin, 2004; Laird & De Los Reyes, 2013). For example, a difference score of 0 from two *high* acculturation scores in a parent-child dyad could yield the same 0 score as two *low* acculturation scores in a different parent-child dyad. The low acculturation gap score of 0 representing both sets of these parent-child dyads would be misleading, as the type of family functioning in a dyad with two high scores is unlikely to be identical to that of the dyad with two low scores.

The interaction approach is preferred because it takes into account both the parents' and the children's acculturation score simultaneously, by creating an interaction term of the acculturation score for parents and children in a study (Birman, 2006). Using this method, a simple slope analysis (Aiken & West, 1991) is conducted to determine how a child's acculturation level on the x-axis and a dependent variable of interest (e.g., depression) varies by the moderating variables (i.e., parent's acculturation level). For example, in Chinese Canadian immigrant families, when parents reported high levels of Chinese language use, children's Chinese language use related to lower levels of depressive symptoms (Costigan & Dokis, 2006). Such findings highlight how a match in acculturation in Chinese Canadian immigrant parents and their children can result in lower depressive symptoms in children.

The multilevel modeling approach to assessing acculturation gap takes into account the dyadic nature of the parent-child relationship being nested within a family (Kim, Chen, et al., 2013). This approach is more advantageous than the interaction approach, which models the acculturation gap of the entire sample of parents and the entire sample of children to assess acculturation gaps and their influence on child adjustment. The multilevel approach is able to distinguish the variance components attributable to the dyad versus to individual members of the dyad. More precise measurements assist researchers in making better estimates of the acculturation gap and its resulting influence on child adjustment (Kim, Chen, et al., 2013).

The actor-partner interdependence model of acculturation gap also accounts for the dyadic nature of parent-child relationships in modeling acculturation gap. Specifically, this model recognizes the interdependence of parents and children by modeling the child's effects on adjustment based on the actor effect (child) as well as the partner effect (parent) of acculturation (Wang-Schweig & Miller, 2018). The reverse direction, the actor effect (parent) as well as the partner effect (child) of acculturation is also tested simultaneously in the same actor-partner interdependence model (Wang-Schweig & Miller, 2018). Using a sample of Chinese American families, better adjustment was demonstrated when adolescents were more acculturated and when parents were more acculturated, supporting the hypothesis that better adjustment results from an acculturation match between parents and children (Wang-Schweig & Miller, 2018). From the parents' perspective, better adjustment was demonstrated when their children scored higher on both acculturation and heritage cultural orientation, supporting the value of bicultural orientation in the adjustment of children (Wang-Schweig & Miller, 2018).

We advocate using a person-centered methodology, such as latent profile analysis, which has the ability to consider the multidimensionality of acculturation dimensions simultaneously, to capture a more accurate picture of the generational dissonance that occurs in immigrant families. In fact, a study comparing studies using the difference score, interaction, and person-centered approaches when assessing acculturation gap demonstrated the superiority of the latent profile analysis approach when assessing acculturation gap as a means to understand adolescent mental health outcomes (Bámaca-Colbert & Gayles, 2010). In a sample of Mexican-origin adolescent girls and their mothers, a latent profile characterized by cultural dissonance between mothers and adolescents, together with high conflict and low maternal supportive parenting, related to poor adjustment in girls (Bámaca-Colbert & Gayles, 2010).

Another example of a latent profile approach to assessing acculturation gap is demonstrated by Weaver and Kim (2008), who used a person-centered approach to identify three profiles of acculturation in a Chinese American sample (bicultural, more American, and more Chinese), based on five indicators of acculturation (American and Chinese orientations, English and Chinese proficiency, and family obligation). They revealed that different combinations of adolescents' and parents' acculturation profiles had different implications for adolescent outcomes, findings that largely support the acculturation gap-distress model. In fact, relative to other combinations, parent-child dyads with an acculturation match—specifically, bicultural adolescents with bicultural parents—experienced more supportive parenting, which then related to fewer adolescent depressive symptoms. In addition, dyads with an acculturation mismatch (or acculturation gap)—specifically, American-oriented adolescents with Chinese-oriented parents—reported the least supportive parenting and the most depressive symptoms.

Still, other scholars demonstrate the need to go beyond assessing acculturation gap from scores derived from parent and child. A measure that assesses the acculturation gap via *acculturative family distancing* has been proposed and empirically supported (Nair, Roche, & White, 2018). *Acculturative family distancing* refers to communication challenges and cultural value incongruence between parent and child that create a distance between the two individuals (Hwang, Wood, & Fujimoto, 2010). *Acculturative family distancing* relates to increased risk for depression in Chinese American high school students via increased family conflict (Hwang et al., 2010). *Acculturative family distancing* also relates to changes in alcohol use through increased parent-child conflict in Latinx adolescents (Nair et al., 2018). One advantage of measuring *acculturative family distancing* is that this approach avoids the drawbacks of using acculturation scores from two different informants. Specifically, the measure assessing the acculturation status of parent and child as two different informants would need to demonstrate measurement equivalence (Nair et al., 2018). However, this is rarely done, which raises questions about the validity of acculturation gap scores that rely on assessments from two different informants. Acculturative family distancing has the advantage of using a single measure to gather perceptions of agreement on items that may indicate the acculturation gap in parent-child dyads (Nair et al., 2018). An example item would be, "My parent and I agree on whether to spend free time with friends or family." Questions like this can also provide useful data when only a single informant is available to assess acculturation gap.

In summary, we have shown that variation in family members' acculturation levels can result in various forms of acculturation gap. Depending on the type of acculturation gap, it can relate to the quality of parent-child relationships and adolescent outcomes in ways that are supportive or unsupportive. We also offered methodological considerations in the assessment of acculturation gap in examining its links to the mental health of adolescents. In the next section, we describe how varying linguistic acculturation levels between parents and children can result in children functioning as language brokers for their families, and how this activity influences family processes and mental health outcomes.

Language brokering

An acculturation challenge facing Chinese and Mexican immigrants is that they speak a heritage language other than English. Attending public school facilitates acculturation for children in immigrant families, such that many become more oriented to the US culture and language than their parents. This can result in children functioning as interpreters and translators (i.e., language brokers) for their English-limited parents (Wu & Kim, 2009). As language brokers, children play an important role as intermediaries between their parents and the host society (Kim, Hou, & Gonzalez, 2017). Between 71% and 89% of children in immigrant families are language brokers (Chao, 2006).

Language brokering represents an example of the *adaptive cultural system* advanced by Garcia Coll et al. (1996), which can either promote or undermine developmental outcomes among children in immigrant families (White, Nair, & Bradley, 2018). As a component of bilingualism, language brokering can enhance cognitive and language skills, by reducing processing time when switching between languages (Dorner, Orellana, & Li-Grining, 2007) and by utilizing skills critical for reading (e.g., vocabulary development, chunking text) and achievement (Dorner et al., 2007). Being asked to provide family assistance, such as by language brokering, can be a source of pride as well as a source of stress for children (Telzer & Fuligni, 2009; Wu & Kim, 2009). While language brokers report feeling helpful for providing assistance to their families (Roche, Lambert, Ghazarian, & Little, 2015), language brokering has also been linked to more depressive symptoms and substance use in Latinx adolescents (Kam & Lazarevic, 2014; Kim, Hou, & Gonzalez, 2017).

We propose that whereas research examining language brokering frequency has resulted in a mixed picture of positive and negative consequences, considering children's subjective appraisals of the language brokering experience (e.g., feeling a sense of burden or feeling proud) provides clearer linkages to positive or negative outcomes. Advances in the measurement of subjective experiences of language brokering have greatly facilitated an examination of how appraisal of this experience can inform developmental outcomes among language brokers. Measurements of language brokering now include examining the extent of, and attitudes toward, language brokering (Shen, Seo, Hu, Zhang, & Chao, 2019); the positive and negative feelings attached to language brokering, along with parent-child relationship implications of language brokering (Kim et al., 2014; Kim, Hou, Shen, & Zhang, 2017); and parent-child interaction goals during language brokering (Guntzviller, 2016).

One of the earliest studies that showed the mixed effects of language brokering was by Chao (2006). This study found that more frequent language brokering was associated with higher respect for parents, but also more internalizing problems among adolescents. Considering subjective appraisals of the language brokering experience can help reveal the conditions that may relate to the disparate findings in previous research on parent-child relationship quality and adolescent outcomes. For example, higher frequency of language brokering related to more respect for parents in Chinese American adolescents because adolescents perceived that their parents were making sacrifices for them (Shen, Kim, Wang, & Chao, 2014). Other positive perceptions (feeling happy, proud, useful) around language brokering were also found to be associated with better adolescent outcomes, such as higher self-esteem, in Mexican American adolescents (Weisskirch, 2007). In terms of negative perceptions, when adolescents perceived their language brokering as burdensome, this instigated family-based acculturation stress to relate to more substance use in a mostly Mexican American adolescent sample (Kam & Lazarevic, 2014). Similarly, adolescents' negative feelings and a sense of brokering burden were associated with parent-child conflict and depressive symptoms in a Chinese American sample (Kim, Wang, et al., 2014).

We also see evidence that acculturation and culture-related stressors function as predictors of positive and negative language brokering experiences. Using a sample of Mexican American adolescents in immigrant families, one study found that adolescents who are more bicultural in their acculturation status, with parents who are less acculturated, reported more positive and less negative language brokering experiences (Zhang, Kim, Hou, & Shen, 2019). Low heritage cultural orientation and a weak sense of family obligation also function as precursors to negative feelings about language brokering behaviors (Wu & Kim, 2009). Similarly, adolescents' positive personal characteristics, such as resilience, are precursors to positive feelings about brokering (Kim, Hou, & Gonzalez, 2017). These studies suggest that focusing on the conditions under which language brokering behaviors relate to positive versus negative subjective appraisals is fruitful, in order to understand better the impact of language brokering on parent-child relationships and adolescent developmental outcomes.

There are three recent advances in the study of language brokering and mental health outcomes among adolescents in immigrant families. First, studies are using latent profile approaches to recognize the multitude of language brokering experiences and their relationship to adolescent mental health. In a sample of Chinese American adolescents, two profiles of burdened and efficacious language brokers emerged (Shen, Kim, & Benner, 2019). These profiles were derived by using four measures of language brokering subjective experiences, including brokering burden, negative feelings, brokering efficacy, and positive feelings. The efficacious brokers were predicted by higher levels of bilingualism in English and Chinese. The burdened brokers showed high levels of parent-child alienation and in turn, more depressive symptomatology relative to non-brokers and efficacious brokers (Shen, Kim et al., 2019).

Second, studies are considering the experiences of language brokering within the contextual demands of the environment in which language brokers are embedded, showing the conditions under which language brokering can have positive or negative mental health outcomes in children (Kim et al., 2018). In Kim et al.'s study, three sociocultural stressors were selected to represent the contextual stressors facing Mexican American adolescent language brokers: economic stress, discrimination, and foreigner stress. These three sociocultural stressors were selected because fulfilling family responsibilities, such as by language brokering for their parents, may exacerbate adolescents' perceptions of economic stress, discrimination, and foreigner stress. For example, language brokers may be privy to the family's financial situation, making the family's economic stress more apparent. Performing an activity not practiced by children of native-born parents can also invite discriminatory treatment. Despite the fact that the majority of Mexican-origin language brokers are US-born, they may still be perceived as foreigners for speaking Spanish and engaging in Mexican cultural practices as a way to communicate and interact with their English-limited immigrant parents. These sociocultural stressors (economic stress, discrimination, foreigner stress) were also selected because of a strong empirical basis for their effects on mental health and developmental outcomes of adolescents. Economic stress and discrimination are consistently linked to poor adolescent mental health (Benner & Kim, 2009; Conger & Donnellan, 2007). Foreigner stress is linked to depressive symptoms and life satisfaction (Armenta et al., 2013; Kim, Hou, & Gonzalez, 2017). The study's goal was to determine how the focal sociocultural stressors, together with positive and negative language brokering experiences, form profiles to influence adolescent mental and physical health.

Latent profile analysis on language brokering adolescents in Mexican immigrant families identified three types of sociocultural stress profiles: *moderate, protective,* and *risk* (Kim et al., 2018). Adolescents in the *moderate* profile group showed medium levels of all stressors (daily discrimination, foreigner stress, economic stress, and language brokering experiences). Adolescents in the *protective* profile group also showed medium levels of three of the stressors, but they reported their language brokering experiences as being beneficial. Those with a *risk* profile showed high levels of all stressors, including negative language brokering experiences.

Relative to the *moderate* profiles, Kim et al. (2018) found that the *protective* profiles related to lower levels of delinquent behaviors and better self-reported sleep quality, whereas the *risk* profiles showed worse outcomes including more depressive symptoms. As posited by the accumulation model of risk (Walsemann, Goosby, & Farr, 2016), negative language brokering experiences—when combined with others stressors in the environment, as in the case of the stable *risk* profile—are associated with adverse developmental outcomes in adolescents. The results also suggest that positive language brokering experiences (as seen in the *protective* profiles) are beneficial for adolescents' development, protecting brokers from the detrimental effects of other stressors that occur at moderate levels.

Third, studies are recognizing parents as actors in the language brokering process, and are assessing parent-child interaction goals while language brokering from the perspective of both parent and child (Guntzviller, 2016). Mutual goal setting between parent and child while language brokering relates to relationship satisfaction (Guntzviller, 2017). In Latinx families, various profiles of coping with language brokering in parents and children also have implications for mental health outcomes, such as depressive symptoms in parents and children (Kam, Basinger, & Guntzviller, 2017). Specifically, mothers with more communal coping related to language brokering—who tend to perceive stressors as shared problems and cope with the stressors with their children as a team—experience fewer depressive symptoms, whereas children expressing more independent coping related to language brokering experiences—who tend to consider stressors as their own problems and cope with them alone—show more depressive symptoms (Kam et al., 2017).

To recapitulate, language brokering can result from disparate linguistic acculturation levels among immigrant family members, especially when immigrant parents are English-limited relative to their adolescents. Subjective experiences of language brokering can be either positive or negative, influencing parent-child relationships and adolescent outcomes accordingly. More recent scholarship is also recognizing the social context in which language brokering occurs to determine its mental health outcomes in children.

Conclusion

Garcia Coll et al.'s (1996) integrative model provides a useful overarching framework to understand minority children's development. We have focused on children in immigrant families more specifically, by reviewing two aspects of their conceptual framework, *adaptive culture* (acculturation), and *family* (parent-child relationship). We recognize that the acculturation of parents and children in immigrant families can influence their cultural values, parent-child relationships, and adolescent outcomes. The acculturation challenges facing Chinese and Mexican immigrant families can manifest as an acculturation gap between children and parents, with children functioning as language brokers for their families. This review examined the conditions under which parenting, acculturation gap, and language brokering may represent sources of risk or protection in the mental health and developmental outcomes of adolescents (Perez-Brena et al., 2018). While our focus was on Chinese and Mexican immigrant families, we invite readers to apply our conceptual review to other immigrant groups of interest.

As immigrants continue to drive population growth in the United States (Lopez et al., 2015), children of these immigrants will make up a significant portion of the US' population. Continued research on the interrelationships among the constructs described in this chapter would be helpful, as a better understanding of immigrant children's development will be important in improving the health and well-being of America's children more generally.

References

Aiken, L. S., & West, S. G. (1991). *Multiple regression: Testing and interpreting interactions*. Thousand Oaks, CA: Sage Publications, Inc.

Armenta, B. E., Lee, R. M., Pituc, S. T., Jung, K.-R., Park, I. J. K., Soto, J. A., et al. (2013). Where are you from? A validation of the foreigner objectification scale and the psychological correlates of foreigner objectification among Asian Americans and Latinos. *Cultural Diversity and Ethnic Minority Psychology*, *19*, 131–142. https://doi.org/10.1037/a0031547.

Bámaca-Colbert, M. Y., & Gayles, J. G. (2010). Variable-centered and person-centered approaches to studying Mexican-origin mother–daughter cultural orientation dissonance. *Journal of Youth and Adolescence*, *39*, 1274–1292. https://doi.org/10.1007/s10964-009-9447-3.

Bámaca-Colbert, M. Y., Umaña-Taylor, A. J., Espinosa-Hernández, G., & Brown, A. M. (2012). Behavioral autonomy age expectations among Mexican-origin mother–daughter dyads: An examination of within-group variability. *Journal of Adolescence*, *35*, 691–700. https://doi.org/10.1016/j.adolescence.2011.10.005.

Benner, A. D., & Kim, S. Y. (2009). Experiences of discrimination among Chinese American adolescents and the consequences for socioemotional and academic development. *Developmental Psychology*, *45*, 1682–1694. https://doi.org/10.1037/a0016119.

Birman, D. (2006). Measurement of the 'Acculturation Gap' in immigrant families and implications for parent-child relationships. In M. H. Bornstein & L. R. Cote (Eds.), *Acculturation and parent-child relationships: Measurement and development* (pp. 113–134). Mahwah, NJ: Lawrence Erlbaum Associates Publishers.

Calzada, E., Barajas-Gonzalez, R. G., Huang, K.-Y., & Brotman, L. (2017). Early childhood internalizing problems in Mexican- and Dominican-origin children: The role of cultural socialization and parenting practices. *Journal of Clinical Child and Adolescent Psychology*, *46*, 551–562. https://doi.org/10.1080/15374416.2015.1041593.

Calzada, E. J., Huang, K.-Y., Anicama, C., Fernandez, Y., & Brotman, L. M. (2012). Test of a cultural framework of parenting with Latino families of young children. *Cultural Diversity and Ethnic Minority Psychology*, *18*, 285–296. https://doi.org/10.1037/a0028694.

Ceballo, R., Kennedy, T. M., Bregman, A., & Epstein-Ngo, Q. (2012). Always aware (Siempre pendiente): Latina mothers' parenting in high-risk neighborhoods. *Journal of Family Psychology*, *26*, 805–815. https://doi.org/10.1037/a0029584.

Céspedes, Y. M., Huey, S. J., Jr. (2008). Depression in Latino adolescents: A cultural discrepancy perspective. *Cultural Diversity and Ethnic Minority Psychology*, *14*, 168–172. https://doi.org/10.1037/1099-9809.14.2.168.

Chao, R. K. (1994). Beyond parental control and authoritarian parenting style: Understanding Chinese parenting through the cultural notion of training. *Child Development*, *65*, 1111–1119. https://doi.org/10.2307/1131308.

Chao, R. K. (2006). The prevalence and consequences of adolescents' language brokering for their immigrant parents. In M. H. Bornstein & L. R. Cote (Eds.), *Acculturation and parent–child relationships: Measurement and development* (pp. 271–296). Mahwah, NJ: Erlbaum.

Chua, A. (2011). *Battle hymn of the tiger mother*. New York: Penguin Books.

Conger, R. D., & Donnellan, M. B. (2007). An interactionist perspective on the socioeconomic context of human development. *Annual Review of Psychology*, *58*, 175–199. https://doi.org/10.1146/annurev.psych.58.110405.085551.

Costigan, C. L., & Dokis, D. P. (2006). Relations between parent-child acculturation differences and adjustment within immigrant Chinese families. *Child Development*, *77*, 1252–1267. https://doi.org/10.1111/j.1467-8624.2006.00932.x.

De Los Reyes, A., & Kazdin, A. E. (2004). Measuring informant discrepancies in clinical child research. *Psychological Assessment*, *16*, 330–334. https://doi.org/10.1037/1040-3590.16.3.330.

Domenech Rodríguez, M. M., Donovick, M. R., & Crowley, S. L. (2009). Parenting styles in a cultural context: Observations of 'protective parenting' in first-generation Latinos. *Family Process*, *48*, 195–210. https://doi.org/10.1111/j.1545-5300.2009.01277.x.

Dornbusch, S. M., Ritter, P. L., Leiderman, P. H., Roberts, D. F., & Fraleigh, M. J. (1987). The relation of parenting style to adolescent school performance. *Child Development*, *58*, 1244–1257. https://doi.org/10.2307/1130618.

Dorner, L. M., Orellana, M. F., & Li-Grining, C. P. (2007). 'I helped my Mom,' and it helped me: Translating the skills of language brokers into improved standardized test scores. *American Journal of Education*, *113*, 451–478. https://doi.org/10.1086/512740.

Garcia Coll, C., Lamberty, G., Jenkins, R., McAdoo, H. P., Crnic, K., Wasik, B. H., et al. (1996). An integrative model for the study of developmental competencies in minority children. *Child Development*, *67*, 1891–1914. https://doi.org/10.2307/1131600.

Gassman-Pines, A., & Skinner, A. T. (2018). Psychological acculturation and parenting behaviors in Mexican-immigrant families. *Journal of Family Issues*, *39*, 1139–1164. https://doi.org/10.1177/0192513x16687001.

Guntzviller, L. M. (2016). Mother-child communication quality during language brokering: Validation of four measures of brokering interaction goals. *Hispanic Journal of Behavioral Sciences*, *38*, 1–23. https://doi.org/10.1177/0739986315613053.

Guntzviller, L. M. (2017). Testing multiple goals theory with low-income, mother-child Spanish-speakers: Language brokering interaction goals and relational satisfaction. *Communication Research, 44*, 717–742. https://doi.org/10.1177/0093650215608238.

Hagelskamp, C., & Hughes, D. L. (2014). Workplace discrimination predicting racial/ethnic socialization across African American, Latino, and Chinese families. *Cultural Diversity and Ethnic Minority Psychology, 20*, 550–560. https://doi.org/10.1037/a0035321.

Halgunseth, L. C., Ispa, J. M., & Rudy, D. (2006). Parental control in Latino families: An integrated review of the literature. *Child Development, 77*, 1282–1297. https://doi.org/10.1111/j.1467-8624.2006.00934.x.

Hou, Y., Kim, S. Y., & Wang, Y. (2016). Parental acculturative stressors and adolescent adjustment through interparental and parent–child relationships in Chinese American families. *Journal of Youth and Adolescence, 45*, 1466–1481. https://doi.org/10.1007/s10964-016-0441-2.

Hwang, W.-C., Wood, J. J., & Fujimoto, K. (2010). Acculturative family distancing (AFD) and depression in Chinese American families. *Journal of Consulting and Clinical Psychology, 78*, 655–667. https://doi.org/10.1037/a0020542.

Juang, L. P., Shen, Y., Kim, S. Y., & Wang, Y. (2016). Development of an Asian American parental racial–ethnic socialization scale. *Cultural Diversity and Ethnic Minority Psychology, 22*, 417–431. https://doi.org/10.1037/cdp0000083.

Kam, J. A., Basinger, E. D., & Guntzviller, L. M. (2017). Communal coping among Spanish-speaking mother–child dyads engaging in language brokering: A latent class analysis. *Communication Research, 44*, 743–769. https://doi.org/10.1177/0093650216684927.

Kam, J. A., & Lazarevic, V. (2014). The stressful (and not so stressful) nature of language brokering: Identifying when brokering functions as a cultural stressor for Latino immigrant children in early adolescence. *Journal of Youth and Adolescence, 43*, 1994–2011. https://doi.org/10.1007/s10964-013-0061-z.

Kim, S. Y., Chen, S., Hou, Y., Zeiders, K. H., & Calzada, E. J. (2019). Parental socialization profiles in Mexican-origin families: Considering cultural socialization and general parenting practices. *Cultural Diversity and Ethnic Minority Psychology, 25*, 439–450. https://doi.org/10.1037/cdp0000234.

Kim, S. Y., Chen, Q., Li, J., Huang, X., & Moon, U. J. (2009). Parent–child acculturation, parenting, and adolescent depressive symptoms in Chinese immigrant families. *Journal of Family Psychology, 23*, 426–437. https://doi.org/10.1037/a0016019.

Kim, S. Y., Chen, Q., Wang, Y., Shen, Y., & Orozco-Lapray, D. (2013). Longitudinal linkages among parent–child acculturation discrepancy, parenting, parent–child sense of alienation, and adolescent adjustment in Chinese immigrant families. *Developmental Psychology, 49*, 900–912. https://doi.org/10.1037/a0029169.

Kim, S. Y., Hou, Y., & Gonzalez, Y. (2017). Language brokering and depressive symptoms in Mexican-American adolescents: Parent–child alienation and resilience as moderators. *Child Development, 88*, 867–881. https://doi.org/10.1111/cdev.12620.

Kim, S. Y., Hou, Y., Shen, Y., & Zhang, M. (2017). Longitudinal measurement equivalence of subjective language brokering experiences scale in Mexican American adolescents. *Cultural Diversity and Ethnic Minority Psychology, 23*, 230–243. https://doi.org/10.1037/cdp0000117.

Kim, S. Y., Hou, Y., Song, J., Schwartz, S. J., Chen, S., Zhang, M., et al. (2018). Profiles of language brokering experiences and contextual stressors: Implications for adolescent outcomes in Mexican immigrant families. *Journal of Youth and Adolescence, 47*, 1629–1648. https://doi.org/10.1007/s10964-018-0851-4.

Kim, S. Y., Shen, Y., Huang, X., Wang, Y., & Orozco-Lapray, D. (2014). Chinese American parents' acculturation and enculturation, bicultural management difficulty, depressive symptoms, and parenting. *Asian American Journal of Psychology*, *5*, 298–306. https://doi.org/10.1037/a0035929.

Kim, S. Y., Wang, Y., Orozco-Lapray, D., Shen, Y., & Murtuza, M. (2013). Does 'tiger parenting' exist? Parenting profiles of Chinese Americans and adolescent developmental outcomes. *Asian American Journal of Psychology*, *4*, 7–18. https://doi.org/10.1037/a0030612.

Kim, S. Y., Wang, Y., Shen, Y., & Hou, Y. (2015). Stability and change in adjustment profiles among Chinese American adolescents: The role of parenting. *Journal of Youth and Adolescence*, *44*, 1735–1751. https://doi.org/10.1007/s10964-015-0303-3.

Kim, S. Y., Wang, Y., Weaver, S. R., Shen, Y., Wu-Seibold, N., & Liu, C. H. (2014). Measurement equivalence of the language-brokering scale for Chinese American adolescents and their parents. *Journal of Family Psychology*, *28*, 180–192. https://doi.org/10.1037/a0036030.

Laird, R. D., & De Los Reyes, A. (2013). Testing informant discrepancies as predictors of early adolescent psychopathology: Why difference scores cannot tell you what you want to know and how polynomial regression may. *Journal of Abnormal Child Psychology*, *41*, 1–14. https://doi.org/10.1007/s10802-012-9659-y.

Lau, A. S., McCabe, K. M., Yeh, M., Garland, A. F., Wood, P. A., & Hough, R. L. (2005). The acculturation gap-distress hypothesis among high-risk Mexican American families. *Journal of Family Psychology*, *19*, 367–375. https://doi.org/10.1037/0893-3200.19.3.367.

Lopez, M. H., Passel, J., & Rohal, M. (2015). *Modern immigration wave brings 59 million to U.S., driving population growth and change through 2065: Views of immigration's impact on U.S. society mixed*. Washington, DC: Pew Research Center.

López-Zerón, G., Parra-Cardona, J. R., & Yeh, H.-H. (2019). Addressing immigration-related stress in a culturally adapted parenting intervention for Mexican-origin immigrants: Initial positive effects and key areas of improvement. *Family Process*, https://doi.org/10.1111/famp.12481.

Lui, P. P. (2015). Intergenerational cultural conflict, mental health, and educational outcomes among Asian and Latino/a Americans: Qualitative and meta-analytic review. *Psychological Bulletin*, *141*, 404–446. https://doi.org/10.1037/a0038449.

Lui, P. P. (2018). Rethinking the acculturation gap-distress theory among Asian Americans: Testing bidirectional indirect relations. *American Journal of Orthopsychiatry*, https://doi.org/10.1037/ort0000322.

Maccoby, E. E., & Martin, J. A. (1983). Socialization in the context of the family: Parent-child interaction. In P. H. Mussen & E. M. Hetherington (Eds.), *Handbook of child psychology: Vol. 4. Socialization, personality, and social development*. (4th ed., pp. 1–101). New York, NY: Wiley.

Miao, S. W., Costigan, C. L., & MacDonald, S. W. S. (2018). Spillover of stress to Chinese Canadian immigrants' parenting: Impact of acculturation and parent–child stressors. *Asian American Journal of Psychology*, *9*, 190–199. https://doi.org/10.1037/aap0000105.

Nair, R. L., Roche, K. M., & White, R. M. B. (2018). Acculturation gap distress among Latino youth: Prospective links to family processes and youth depressive symptoms, alcohol use, and academic performance. *Journal of Youth and Adolescence*, *47*, 105–120. https://doi.org/10.1007/s10964-017-0753-x.

Perez-Brena, N. J., Rivas-Drake, D., Toomey, R. B., & Umaña-Taylor, A. J. (2018). Contributions of the integrative model for the study of developmental competencies in minority children: What have we learned about adaptive culture? *American Psychologist*, *73*, 713–726. https://doi.org/10.1037/amp0000292.

Roche, K. M., Lambert, S. F., Ghazarian, S. R., & Little, T. D. (2015). Adolescent language brokering in diverse contexts: Associations with parenting and parent–youth relationships in a new immigrant destination area. *Journal of Youth and Adolescence*, *44*, 77–89. https://doi.org/10.1007/s10964-014-0154-3.

Santisteban, D. A., Coatsworth, J. D., Briones, E., Kurtines, W., & Szapocznik, J. (2012). Beyond acculturation: An investigation of the relationship of Familism and parenting to behavior problems in Hispanic youth. *Family Process*, *51*, 470–482. https://doi.org/10.1111/j.1545-5300.2012.01414.x.

Schofield, T. J., Parke, R. D., Kim, Y., & Coltrane, S. (2008). Bridging the acculturation gap: Parent-child relationship quality as a moderator in Mexican American families. *Developmental Psychology*, *44*, 1190–1194. https://doi.org/10.1037/a0012529.

Schwartz, S. J., Unger, J. B., Zamboanga, B. L., & Szapocznik, J. (2010). Rethinking the concept of acculturation: Implications for theory and research. *American Psychologist*, *65*, 237–251. https://doi.org/10.1037/a0019330.

Shen, Y., Kim, S. Y., & Benner, A. D. (2019). Burdened or efficacious? Subgroups of Chinese American language brokers, predictors, and long-term outcomes. *Journal of Youth and Adolescence*, *48*, 154–169. https://doi.org/10.1007/s10964-018-0916-4.

Shen, Y., Kim, S. Y., Wang, Y., & Chao, R. K. (2014). Language brokering and adjustment among Chinese and Korean American adolescents: A moderated mediation model of perceived maternal sacrifice, respect for the mother, and mother–child open communication. *Asian American Journal of Psychology*, *5*, 86–95. https://doi.org/10.1037/a0035203.

Shen, Y., Seo, E., Hu, Y., Zhang, M., & Chao, R. K. (2019). Measurement invariance of language brokering extent and attitudes in linguistic minority adolescents: Item response theory analyses. *Cultural Diversity and Ethnic Minority Psychology*, *25*, 170–178. https://doi.org/10.1037/cdp0000224.

Sue, S., & Okazaki, S. (1990). Asian-American educational achievements: A phenomenon in search of an explanation. *American Psychologist*, *45*, 913–920. https://doi.org/10.1037/0003-066x.45.8.913.

Telzer, E. H., & Fuligni, A. J. (2009). Daily family assistance and the psychological well-being of adolescents from Latin American, Asian, and European backgrounds. *Developmental Psychology*, *45*, 1177–1189. https://doi.org/10.1037/a0014728.

Telzer, E. H., Yuen, C., Gonzales, N., & Fuligni, A. J. (2016). Filling gaps in the acculturation gap-distress model: Heritage cultural maintenance and adjustment in Mexican–American families. *Journal of Youth and Adolescence*, *45*, 1412–1425. https://doi.org/10.1007/s10964-015-0408-8.

Umaña-Taylor, A. J., O'Donnell, M., Knight, G. P., Roosa, M. W., Berkel, C., & Nair, R. (2014). Mexican-origin early adolescents' ethnic socialization, ethnic identity, and psychosocial functioning. *The Counseling Psychologist*, *42*, 170–200. https://doi.org/10.1177/0011000013477903.

Umaña-Taylor, A. J., Zeiders, K. H., & Updegraff, K. A. (2013). Family ethnic socialization and ethnic identity: A family-driven, youth-driven, or reciprocal process? *Journal of Family Psychology*, *27*, 137–146. https://doi.org/10.1037/a0031105.

Walsemann, K. M., Goosby, B. J., & Farr, D. (2016). Life course SES and cardiovascular risk: Heterogeneity across race/ethnicity and gender. *Social Science & Medicine*, *152*, 147–155. https://doi.org/10.1016/j.socscimed.2016.01.038. 1982.

Wang-Schweig, M., & Miller, B. A. (2018). Examining the interdependence of parent–adolescent acculturation gaps on acculturation-based conflict: Using the actor-partner interdependence model. *Journal of Youth and Adolescence*, https://doi.org/10.1007/s10964-018-0948-9.

Weaver, S. R., & Kim, S. Y. (2008). A person-centered approach to studying the linkages among parent-child differences in cultural orientation, supportive parenting, and adolescent depressive symptoms in Chinese American families. *Journal of Youth and Adolescence*, *37*, 36–49. https://doi.org/10.1007/s10964-007-9221-3.

Weisskirch, R. S. (2007). Feelings about language brokering and family relations among Mexican American early adolescents. *The Journal of Early Adolescence*, *27*, 545–561. https://doi.org/10.1177/0272431607302935.

White, R. M. B., Liu, Y., Gonzales, N. A., Knight, G. P., & Tein, J. Y. (2016). Neighborhood qualification of the association between parenting and problem behavior trajectories among Mexican-origin father–adolescent dyads. *Journal of Research on Adolescence*, https://doi.org/10.1111/jora.12245.

White, R. M. B., Liu, Y., Nair, R. L., & Tein, J.-Y. (2015). Longitudinal and integrative tests of family stress model effects on Mexican origin adolescents. *Developmental Psychology*, *51*, 649–662. https://doi.org/10.1037/a0038993.

White, R. M. B., Nair, R. L., & Bradley, R. H. (2018). Theorizing the benefits and costs of adaptive cultures for development. *American Psychologist*, *73*, 727–739. https://doi.org/10.1037/amp0000237.

White, R. M. B., Pasco, M. C., Gonzales, N. A., Knight, G. P., & Burleson, E. (2019). US Mexican parents' use of harsh parenting in the context of neighborhood danger. *Journal of Family Psychology*, *33*, 77–87. https://doi.org/10.1037/fam0000447.

White, R. M. B., Roosa, M. W., Weaver, S. R., & Nair, R. L. (2009). Cultural and contextual influences on parenting in Mexican American families. *Journal of Marriage and Family*, *71*, 61–79. https://doi.org/10.1111/j.1741-3737.2008.00580.x.

White, R. M. B., Zeiders, K. H., Gonzales, N. A., Tein, J.-Y., & Roosa, M. W. (2013). Cultural values, U.S. neighborhood danger, and Mexican American parents' parenting. *Journal of Family Psychology*, *27*, 365–375. https://doi.org/10.1037/a0032888.

Wu, N. H., & Kim, S. Y. (2009). Chinese American adolescents' perceptions of the language brokering experience as a sense of burden and sense of efficacy. *Journal of Youth and Adolescence*, *38*, 703–718. https://doi.org/10.1007/s10964-008-9379-3.

Zhang, M., Kim, S. Y., Hou, Y., & Shen, Y. (2019). Parent–adolescent acculturation profiles and adolescent language brokering experiences in Mexican immigrant families. *Journal of Youth and Adolescence*, https://doi.org/10.1007/s10964-019-01064-5.

Chapter 3

Acculturation, enculturation, and bicultural orientations: Conceptualizations and links to alcohol use

Byron L. Zamboanga[a], P. Priscilla Lui[b] and Savannah Pham[b]
[a]*Smith College, Northampton, MA, United States,* [b]*Southern Methodist University, Dallas, TX, United States*

The immigrant population in the United States has been growing substantially since 1965 when the immigration laws replaced a quota system. Immigrants to the United States who are born outside of the country currently account for approximately 15% of the overall population (Radford, 2019). Recent data from 2017 show that the share of immigrants in the United States is close to historic highs, just second to that in the 1890s. At least 25% of all children in the United States are foreign- or native-born to immigrant parents (Child Trends, 2018). Asian and Hispanic/Latinx Americans make up the largest immigrant groups, particularly individuals who come from Mexico, China, India, and the Philippines (Radford, 2019). Although Hispanic Americans make up the largest ethnic group in the United States, the composition of the immigrant population is shifting drastically (Census Bureau, 2011). Hispanic women no longer account for the majority of immigrant births; rather, the Asian population continues to grow exponentially (Livingston, 2019; Pew Research Center, 2013). Thus, there is a large US population who come from immigrant family background, and their mental health and behavioral health are important concerns for the public.

Alcohol use and misuse mark one area of concern of immigrant mental and behavioral health. Four out of five adults in the United States consume alcohol, and one in three adults is diagnosed with alcohol use disorder at some point in their lives (Grant et al., 2015). Alcohol misuse is linked to a host of adverse health, personal, and social consequences, such as liver diseases, lost work productivity and school dropouts, and heightened healthcare costs (Sacks, Gonzales, Bouchery, Tomedi, & Brewer, 2015). Disparities are

Mental and Behavioral Health of Immigrants in the United States
https://doi.org/10.1016/B978-0-12-816117-3.00003-8

reflected in differences in alcohol use outcomes across individuals of Asian and Hispanic heritage and immigrant backgrounds. Although immigrant and native-born Asian and Hispanic Americans are less likely to consume alcohol, they experience disproportionately greater burden associated with alcohol use disorder than their Euro American counterparts (Chartier & Caetano, 2010). In the Hispanic population, 45% engage in alcohol use whereas 25% engage in past-month binge drinking. By contrast, Asian Americans show much lower rates of alcohol use and misuse: 38% and 13% engage in past-month alcohol use and binge drinking, respectively (see Lui & Zamboanga, 2019). With the steep rise in the Asian immigrant population, there is also a steep increase in alcohol use and alcohol use disorder among Asians in immigrant families (Grant et al., 2017). Compared to their immigrant counterparts, native-born Asian and Hispanic individuals are at greater risk for experiencing more alcohol-related problems. For example, across three generations of Mexican Americans, frequency and intensity of alcohol consumption increased by immigration generational status (Markides, Krause, & Leon, 1988). These patterns have galvanized the field in identifying and understanding sociocultural determinants of alcohol-related outcomes that underlie disparities across ethnic groups and immigration generational statuses.

For individuals of immigrant backgrounds, adapting to new societal and cultural environments often is a salient experience. The process of acculturation, then, holds promise in illuminating foreign- and native-born Asian and Hispanic Americans' risk for alcohol use and misuse. Despite extensive research that has aimed to contextualize the impact of acculturation on mental and behavioral health, findings remain inconsistent pertaining to alcohol use outcomes. Existing results also have not yielded concrete recommendations on services that aim to prevent or treat alcohol use disorders in immigrant populations. In order to alleviate the health burden associated with alcohol use disorder, we must first understand the state of the science on alcohol use and misuse in the US immigrant population. As such, a review of the current literature is needed to critique existing knowledge, resolve inconsistencies, identify critical gaps, and provide insight on opportunities to advance basic and applied research. Hence, the goals of the current chapter are to review (a) the definitions of acculturation-related factors, (b) the measurement of cultural orientations, and (c) the evidence on how these are linked to alcohol use in Asian and Hispanic immigrant groups. We will discuss barriers to further advancement in this literature and present recommendations for future research.

Definitions of acculturation, enculturation, and bicultural orientations

For immigrants and their children, the psychological process of acculturation can be inherently challenging when it comes to navigating bicultural contexts. Many individuals experiencing cultural transition or intercultural contact acculturate to the host society and adjust their behavioral practices, values, and self-identity in order to fit in. In some instances, expectations and demands from their ethnic heritage culture and family of origin require them to retain or relearn behavioral repertoires and value orientations (Berry & Sam, 1997; Schwartz, Unger, Zamboanga, & Szapocznik, 2010). Recognizing that these cultural influences can take place separately and simultaneously, research focusing on the acculturation process has considered both acculturation and enculturation orientations to be independent of each other. Immigrant populations can adhere to mainstream American ways of life and can also be well immersed in their ethnic heritage ways of life. Individuals who are more acculturated to the US mainstream are typically fluent in English, comfortable socializing with majority group members of the host society, and endorse individualistic ideologies. On the other hand, individuals who are more enculturated to their ethnic heritage are usually fluent in their native languages, knowledgeable of historic and current events, comfortable with same-ethnic peers, and hold collectivistic beliefs.

To the extent that acculturation and enculturation orientations do not occur in isolation and that individuals can simultaneously exhibit behavioral repertoires and values along both cultural dimensions, Berry's (1997) conceptual model of bicultural orientation helps to frame these individual differences. Considering individuals in a US cultural context and placing acculturation and enculturation orientations at 90 degrees as perpendicular axes, bicultural orientations can be classified into four distinct profiles. The integrated profile is characterized by high US orientation and also high heritage orientation. Individuals with a separated profile are characterized as being highly immersed in their heritage culture but not the mainstream US culture. Individuals with an assimilated profile are characterized as highly oriented toward the mainstream US culture but not their heritage culture. Individuals who have a marginalized profile are detached from both their heritage and mainstream US cultures. This typological categorization of bicultural orientation does not necessarily discredit acculturation or enculturation as viable cultural dimensions; rather, it provides the opportunity to discern their mutual influences and mechanisms that relate to mental and behavioral health outcomes. Furthermore, along these cultural dimensions, acculturation, enculturation, and bicultural orientations may be manifested across three key life domains: behavioral practices, values, and identification (Schwartz et al., 2010). These advancements in the conceptualization of cultural orientations as determinants of alcohol use and other health behaviors is critical because it moves the field toward using psychologically relevant and potentially malleable variables to understand behavioral and mental health (Lui & Rollock, 2012; Wallace, Pomery, Latimer, Martinez, & Salovey, 2010). Specifically, examining acculturation as a culture-learning process can isolate concrete beliefs, emotions, stress, and other psychological processes that explain individual differences in how acculturation-related factors may impact alcohol (mis)use (Chun, Balls Organista, & Marín, 2003; Lazarus, 1997).

Measurement of acculturation, enculturation, and bicultural orientations

Focusing specifically on studies on alcohol use and broadly on other health outcomes, a review of the literature indicates that there is a great deal of variability in how acculturation, enculturation, and bicultural orientations are being measured. Historically, studies have used demographic proxies to assess acculturation-related factors (see Lui & Zamboanga, 2018a, 2018b; Zamboanga, Tomaso, & Lui, 2017 for review). For example, single-item variables asking about individuals' nativity status, length of residence in the host country, and language preference are common indicators of acculturation status. Yet, these demographic proxies do not capture the psychological impact of acculturation processes or individuals' lived experiences (Cabassa, 2003). Beyond these proxies, there are two main approaches that have been used to assess individual differences in bicultural orientations. The first measurement approach involves the use of self-report measures that tap into acculturation and enculturation dimensions. The second measurement approach involves the use of self-report measures that capture the extent to which individuals are integrated into bicultural contexts and possible stresses that underlie such integration. Existing measures also vary in the domains of cultural orientations they cover. Most assess behavioral practices (including language competency and cultural knowledge), and few assess cultural values and self-identification. Some of these measures have been designed for multigroup use, whereas others have been developed for specific ethnic groups. Table 1 summarizes features of these key measures.

Acculturation profiles

In the first measurement approach, bicultural orientations are examined as discrete acculturation profiles. Acculturation and enculturation orientations typically are assessed as separate dimensions, and four acculturation profiles are derived from these two scale scores. This approach is commonly used in studies with immigrant populations (e.g., Asian Americans, Hispanic Americans). Drawing from Berry's (1997) model, individuals' scores on acculturation and enculturation measures can inform their classifications into integrated, separated, assimilated, and marginalized profiles. The integrated profile is typically indicated by higher scores on both acculturation and enculturation scales. The separated profile is typically indicated by lower scores on measures of acculturation and higher scores on measures of enculturation. The assimilated profile is typically indicated by higher scores on measures of acculturation and lower scores on measures of enculturation. Finally, the marginalized profile is typically indicated by lower scores on both acculturation and enculturation scales. When classifying these bicultural orientations using acculturation and enculturation measures, researchers tend to use midpoints on the range of possible scores (e.g., Coatsworth, Maldonado-Molina, Pantin, & Szapocznik, 2005) or sample-specific median scores (e.g., Giang & Wittig, 2006) to determine high and low levels of acculturation and enculturation orientations.

TABLE 1 Overview of key measures of bicultural orientations.

Measure and authors	Multigroup (MG) or group-specific (GS)	Dimension and domain of cultural orientations with sample item	Psychometric properties	
			Cronbach's α	Evidence for validity
Acculturation profiles				
Acculturation Scale (Caetano, 1987)	GS: Hispanic Americans	Acculturation; Behavioral: "Ability to speak English" Enculturation; Behavioral: "Use of Spanish on a daily basis"	0.91	A principal components factor analysis yielded one primary component of language. The Acculturation Scale demonstrated construct validity with its association with nativity status ($r=0.58$). The AS has demonstrated criterion-related validity with alcohol use outcomes (e.g., Karriker-Jaffe & Zemore, 2009).
Acculturation Rating Scale for Mexican Americans (ARSMA-II; Cuellar, Arnold, & Maldonado, 1995)	GS: Latino immigrant populations	Anglo Orientation Scale (AOS); Behavioral: "I associate with Anglos" Identification: "I like to identify myself as an Anglo American" Mexican Orientation Scale (MOS); Behavioral: "I enjoy listening to Spanish language music" Identification: "I like to identify myself as Mexican"	0.83 (AOS) 0.88 (MOS)	A factor analysis yielded three factors: language, ethnic identity, and ethnic interaction/distance. Concurrent validity was established with the original ARSMA ($r=0.89$). The ARSMA-II has demonstrated criterion-related validity in with alcohol use severity (e.g., Cano et al., 2015; $r=0.20$).

Continued

TABLE 1 Overview of key measures of bicultural orientations—cont'd

Measure and authors	Multigroup (MG) or group-specific (GS)	Dimension and domain of cultural orientations with sample item	Psychometric properties: Cronbach's α	Psychometric properties: Evidence for validity
Asian American Multidimensional Acculturation Scale (AAMAS; Chung, Kim, & Abreu, 2004)	GS: Asian Americans	European American (EA); Behavioral: "How well do you read and write in [English]" Identification: "How much do you feel you have in common with [European Americans]" Culture of Origin (CO); Behavioral: "How often do you actually eat the food of [culture of origin]" Identification: "How proud are you to be a part of [culture of origin]" Asian American (AA); Behavioral: "How knowledgeable are you about the history of [Asian Americans]" Identification: "How much do you identify with [Asian Americans]"	0.81 (EA) 0.89 (CO) 0.83 (AA)	A factor analysis suggested a four-factor structure for each scale: language, cultural identity, cultural knowledge, and food consumption. Criterion-related validity was established as CO scores negatively correlated with generational status ($r = -0.36$). Test-retest reliability was established over a 2-week period: 0.78 (EA), 0.75 (AA), 0.89 (CO). Divergent validity was established through nonsignificant correlations between AAMAS scores and ICI (Intergenerational Conflict Inventory) scores.
Short Acculturation Scale for Hispanics (SASH; Marín, Sabogal, VanOss Marín, Otero-Sabogal, & Pérez-Stable, 1987)	GS: Hispanic	Behavior: "In what language do you usually think?"	0.92	A principal components factor analysis suggested a three-component solution: language use and ethnic loyalty, media, and ethnic social relations. The SASH demonstrated external validity by its correlation with generational status ($r = 0.65$). Criterion-related validity has been demonstrated with alcohol use (e.g., Myers et al., 2009).

Stephenson Multigroup Acculturation Scale (SMAS; Stephenson, 2000)	MG	Dominant Society Immersion (DSI); Behavioral: "I am familiar with important people in American history" Ethnic Society Immersion (ESI); Behavioral: "I eat traditional foods from my native culture"	0.78 (DSI) 0.94 (ESI)	A principal components analysis suggested a two-component solution: Dominant Society Immersion and Ethnic Society Immersion. The SMAS DSI was validated in its positive correlation with the ARSMA-II AOS scale. The DSI was validated in its positive correlation with the ARSMA-II MOS scale and Hispanic Domain Scale of the Bidimensional Acculturation Scale for Hispanics (BAS). Criterion-related validity has been demonstrated with alcohol use outcomes (e.g., Pham & Lui, 2019a, 2019b).
Bicultural identity integration and bicultural stress				
Bicultural Identity Integration Scale-Version II (BII-2; Huynh, Nguyen, & Benet-Martínez, 2011)	MG	Blendedness versus compartmentalization; Identification: "I feel part of a combined culture" "I keep [heritage] and American cultures separate" Harmony versus conflict; Identification: "I rarely feel conflicted about being bicultural" "I feel caught between the [heritage] and American cultures"	0.81 (blendedness) 0.86 (harmony)	A confirmatory factor analysis yielded a two-factor structure: cultural blendedness vs compartmentalization and cultural harmony vs conflict. Convergent validity was established with positive correlations between cultural harmony and ethnic identity affirmations, as well as negative correlations with acculturation-related stressors. Test-retest reliability was established over a 2-week period: 0.73 (blendedness), 0.77 (harmony).
Bicultural Involvement Questionnaire-Short Version (BIQ-S; Szapocznik, Kurtines, & Fernandez, 1980)	GS: Hispanics	Hispanic Orientation Scale (HOS); Behavior: "How comfortable are you speaking Spanish at home?" American Orientation Scale (AOS); Behavior: "I enjoy American-type recreations"	0.93 (HOS) 0.89 (AOS)	A confirmatory factor analysis revealed a four-factor model: comfort with use of Spanish language, enjoyment of Spanish cultural activities, comfort with use of English language, and enjoyment of American cultural activities.

Continued

TABLE 1 Overview of key measures of bicultural orientations—cont'd

Measure and authors	Multigroup (MG) or group-specific (GS)	Dimension and domain of cultural orientations with sample item	Psychometric properties	
			Cronbach's α	Evidence for validity
Bicultural Self-Efficacy Scale (BSES; David, Okazaki, & Saw, 2009)	MG	Social groundedness; Identification: "I feel like I fit in when I am with mainstream Americans as well as people from the same heritage culture as myself" Communication ability; Behavior: "I am proficient in both standard English and the language of my heritage culture" Positive attitudes toward both groups; Identification: "I take pride in both the mainstream American culture and my heritage culture" Knowledge of cultural beliefs and values; Behavior: "I am knowledgeable about the history of both mainstream America and my cultural group" Role repertoire; Behavior: "I can choose the degree and manner to which I affiliate with each culture" Bicultural beliefs; Identification: "Being bicultural does not mean I have to compromise my sense of cultural identity"	91 (social groundedness) 0.79 (communication ability) 0.89 (positive attitudes) 0.80 (knowledge) 0.69 (role repertoire) 0.77 (beliefs)	A confirmatory factor analysis suggested a six-factor solution. Criterion-related validity has been demonstrated with depression.

Bicultural Stress Scale (BSS; Romero & Roberts, 2003)	MG	Family stressors; Behavior: "Argue with family about traditions" Discrimination stressors; Behavior: "Don't understand different cultures" Monolingual stressors; Behavior: "Need better Spanish" Peer stressors; Behavior: "Belong to gang for ethnicity"	0.93	The BSS has demonstrated criterion validity with alcohol use outcomes (e.g., Meca et al., 2019).
Hispanic Stress Inventory Version 2 (HSI2; Cervantes, Fisher, Padilla, & Napper, 2016)	GS: Hispanics (Immigrant version and US-born versions)	Parental; Behavior: "I had difficulties motivating my child about school" Occupational/Economic; Behavior: "I have been forced to accept low paying jobs" Marital; Behavior: "My spouse and I talked about divorce" Discrimination; Behavior: "I experienced discrimination because of the color of my skin" Immigrant-related; Behavior: "My legal status has been a problem in getting a good job" Marital acculturation gap; Behavior: "My spouse and I have disagreed on which language is spoken by our children at home" Health; Behavior: "I did not have health insurance to cover my illness" Language-related; Behavior: "Because of language barriers, I could not communicate with others" Premigration; Behavior: "I was forced to leave my home country due to poverty" Family-related; Behavior: "I had serious arguments with family members"	0.97 (Immigrant version total scale) 0.93 (US-born version total scale)	A factor analysis yielded 10 factors for the Immigrant version and 7 factors for the US-born version. Concurrent validity was established; both versions of the HSI2 were correlated with measures of psychological distress (e.g., depression and anxiety).

Within this measurement approach, there are multigroup and group-specific instruments. One commonly used multigroup measure is the Stephenson Multigroup Acculturation Scale (SMAS; Stephenson, 2000). The SMAS contains two subscales assessing respondents' host society immersion (e.g., "I am informed about current affairs in the United States") and ethnic society immersion (e.g., "I know how to speak my native language"). Respondents are asked to describe their comfort in language and behavioral practices in relation to their native/heritage country and the United States. These items are not specific to any group membership and have been used across ethnic groups including Euro Americans (e.g., Lui, Berkley, & Zamboanga, 2019; Stephenson, 2000). In contrast to multigroup measures, other available instruments have been designed to tap into cultural experiences that are unique to distinct ethnic populations. For example, the Acculturation Rating Scale for Mexican Americans (ARSMA-II; Cuellar et al., 1995) contains subscales for Anglo Orientation (e.g., "I associate with Anglos") and Mexican Orientation (e.g., "I enjoy listening to Spanish language music"). This measure contains items focusing on language, behavioral practices, and ethnic identity. Although this measure was initially intended to capture acculturation and enculturation orientations among Mexican Americans, it has been adapted for use in other Hispanic immigrant groups, including Puerto Ricans, Dominicans, and Guatemalans (e.g., Jimenez, Gray, Cucciare, Kumbhani, & Gallagher-Thompson, 2010; Wallace et al., 2010). Among Asian Americans, the Suinn-Lew Asian Self-Identity Acculturation Scale (SL-ASIA) is commonly used to indicate individuals' acculturation and enculturation statuses (Suinn, Ahuna, & Khoo, 1992). This scale assesses language, behavior, and social orientations (e.g., "What language do you speak?" and "If you could pick, whom would you prefer to associate with in the community?"). The SL-ASIA was developed to assess acculturation as a unidimensional construct; more recently, it has been adapted to be a multidimensional measure to capture aspects of traditionalism (enculturation), assimilation (acculturation), and biculturalism (Suinn et al., 1992; Suinn, Khoo, & Ahuna, 1995). Specifically, lower scores are indicative of higher levels of traditionalism, higher scores indicate higher levels of assimilation, and mid-range scores indicate biculturalism.

Bicultural integration and bicultural stress

In the second measurement approach, bicultural orientations and related factors are directly assessed using self-report instruments. These factors include bicultural competence, bicultural identity integration, and bicultural stress. Similar to the conceptualization of the integrated acculturation profile, individuals with bicultural competence are characterized by their strong and equal involvement with both mainstream and heritage cultures. This involvement is typically measured in terms of behavioral repertoires and self-identification (LaFromboise, Coleman, & Gerton, 1993). One commonly used instrument of bicultural behavioral competence is the Bicultural Self-Efficacy Scale (BSES; David et al.,

2009). It contains six subscales: social groundedness (e.g., "I can count on mainstream Americans and people from the same heritage culture as myself"), communication ability, positive attitude, knowledge, role repertoire, and bicultural beliefs. This measure has been validated among Asian Americans, African Americans, and Hispanic Americans. There are also scales that focus more specifically on self-identification within a bicultural context, such as the Bicultural Identity Integration Scale-Version 2 (BII-2). Bicultural identity integration reflects how individuals conceptualize their cultural identities and feel about the integration of their mainstream and ethnic heritage cultural orientations (Benet-Martínez & Haritatos, 2005). The BII-2 assesses the extent to which individuals feel that their two cultures are blended or disconnected (e.g., "I feel [heritage culture] and American at the same time"). The BII-2 also assesses the extent to which individuals feel conflicted about their cultural identities (e.g., "I find it easy to balance both [heritage] and American cultures"; Huynh, Benet-Martínez, & Nguyen, 2018). Designed to be a multigroup measure, the BII-2 has been used across Asian Americans, African Americans, and Hispanic Americans (Huynh et al., 2018; Schwartz et al., 2019).

To the extent that navigating a bicultural context can be stressful when individuals lack sufficient resources to adapt to their cultural environments, bicultural stress has been studied as a construct closely related to bicultural orientations. The Bicultural Stress Scale (BSS) measures stress that may be experienced as a result of intergenerational conflict (e.g., "family obligations"), discrimination (e.g., "harder to succeed because of ethnicity"), monolingualism (e.g., "problems at school because of poor English"), and peer relationships (e.g., "not accepted because of ethnicity"; Romero & Roberts, 2003). The BSS has been used with diverse Hispanic ethnic groups and Asian Americans (e.g., Romero, Carvajal, Valle, & Orduña, 2007). Additional measures have been created to tap into group-distinct stress experiences frequently facing immigrant and ethnic minority individuals. For example, the Hispanic Stress Inventory Version 2 (HSI2) assesses the frequencies and stressfulness of minority-related events among Hispanic individuals; these stressors are related to parental and marital relationships, occupation and economic difficulties, discrimination, immigration, marital acculturation gap, health, language, premigration challenges, and family conflict (Cervantes et al., 2016). There are distinct sets of items for Hispanic immigrants (e.g., "I was called names and treated badly because I am an immigrant") and US-born Hispanic Americans (e.g., "I was treated 'less than' other Americans because I am Hispanic"). This measure has been validated across Hispanic subgroups, including Mexican Americans, Puerto Ricans, and Cuban Americans.

Strengths and limitations of existing measures

Our review of the literature identifies several key measures of bicultural orientations and shows that each measurement approach has strengths and limitations.

The acculturation profile approach utilizes measures that separately examine acculturation and enculturation. These measures typically assess behaviors as indicators of individuals' comfort in a bicultural context. There is value in understanding the extent to which individuals are immersed in their mainstream and heritage cultures and how they are distinctly influenced by them. Yet, it is also important to note that this approach has received criticism (Rudmin, 2003; Schwartz et al., 2010). Reliance on sample-specific scores makes it difficult to replicate study results across samples and to generalize them to the population. Additionally, the four theory-defined acculturation profiles are not consistently classified across studies; for example, one study found six, rather than four profiles (Schwartz & Zamboanga, 2008). If this acculturation profiles approach is used, then a dimensional approach to classification would ameliorate some of these methodological limitations. A dimensional approach to acculturation profiles has two advantages. First, it likely yields deepened and replicable knowledge regarding bicultural orientations across samples (see Pham & Lui, 2019b). Second, it bridges the currently separated research areas on acculturation/enculturation and on biculturalism.

The second approach to biculturalism, which directly measures bicultural orientations and related factors, is less frequently used among immigrant populations especially in the context of alcohol use. Arguably, measures of competence and integration more directly tap into the psychological experiences associated with a bicultural identity than simply acculturation and enculturation orientations alone. Measures of bicultural competence and identity integration directly assess individuals' feelings and psychological experiences in navigating and adapting to two sets of cultural expectations. Additionally, with the conceptual understanding that learning how to adapt to two separate cultures may be stressful, measures of bicultural stress likely show added value in capturing individuals' experiences with biculturalism. Considering that an acculturation profile measurement approach to studying bicultural orientation partly draws from stress theory (i.e., being marginalized from both sets of cultures can yield stress and negative psychological impact), direct measurement of bicultural stress can provide greater precision in assessing individuals' (dis) comfort levels in bicultural contexts. More research needs to be done in order to validate these measures among immigrant populations, especially in the context of alcohol use.

State of the science on relations between alcohol use and acculturation, enculturation, and bicultural orientations

To some extent, acculturation can help shed some light on how immigrant individuals and their descendants navigate through the cultural drinking norms of the host society. Researchers have recently examined the strength of the association between acculturation and alcohol use among US Latinx/Hispanics and Asian Americans. Alvarez, Frietze, Ramos, Field, and Zarate (2017) conducted a meta-analysis of 31 studies with Latinx/Hispanic adults. They found that the weighted mean correlation between acculturation and alcohol use was 0.16, and the association between these variables was larger among women ($r=0.18$) compared to men ($r=0.10$). Lui and Zamboanga (2018b) conducted an expanded follow-up meta-analysis of 68 studies with Latinx/Hispanic adolescents and adults. They found statistically significant but modest effects in the weighted mean correlation between acculturation and overall alcohol use ($r=0.09$), drinking intensity ($r=0.09$), binge drinking ($r=0.05$), and drinking problems ($r=0.06$). Acculturation was also positively associated with binge drinking and drinking problems among women but not men. Finally, in a recent meta-analysis of 31 studies with Asian American adolescents and adults, the weighted mean correlation between acculturation and alcohol consumption was 0.07 (Lui & Zamboanga, 2018a). Enculturation was also modestly and negatively associated with alcohol use ($r=-0.05$). The association between acculturation and alcohol use was in a positive direction for women whereas the opposite was found for men.

Reviews of the literature on acculturation and alcohol use among US Hispanics and Asian Americans also indicate a lack of consensus in the direction of associations (except among women where the direction tends to be positive). Some studies indicate that acculturation is positively associated with alcohol use; these findings are usually conceptualized in the context of drinking norms and/or stress. A norms perspective posits that as immigrants and their descendants become more immersed in mainstream US culture, they are socialized to develop the drinking norms and behaviors of US society (Pinedo, Zemore, Cherpitel, & Caetano, 2017; Vaeth, Wang-Schweig, & Caetano, 2017). A stress perspective posits that the process of adopting mainstream US culture can lend itself to stressful life experiences (e.g., family acculturation mismatch and intergenerational cultural conflict; Lui, 2015; discrimination and microaggression; Lui & Quezada, 2019; Meca et al., 2019; Pinedo et al., 2017; Torres, Driscoll, & Voell, 2012; Vaeth et al., 2017), which conceivably can increase the risk for alcohol use as a means to cope among individuals of immigrant backgrounds. Relinquishing heritage cultural orientations can also result in greater stress and alienation within the family, thereby increasing one's risk for alcohol use to cope. This stress perspective also is consistent with the observation that lower levels of enculturation are associated with more alcohol use. The stress perspective implies that acculturation orientations can serve as a proxy for levels of acculturative stress (Abraído-Lanza, Armbrister, Flórez, & Aguirre, 2006; Pinedo et al., 2017; Vaeth et al., 2017).

Other studies indicate that higher levels of enculturation are associated with less, and in some cases, more alcohol use. Consistent with a norms perspective, for example, adherence to cultural norms that encompass conformity, harmony, interdependence, and responsibility for others can facilitate moderate use of alcohol among racial/ethnic minorities (Caetano, Clark, & Tam, 1998). Finally, a gender role norms perspective has also been used to explain findings where gender differences in the associations between acculturation/enculturation and alcohol use are observed. For instance, research indicates that in some Latinx/Hispanic immigrant groups, conformity to gender role norms can promote positive or negative attitudes toward alcohol use. This gender role difference, in turn, can influence individuals to drink or abstain (see Perrotte & Zamboanga, 2019 for a review).

In summary, research on the relations between acculturation and alcohol use among US Latinx/Hispanics and Asian Americans suggests that the direction of the associations tends to be positive, and it appears that women's drinking behaviors are more affected by acculturation than men. The effects are also quite small and suggest that acculturation is a weak proxy—and arguably a distal—determinant of alcohol use. Because immigrants and their descendants can simultaneously endorse their heritage culture and the mainstream culture, it is also important to consider how bicultural orientations are associated with alcohol use in these populations.

Bicultural orientations have been examined in relation to alcohol use outcomes among immigrant populations, such as Hispanic Americans and Asian Americans, but also among Native Americans. A study with a large, multisite sample of Hispanic American college students examined the relationship between biculturalism and alcohol use with a multidimensional approach to acculturation profiles (Des Rosiers, Schwartz, Zamboanga, Ham, & Huang, 2013). In this study, biculturalism was measured using the SMAS. Researchers found five separate acculturation profiles: separated, assimilated, separated bicultural (elevated Hispanic orientations), high bicultural (both Hispanic and American orientations highly endorsed), and low bicultural (both Hispanic and American orientations moderately endorsed). The three distinct "bicultural" profiles show support for prior research: integration is likely the most common form of acculturation profile across individuals because it is difficult for individuals to adjust well to a pluralistic host society without internalizing influences from either heritage or mainstream culture (Berry, Phinney, Sam, & Vedder, 2006). Results on these classifications also highlight individual differences in the degree to which they navigate bicultural contexts and how these cultural orientations are linked to alcohol-related behaviors (Des Rosiers et al., 2013). Individuals with a separated bicultural profile engaged in less frequent binge drinking, whereas individuals with a low bicultural profile were less likely to engage in binge drinking. These findings extended scientific understanding of how bicultural orientations may be associated with alcohol use outcomes.

Another study examining Hispanic individuals' bicultural orientations yielded different classifications of bicultural orientations and results regarding their relations to alcohol use (Salas-Wright, Clark, Vaughn, & Córdova, 2015). The researchers measured language, social orientation, and Hispanic identity, and used these variables to classify individuals into five acculturation profiles: Spanish-dominant/strongly separated; Spanish-dominant/separated; English-dominant/bicultural; bilingual/bicultural; and English-dominant/assimilated.

They then examined group differences in alcohol use across these five acculturation profiles. Results indicated that individuals in the English-dominant/assimilated group were at the highest risk for alcohol use disorder. In contrast, those who were predominantly Spanish speakers and strongly immersed in their ethnic culture were at the lowest risk for alcohol use disorders. In contrast to assimilated and separated profiles, there were no differences in the prevalence of alcohol use disorders across bicultural subgroups.

Another study specifically examined bicultural orientations among Vietnamese and Cambodian Americans (Kane et al., 2016). Using scores from the SL-ASIA, only three of the four acculturation profiles were identified in this sample. The authors referred to these classifications as biculturalism (i.e., integrated), assimilation, and traditionalism (i.e., separated). Researchers showed that biculturalism was not associated with whether someone was a drinker or abstainer, and bicultural/integrated profile was linked to alcohol use patterns—including frequency and quantity of drinking behavior—among drinkers. Furthermore, higher degrees of separation and integration were associated with lower levels of alcohol consumption among drinkers. In contrast to prior research, there was no association between assimilation and drinking behaviors. These findings suggested that not only was immersion in both mainstream US and heritage cultures protective against alcohol misuse, but that there appeared to be no inherent risk associated with identifying with the US and being more assimilated. Rather, the researchers indicated the loss of socialization to traditional heritage culture might be the risk factor for increased alcohol use and related consequences.

To the extent that studies using a typological approach of acculturation have yielded different classifications of bicultural orientations and shown inconsistent associations with alcohol involvement, there is a need to use a dimensional approach to examine the relations between biculturalism and alcohol use. For example, more recent studies have examined the interaction between acculturation and enculturation orientations as determinants of drinking outcomes in immigrant groups. This analytic approach presents an opportunity to better understand individual differences in bicultural orientations, and identify those in the population who may be at greater risk for alcohol use and misuse. In an Asian American sample of undergraduate and graduate students, for example, researchers found that bicultural orientations were associated with alcohol use outcomes above and beyond dimensions of acculturation and enculturation alone. Asian Americans with greater marginalized tendencies reported higher levels of drinking-related consequences whereas those with more integrated tendencies appeared to be protected against drinking-related consequences (Pham & Lui, 2019b). These results suggest that Asian Americans with more integrated tendencies may glean protection and receive support from both sets of cultures. In a Hispanic American sample, bicultural orientations were found to be associated with alcohol consumption above and beyond dimensions of acculturation and enculturation. Individuals with greater marginalized tendencies reported lower levels of alcohol consumption. It is possible that being marginalized from both sets of cultures would decrease the likelihood of having social situations where an individual is drinking (Pham & Lui, 2019a).

Although research on bicultural orientations with immigrant groups has relied on the acculturation and enculturation literatures and the typological measurement approach, there are new opportunities in examining how biculturalism is linked to alcohol use outcomes by directly assessing bicultural competence and integration. This latter approach has been studied less frequently among Asian Americans and Hispanic Americans but is more commonly researched among Native American populations. For example, among Native Americans, research has shown promising effectiveness in preventing alcohol and substance misuse by promoting youth's bicultural competence skills (LaFromboise et al., 1993; Schinke et al., 1988). Native American youth who received bicultural competence skills training reported less alcohol use than individuals who did not receive the preventive intervention. Compared to individuals who are not considered bicultural, individuals with greater bicultural competence likely have the efficacy and behavioral skills to navigate both mainstream Euro American and heritage cultural contexts. They may, therefore, receive more emotional and social support, and experience less bicultural stress, and in turn, they will less likely consume alcohol to cope with minority-related and life stresses.

Consistent with a bicultural integration conceptualization, bicultural stress has been shown to be positively associated with high-risk drinking among Hispanic Americans (e.g., Romero, Martinez, & Carvajal, 2007). Research has suggested that higher levels of bicultural stress in adolescence are linked to cognitive vulnerabilities—including positive alcohol expectancies—that may heighten risky drinking behaviors (Oshri et al., 2014). In one study that focused on predictive roles of bicultural stress, acculturation, and enculturation on alcohol initiation among Hispanic adolescents (Meca et al., 2019), bicultural stress accounted for trajectories in alcohol initiation above and beyond acculturation and enculturation orientations. The stress associated with having to navigate a bicultural context—where norms and values differ greatly between both cultures—was found to place individuals at greater risk for alcohol initiation.

The state of the science on the relations between bicultural orientations and alcohol use outcomes among immigrant populations reflects the psychometric properties and utility of current measurement approaches and instruments of biculturalism. Evidence indicates that measuring biculturalism is important, given the construct reflects the cultural realities of many immigrants. Therefore, understanding individual variations in bicultural orientations and their associations with alcohol use outcomes can better inform who are at greater risk for alcohol misuse. There is a utility in the first measurement approach of acculturation profiles and being able to understand the extent to which individuals are immersed in heritage and mainstream cultures. Thus far, this has been the main approach in the alcohol use literature and has informed scientific understanding of bicultural orientations. Yet, the literature shows mixed results. In general, being immersed in one's heritage culture and integrated into both mainstream American and heritage cultures appear to be protective against alcohol misuse. In some studies, however, individuals with marginalized tendencies and separated tendencies appear to be at the lowest risk for developing alcohol use disorder or engaging in alcohol misuse (e.g., Kane et al., 2016; Pham & Lui, 2019a; Salas-Wright et al., 2015). These findings are in direct contrast to findings from those in a meta-analysis on biculturalism and psychological adjustment, where individuals with marginalized and separated profiles are shown to experience worse psychological adjustment outcomes (e.g., higher levels of depression, anxiety, and distress) than individuals with an integrated profile (Nguyen & Benet-Martínez, 2013). Collectively, the evidence underscores the importance of examining how bicultural orientations are related to different mental health outcomes. Considering specific health-related behaviors can show how biculturalism may be adaptive or detrimental across different health and mental health domains. What is lacking in the acculturation profile approach to alcohol research can be addressed in research that taps into bicultural identity integration and bicultural stress. Yet, there is currently a lack of knowledge regarding how bicultural comfort, behavioral competence, and stress are linked to alcohol use among immigrant populations. By integrating acculturation and biculturalism literatures, research can advance knowledge pertaining to the risk and protective factors for alcohol use and misuse in immigrant groups.

Limitations of this literature and recommendations for future research

Although existing studies on acculturation, enculturation, and biculturation orientations and alcohol use have advanced both multicultural psychology and alcohol research fields, several critical research inquiries remain unanswered. First, the present conceptualization of intercultural contact and acculturation process assumes that the drinking-related beliefs, norms, and expectations are different in the societies from and to which individuals move. For example, there are immigrants who have been enculturated to drink moderately or to abstain from alcohol use. When these individuals move to a community where drinking is widely accepted and encouraged, they may adopt these new cultural drinking norms, which in turn can give rise to changes in their drinking behaviors in ways that mirror the consumption patterns of the host community. Still, there are immigrants who move to a community where the cultural drinking norms and behaviors of that society match their heritage cultural drinking norms. Because these immigrants would not be acculturating to any "new" drinking norms, the concepts of acculturation, enculturation, and bicultural orientations may not be as applicable in this context. Hence, when conducting any research on acculturation, enculturation, and bicultural orientations and alcohol use with immigrant groups, we strongly recommend that researchers pay close attention to the extent to which the drinking norms and behaviors of the heritage and receiving cultures are similar or different (Bornstein, 2017; Fox, Thayer, & Wadhwa, 2017; Hunt, Schneider, & Comer, 2004; Salas-Wright, Vaughn, Clark Goings, Córdova, & Schwartz, 2018). Future researchers will benefit greatly by examining specifically the process by which immigrants' attitudes toward alcohol use change over time, and the extent to which these changes are directly tied to increased or decreased risk for alcohol use and misuse. There is also a need to examine how their adherence to heritage cultural drinking norms and behaviors might increase or decrease their risk for alcohol use. Finally, when it comes to bicultural orientation, researchers could examine how and why immigrants' involvement in their heritage culture and the mainstream culture increases or decreases their risk for alcohol use.

As shown in our review, existing literature on cultural orientations and alcohol use continues to be fraught with theoretical and methodological challenges. These challenges include not only a lack of measurement precision of acculturation-related factors and small effect sizes linking cultural orientations and alcohol use outcomes, but also a lack of domain specificity and direct relevance to drinking behaviors. The present measures of acculturation-related factors assess general cultural values, behavioral practices and preferences, and language use; none of these measures taps into drinking-related cognitions and values across cultural contexts. It would be more precise to measure immigrant groups' heritage and mainstream cultural norms around alcohol use. Specifically, these may include but are not limited to: individuals and cultural expectations about the effects of alcohol consumption, motivations to drink, willingness to engage in behavior practices that are designed to protect them from drinking harms, and consumption behaviors upon arrival (cf. Cooper, Kuntsche, Levitt, Barber, & Wolf, 2016; Monk & Heim, 2013; Pearson, 2013). Pre- and postassessment of these constructs will enable researchers to examine what changes—and how such changes—are related to drinking behaviors. Such research endeavors can illuminate the mechanisms by which intercultural contact affects immigrants' and their family members' drinking norms, attitudes toward consumption, and ultimately alcohol use behaviors.

Second, to the extent that a stress perspective is often used to help explain findings regarding the association between acculturation/enculturation and alcohol use, being marginalized from both mainstream and heritage cultures can result in a lack of social support and higher levels of stress (Berry, 2005). In order to move the field forward, we recommend that researchers directly measure the extent to which immigrants might be motivated to drink alcohol in order to cope with their bicultural stresses or any conflicts they might be experiencing regarding their cultural identities. It is critical that researchers also examine how drinking to cope specifically with bicultural stressors are associated with alcohol consumption and risk for experiencing negative drinking consequences while accounting for general life stressors.

Third, another promising avenue for research involves the interactive roles of acculturation-related factors and gender role norms on alcohol use (for review, see Perrotte & Zamboanga, 2019). Results from the World Mental Health Surveys (Degenhardt et al., 2008) indicated that across all countries, men were more likely than women to report lifetime alcohol use, and the same was true for younger adults compared to older adults. Narrative reviews and meta-analytic studies with Asian Americans and US Latinx/Hispanics also indicate that the association between acculturation and alcohol use is stronger for women compared to men (Alvarez et al., 2017; Lui & Zamboanga, 2018a, 2018b; Zamboanga et al., 2017; Zemore, 2007). Although it has been hypothesized that this gender difference may be linked to gender role norms around alcohol use (Iwamoto, Kaya, Grivel, & Clinton, 2016; Kaya, Iwamoto, Grivel, Clinton, & Brady, 2016; Perrotte & Zamboanga, 2019), no published studies have directly examined heritage culture-specific gender role drinking norms and their associations with alcohol use. A rich understanding of gender role norms that are specific to alcohol use in the context of the heritage culture and the mainstream culture among immigrant groups is needed.

Finally, the meaning of "bicultural integration" is not well understood in the alcohol literature. Often referred to as "codeswitching," it is not uncommon for immigrants and their descendants to behave in ways that are consistent with their heritage culture in certain contexts (e.g., at home or around same ethnic peers), while also behave in ways that are consistent with the mainstream host culture in other contexts (e.g., at school or work). Psychological, social, and behavioral "codeswitching," particularly with respect to alcohol use, are not captured in bicultural measures. Researchers have recently begun to study the possible effects of drinking identity on alcohol use outcomes (e.g., Lindgren et al., 2016). Arguably, differences in drinking norms and behaviors between the immigrants' heritage cultures and the mainstream culture can pose additional "codeswitching" challenges. Given the state of the literature, it is unknown whether "alcohol codeswitching" occurs. It is possible that bicultural individuals identify as drinkers in some social contexts where heavy alcohol use is encouraged (e.g., college setting, around people who drink) and identify as nondrinkers in other social contexts where alcohol use is discouraged (e.g., at home with parents, around people who do not drink). In these distinct drinking-related contexts, bicultural individuals may experience a "push-pull" effect. This phenomenon could potentially increase or decrease immigrants' or their descendants' risk for alcohol (mis)use. Pursuing this line of inquiry is needed to better understand the ways in which individual differences in bicultural orientations could impact alcohol use.

Concluding thoughts

For over two decades, researchers have been examining how acculturation, enculturation, and bicultural orientations are associated with alcohol use among immigrant and other ethnic minority populations. There continues to be a great deal of variability in how these constructs are assessed, which makes comparison across studies difficult. It is also common practice for researchers to measure acculturation, enculturation, or bicultural orientations globally, without any specific reference to cultural norms around drinking. These global constructs are correlated with drinking behaviors and then speculations are made about the findings by invoking a norm perspective, a stress perspective, or both. After two decades of research, there is modest progress to elucidating how and why these cultural constructs are associated with drinking attitudes and behaviors among immigrants and other ethnic minority groups in the United States. As evident in our review, three questions remain: What kinds of cultural drinking norms are immigrants and their descendants acculturating into or enculturating from? How do they integrate cultural influences from ethnic and mainstream societies to inform their attitudes toward alcohol use? How might changes in these cultural drinking norms increase or decrease their risk for alcohol use and misuse? We hope that the theoretical insights and the future research recommendations from this chapter will serve as a critical launching point for future work that will generate novel and important research in many years to come.

References

Abraído-Lanza, A. F., Armbrister, A. N., Flórez, K. R., & Aguirre, A. N. (2006). Toward a theory-driven model of acculturation in public health research. *American Journal of Public Health*, *96*(8), 1342–1346. https://doi.org/10.2105/AJPH.2005.064980.

Alvarez, M., Frietze, G., Ramos, C., Field, C., & Zarate, M. A. (2017). A quantitative analysis of Latino acculturation and alcohol use: Myth versus reality. *Alcoholism: Clinical and Experimental Research*, *41*, 1246–1256.

Benet-Martínez, V., & Haritatos, J. (2005). Bicultural identity integration (BII): Components and psychosocial antecedents. *Journal of Personality*, *73*, 1015–1050. https://doi.org/10.1111/j.1467-6494.2005.00337.x.

Berry, J. W. (1997). Immigration, acculturation, and adaptation. *Applied Psychology. An International Review*, *46*, 5–34. https://doi.org/10.1080/026999497378467.

Berry, J. W. (2005). Acculturation: Living successfully in two cultures. *International Journal of Intercultural Relations*, *29*, 697–712. https://doi.org/10.1016/j.ijintrel.2005.07.013.

Berry, J. W., Phinney, J. S., Sam, D. L., & Vedder, P. (2006). Immigrant youth: Acculturation, identity, and adaptation. *Applied Psychology*, *55*, 303–332. https://doi.org/10.1111/j.1464-0597.2006.00256.x.

Berry, J. W., & Sam, D. L. (1997). Acculturation and adaptation. In J. W. Berry, M. H. Segall, & C. Kagitcibasi (Eds.), *Handbook of cross-cultural psychology* (pp. 291–326). Needham Heights, MA: Allyn & Bacon.

Bornstein, M. H. (2017). The specificity principle in acculturation science. *Perspectives on Psychological Science*, *12*(1), 3–45. https://doi.org/10.1177/1745691616655997.

Cabassa, L. J. (2003). Measuring acculturation: Where we are and where we need to go. *Hispanic Journal of Behavioral Sciences*, *25*, 127–146. https://doi.org/10.1177/0739986303025002001.

Caetano, R. (1987). Acculturation and drinking patterns among U.S. Hispanics. *British Journal of Addiction*, *82*, 789–799.

Caetano, R., Clark, C. L., & Tam, T. (1998). Alcohol consumption among racial/ethnic minorities: Theory and research. *Alcohol Health & Research World*, *22*, 233–241.

Cano, M.Á., de Dios, M. A., Castro, Y., Vaughan, E. L., Castillo, L. G., Lorenzo-Blanco, E. I., ... Molleda, L. M. (2015). Alcohol use severity and depressive symptoms among late adolescent Hispanics: Testing associations of acculturation and enculturation in a bicultural transaction model. *Addictive Behaviors*, *49*, 78–82. https://doi.org/10.1016/j.addbeh.2015.06.002.

Census Bureau. (2011). *Overview of race and Hispanic origin: 2010*. Suitland, MD: U.S. Census Bureau.

Cervantes, R. C., Fisher, D. G., Padilla, A. M., & Napper, L. E. (2016). The Hispanic Stress Inventory Version 2: Improving the assessment of acculturation stress. *Psychological Assessment*, *28*, 509–522. https://doi.org/10.1037/pas0000200.

Chartier, K., & Caetano, R. (2010). Ethnicity and health disparities in alcohol research. *Alcohol Research & Health*, *33*, 152–160. Retrieved from PMC.

Child Trends. (2018). *Immigrant children* Retrieved from https://www.childtrends.org/?indicators=immigrant-children.

Chun, K. M., Balls Organista, P., & Marín, G. (Eds.), (2003). *Acculturation: Advances in theory, measurement, and applied research*. Washington, DC: American Psychological Association.https://doi.org/10.1037/10472-000.

Chung, R. H. G., Kim, B. S. K., & Abreu, J. M. (2004). Asian American multidimensional acculturation scale: Development, factor analysis, reliability, and validity. *Cultural Diversity and Ethnic Minority Psychology*, *10*, 66–80. https://doi.org/10.1037/1099-9809.10.1.66.

Coatsworth, J. D., Maldonado-Molina, M., Pantin, H., & Szapocznik, J. (2005). A person-centered and ecological investigation of acculturation strategies in Hispanic immigrant youth. *Journal of Community Psychology*, *33*, 157–174. https://doi.org/10.1002/jcop.20046.

Cooper, L. M., Kuntsche, E., Levitt, A., Barber, L. L., & Wolf, S. (2016). Motivational models of substance use: A review of theory and research on motives for using alcohol, marijuana, and tobacco. In K. J. Sher (Ed.), *The Oxford handbook of substance use and substance use disorders* (pp. 375–421). New York, NY: Oxford University Press.

Cuellar, I., Arnold, B., & Maldonado, R. (1995). Acculturation rating scale for Mexican Americans-II: A revision of the original ARSMA scale. *Hispanic Journal of Behavioral Sciences*, *17*, 275–304. https://doi.org/10.1177/07399863950173001.

David, E. J. R., Okazaki, S., & Saw, A. (2009). Bicultural self-efficacy among college students: Initial scale development and mental health correlates. *Journal of Counseling Psychology*, *56*, 211–226. https://doi.org/10.1037/a0015419.

Degenhardt, L., Chiu, W.-T., Sampson, N., Kessler, R. C., Anthony, J. C., Angermeyer, M., ... Wells, J. E. (2008). Toward a global view of alcohol, tobacco, cannabis, and cocaine use: Findings from the WHO World Mental Health Surveys. *PLoS Medicine*, *5*(7), e141https://doi.org/10.1371/journal.pmed.0050141.

Des Rosiers, S. E., Schwartz, S. J., Zamboanga, B. L., Ham, L. S., & Huang, S. (2013). A cultural and social cognitive model of differences in acculturation orientations, alcohol expectancies, and alcohol-related risk behaviors among Hispanic college students. *Journal of Clinical Psychology*, *69*, 319–340. https://doi.org/10.1002/jclp.21859.

Fox, M., Thayer, Z. M., & Wadhwa, P. D. (2017). Acculturation and health: The moderating role of sociocultural context. *American Anthropologist*, *119*(3), 405–421. https://doi-org.libproxy.smith.edu/10.1111/aman.12867.

Giang, M. T., & Wittig, M. A. (2006). Implications of adolescents' acculturation strategies for personal and collective self-esteem. *Cultural Diversity and Ethnic Minority Psychology*, *12*, 725–739. https://doi.org/10.1037/1099-9809.12.4.725.

Grant, B. F., Chou, S. P., Saha, T. D., Pickering, R. P., Kerridge, B. T., Ruan, W. J., … Hasin, D. S. (2017). Prevalence of 12-month alcohol use, high-risk drinking, and DSM–IV alcohol use disorder in the United States, 2001–2002 to 2012–2013: Results from the National Epidemiologic Survey on Alcohol and Related Conditions. *Journal of the American Medical Association Psychiatry*, *74*, 911–923. https://doi.org/10.1001/jamapsychiatry.2017.2161.

Grant, B. F., Goldstein, R. B., Saha, T. D., Chou, P., Jung, J., Zhang, H., … Hasin, D. S. (2015). Epidemiology of DSM-5 alcohol use disorder: Results from the National Epidemiologic Survey on Alcohol and Related Conditions III. *JAMA Psychiatry*, *72*, 757–766. https://doi.org/10.1001/jamapsychiatry.2015.0584.

Hunt, L. M., Schneider, S., & Comer, B. (2004). Should "acculturation" be a variable in health research? A critical review of research on US Hispanics. *Social Science and Medicine*, *59*(5), 973–986. https://doi-org.libproxy.smith.edu/10.1016/j.socscimed.2003.12.009.

Huynh, Q.-L., Nguyen, A.-M.T.D., & Benet-Martínez, V. (2011). Bicultural identity integration. In (Vols. 1 and 2). *Handbook of identity theory and research* (pp. 827–843). https://doi.org/10.1007/978-1-4419-7988-9_35.

Huynh, Q.-L., Benet-Martínez, V., & Nguyen, A.-M.D. (2018). Measuring variations in bicultural identity across U.S. ethnic and generational groups: Development and validation of the Bicultural Identity Integration Scale—Version 2 (BIIS-2). *Psychological Assessment*, *30*, 1581–1596. https://doi.org/10.1037/pas0000606.

Iwamoto, D. K., Kaya, A., Grivel, M., & Clinton, L. (2016). Under-researched demographics: Heavy episodic drinking on alcohol-related problems among Asian Americans. *Alcohol Research: Current Reviews: 38*, 17–25.

Jimenez, D. E., Gray, H. L., Cucciare, M., Kumbhani, S., & Gallagher-Thompson, D. (2010). Using the revised Acculturation Rating Scale for Mexican Americans (ARSMA-II) with older adults. *Hispanic Health Care International: The Official Journal of the National Association of Hispanic Nurses*, *8*, 14–22. https://doi.org/10.1891/1540-4153.8.1.14.

Karriker-Jaffe, K. J., & Zemore, S. E. (2009). Associations between acculturation and alcohol consumption of Latino men in the United States. *Journal of Studies on Alcohol and Drugs*, *70*, 27–31.

Kaya, A., Iwamoto, D. K., Grivel, M., Clinton, L., & Brady, J. (2016). The role of feminine and masculine norms in college women's alcohol use. *Psychology of Men & Masculinity*, *17*, 206–214. https://doi.org/10.1037/men0000017.

Kane, J. C., Johnson, R. M., Robinson, C., Jernigan, D. H., Harachi, T. W., & Bass, J. K. (2016). Longitudinal effects of acculturation on alcohol use among Vietnamese and Cambodian immigrant women in the USA. *Alcohol and Alcoholism*, *51*, 702–709. https://doi.org/10.1093/alcalc/agw007.

LaFromboise, T., Coleman, H. L. K., & Gerton, J. (1993). Psychological impact of biculturalism: Evidence and theory. *Psychological Bulletin*, *114*, 395–412. https://doi.org/10.1037/0033-2909.114.3.395.

Lazarus, R. S. (1997). Acculturation isn't everything. *Applied Psychology*, *46*, 39–43. https://doi.org/10.1111/j.1464-0597.1997.tb01089.x.

Lindgren, K. P., Gasser, M. L., Werntz, A., Namaky, N., Baldwin, S. A., & Teachman, B. A. (2016). Moderators of implicit and explicit drinking identity in a large U.S. adult sample. *Addictive Behaviors*, *60*, 177–183. https://doi.org/10.1016/j.addbeh.2016.04.022.

Livingston, G. (2019). *Hispanic women no longer account for the majority of immigrant births in the U.S.* Washington, DC: Pew Research Center. Retrieved from https://www.pewresearch.org/fact-tank/2019/08/08/hispanic-women-no-longer-account-for-the-majority-of-immigrant-births-in-the-u-s/.

Lui, P. P. (2015). Intergenerational cultural conflict, mental health, and educational outcomes among Asian and Latino/a Americans: Qualitative and meta-analytic review. *Psychological Bulletin, 141*, 404–446. https://doi.org/10.1037/a0038449.

Lui, P. P., Berkley, S. R., & Zamboanga, B. L. (2019). College alcohol belief and alcohol use: Testing moderations by cultural orientations and ethnicity. *Journal of Counseling Psychology*, Advance online publication. https://doi.org/10.1037/cou0000374.

Lui, P. P., & Quezada, L. (2019). Associations between microaggression and adjustment outcomes: A meta-analytic and narrative review. *Psychological Bulletin, 145*, 45–78. https://doi.org/10.1037/bul0000172.

Lui, P. P., & Rollock, D. (2012). Acculturation and psychosocial adjustment among Southeast Asian and Chinese immigrants: The effects of domain-specific goals. *Asian American Journal of Psychology, 3*, 79–90. https://doi.org/10.1037/a0025411.

Lui, P. P., & Zamboanga, B. L. (2018a). Acculturation and alcohol use among Asian Americans: A meta-analytic review. *Psychology of Addictive Behaviors, 32*, 173–186. https://doi.org/10.1037/adb0000340.

Lui, P. P., & Zamboanga, B. L. (2018b). A critical review and meta-analysis of the associations between acculturation and alcohol use outcomes among Hispanic Americans. *Alcoholism, Clinical and Experimental Research, 42*, 1841–1862. https://doi.org/10.1111/acer.13845.

Lui, P. P., & Zamboanga, B. L. (2019). Ethnocultural diversity in alcohol use and misuse. *American Journal of Orthopsychiatry, 89*, 543–548. https://doi.org/10.1037/ort0000422.

Marín, G., Sabogal, F., VanOss Marín, B., Otero-Sabogal, F., & Pérez-Stable, E. J. (1987). Development of a short acculturation scale for Hispanics. *Hispanic Journal of Behavioral Sciences, 9*, 183–205.

Markides, K. S., Krause, N., & Leon, C.F.M.d. (1988). Acculturation and alcohol consumption among Mexican Americans: A three-generation study. *American Journal of Public Health, 78*, 1178–1181. https://doi.org/10.2105/ajph.78.9.1178.

Meca, A., Zamboanga, B. L., Lui, P. P., Schwartz, S. J., Lorenzo-Blanco, E. I., Gonzales-Backen, M. A., … Lizzi, K. M. (2019). Alcohol initiation among recently immigrated Hispanic adolescents: Roles of acculturation and sociocultural stress. *American Journal of Orthopsychiatry, 89*(5), 569–578. https://doi.org/10.1037/ort0000352.supp. [Supplemental].

Monk, R. L., & Heim, D. (2013). A critical systematic review of alcohol-related outcome expectancies. *Substance Use and Misuse, 48*(7), 539–557. https://doi.org/10.3109/10826084.2013.787097.

Myers, R., Chou, C.-P., Sussman, S., Baezconde-Garbanati, L., Pachon, H., & Valente, T. W. (2009). Acculturation and substance use: Social influence as a mediator among Hispanic alternative high school youth. *Journal of Health and Social Behavior, 50*, 164–179.

Nguyen, A.-M.D., & Benet-Martínez, V. (2013). Biculturalism and adjustment: A meta-analysis. *Journal of Cross-Cultural Psychology, 44*, 122–159. https://doi.org/10.1177/0022022111435097.

Oshri, A., Schwartz, S. J., Unger, J. B., Kwon, J. A., Des Rosiers, S. E., Baezconde-Garbanati, L., … Szapocznik, J. (2014). Bicultural stress, identity formation, and alcohol expectancies and misuse in Hispanic adolescents: A developmental approach. *Journal of Youth and Adolescence, 43*, 2054–2068. https://doi.org/10.1007/s10964-014-0171-2.

Pearson, M. R. (2013). Use of alcohol protective behavioral strategies among college students: A critical review. *Clinical Psychology Review, 33*(8), 1025–1040. https://doi.org/10.1016/j.cpr.2013.08.006.

Perrotte, J. K., & Zamboanga, B. L. (2019). Traditional gender roles and alcohol use among latinas/os: A review of the literature. *Journal of Ethnicity in Substance Abuse*, Advance online publication. https://doi.org/10.1080/15332640.2019.1579142.

Pew Research Center. (2013). *The rise of Asian Americans.* Retrieved from http://www.pewsocialtrends.org/2012/06/19/the-rise-of-asian-americans/.

Pham, S., & Lui, P. P. (2019a). Acculturation profiles and alcohol use among Hispanic Americans. *Journal of Ethnicity in Substance Abuse*, https://doi.org/10.1080/15332640.2019.1679316. Advance online publication.

Pham, S., & Lui, P. P. (2019b). Acculturation and alcohol use outcomes: Incremental roles of bicultural orientations among Asian American undergraduate and graduate students. *Cultural Diversity and Ethnic Minority Psychology*, Advance online publication. https://doi.org/10.1037/cdp0000318.

Pinedo, M., Zemore, S., Cherpitel, C., & Caetano, R. (2017). Acculturation and alcohol use: The role of environmental contexts. In S. J. Schwartz, J. B. Unger, S. J. Schwartz, & J. B. Unger (Eds.), *The Oxford handbook of acculturation and health* (pp. 239–261). New York, NY: Oxford University Press.

Radford, J. (2019). *Key findings about U.S. immigrants.* Washington, DC: Pew Research Center. Retrieved from https://www.pewresearch.org/fact-tank/2019/06/17/key-findings-about-u-s-immigrants/.

Romero, A. J., Carvajal, S. C., Valle, F., & Orduña, M. (2007). Adolescent bicultural stress and its impact on mental well-being among Latinos, Asian Americans, and European Americans. *Journal of Community Psychology*, *35*, 519–534. https://doi.org/10.1002/jcop.20162.

Romero, A. J., Martinez, D., & Carvajal, S. C. (2007). Bicultural stress and adolescent risk behaviors in a community sample of Latinos and non-Latino European Americans. *Ethnicity and Health*, *12*, 443–463. https://doi.org/10.1080/13557850701616854.

Romero, A. J., & Roberts, R. E. (2003). Stress within a bicultural context for adolescents of Mexican descent. *Cultural Diversity and Ethnic Minority Psychology*, *9*, 171–184.

Rudmin, F. W. (2003). Critical history of the acculturation psychology of assimilation, separation, integration, and marginalization. *Review of General Psychology*, *7*, 250. https://doi.org/10.1037/1089-2680.7.3.250.

Sacks, J. J., Gonzales, K. R., Bouchery, E. E., Tomedi, L. E., & Brewer, R. D. (2015). 2010 national and state costs of excessive alcohol consumption. *American Journal of Preventive Medicine*, *49*, e73–e79. https://doi.org/10.1016/j.amepre.2015.05.031.

Salas-Wright, C. P., Clark, T. T., Vaughn, M. G., & Córdova, D. (2015). Profiles of acculturation among Hispanics in the United States: Links with discrimination and substance use. *Social Psychiatry and Psychiatric Epidemiology*, *50*, 39–49. https://doi.org/10.1007/s00127-014-0889-x.

Salas-Wright, C. P., Vaughn, M. G., Clark Goings, T. T., Córdova, D., & Schwartz, S. J. (2018). Substance use disorders among immigrants in the United States: A research update. *Addictive Behaviors*, *76*, 169–173. https://doi.org/10.1016/j.addbeh.2017.08.014.

Schinke, S. P., Orlandi, M. A., Botvin, G. J., Gilchrist, L. D., Trimble, J. E., & Locklear, V. S. (1988). Preventing substance abuse among American-Indian adolescents: A bicultural competence skills approach. *Journal of Counseling Psychology*, *35*, 87–90.

Schwartz, S. J., Meca, A., Ward, C., Szabó, Á., Benet-Martínez, V., Lorenzo-Blanco, E. I., … Zamboanga, B. L. (2019). Biculturalism dynamics: A daily diary study of bicultural identity and psychosocial functioning. *Journal of Applied Developmental Psychology*, *62*, 26–37. https://doi.org/10.1016/j.appdev.2018.12.007.

Schwartz, S. J., Unger, J. B., Zamboanga, B. L., & Szapocznik, J. (2010). Rethinking the concept of acculturation. *The American Psychologist*, *65*, 237–251. https://doi.org/10.1037/a0019330.

Schwartz, S. J., & Zamboanga, B. L. (2008). Testing Berry's model of acculturation: A confirmatory latent class approach. *Cultural Diversity and Ethnic Minority Psychology*, *14*, 275–285. https://doi.org/10.1037/a0012818.

Stephenson, M. (2000). Development and validation of the Stephenson Multigroup Acculturation Scale (SMAS). *Psychological Assessment*, *12*, 77–88.

Suinn, R. M., Ahuna, C., & Khoo, G. (1992). The Suinn-Lew Asian self-identity acculturation scale: Concurrent and factorial validation. *Educational and Psychological Measurement*, *52*, 1041–1046.

Suinn, R. M., Khoo, G., & Ahuna, C. (1995). The Suinn-Lew Asian self-identity acculturation scale: Cross-cultural information. *Journal of Multicultural Counseling and Development*, *23*, 139–148.

Szapocznik, J., Kurtines, W. M., & Fernandez, T. (1980). Bicultural involvement and adjustment in Hispanic-American youths. *International Journal of Intercultural Relations*, *4*, 353–365.

Torres, L., Driscoll, M. W., & Voell, M. (2012). Discrimination, acculturation, acculturative stress, and Latino psychological distress: A moderated mediational model. *Cultural Diversity and Ethnic Minority Psychology*, *18*, 17–25. https://doi.org/10.1037/a0026710.

Vaeth, P. A. C., Wang-Schweig, M., & Caetano, R. (2017). Drinking, alcohol use disorder, and treatment access and utilization among U. S. racial/ethnic groups. *Alcoholism: Clinical and Experimental Research*, *41*(1), 6–19. https://doi.org/10.1111/acer.13285.

Wallace, P. M., Pomery, E. A., Latimer, A. E., Martinez, J. L., & Salovey, P. (2010). A review of acculturation measures and their utility in studies promoting Latino health. *Hispanic Journal of Behavioral Sciences*, *32*, 37–54.

Zamboanga, B. L., Tomaso, C. C., & Lui, P. P. (2017). Acculturation and alcohol use among Hispanic and Asian American college students: What do we know and where could we go? In S. J. Schwartz & J. B. Unger (Eds.), *The Oxford handbook of acculturation and health* (pp. 263–280). New York, NY: Oxford University Press.

Zemore, S. E. (2007). Acculturation and alcohol among Latino adults in the United States: A comprehensive review. *Alcoholism: Clinical and Experimental Research*, *31*, 1968–1990. https://doi.org/10.1111/j.1530-0277.2007.00532.x.

Chapter 4

Acculturation science: Limitations and new directions

Miriam J. Alvarez, Angel D. Armenta and Michael A. Zárate
University of Texas at El Paso, El Paso, TX, United States

The change brought by immigration to the United States is irrefutable. For example, immigrants drive the economic boom in various states (McCann, 2019), produce billions in taxes every year (Joint Economic Committee, 2016; New American Economy, 2017), and incite creative growth (Florida, 2004). As the immigrant population in the United States continues to grow (U.S. Census Bureau, 2012), it is important to understand the processes associated with healthy adaptation. Typically, acculturation has been used as a framework to understand this process. In this chapter, we review acculturation frameworks and review the literature that has applied this framework in the context of health to address two primary questions: is acculturation effectively capturing the process of adaptation immigrants undergo in a new country? What, if any, are new directions in acculturation science?

This chapter has three primary aims. First, in an effort to move forward, this chapter presents a brief history of acculturation and future directions in acculturation theory. In this effort, the chapter discusses metaanalytic research in the field of acculturation and health. Second, special consideration is given to the tools and methods used to understand acculturation. These tools have remained unchanged and static for decades, limiting our understanding of the mechanism that underlies immigrant adaptation. This is particularly important given one basic fact: society is changing. The dynamics and factors that impact daily behaviors, interactions, and environments are key elements in shaping the way in which individuals acculturate. And yet, the dynamic nature of our society is an element that is commonly left out of acculturation frameworks. Here, we propose the cultural inertia framework as a framework that interacts with the acculturative process. The times demand a revitalization of acculturation research.

Mental and Behavioral Health of Immigrants in the United States
https://doi.org/10.1016/B978-0-12-816117-3.00004-X

Paving the way

Culture is defined as a "dynamic system of collective held meanings and practices that are maintained and modified over time" (Halloran & Kashima, 2006, p. 137). In essence, it is the sum of the attitudes, values, norms, beliefs, and practical skills of various members that share a common social identity (Bornstein, 2010; Halloran & Kashima, 2006; Shore, 2002; Triandis, 1995). Cultures help members (and "outsiders") understand their environment, influence self-perceptions, and intergroup relations. One could argue that without migration, cultures would not interact. As globalization increases, migrants bring one culture into contact with another culture at increasing rates (Bornstein, 2017). When such contact occurs, acculturation takes place at two levels—individual and societal. At the individual level, immigrants face various challenges. Acculturation involves engaging in the adjustment of one's customs, language, norms, and values, which means navigating through daily situations with often competing for cultural reference systems. At the societal level, acculturation entails changes to social and service institutions, as well as mainstream practices and norms. These changes often increase tension among immigrants and members of the host society and often lead to negative social consequences, such as prejudice and discrimination. Altogether, acculturation most often involves not only changes to one's environment (i.e., community or city), but also attitudinal changes that may directly or indirectly affect behavior, such that it encompasses individual and societal level adaptation (Pokhrel, Herzog, Sun, Rohrbach, & Sussman, 2013).

Early acculturation theory

One of the first definitions of acculturation was proposed by Redfield, Linton, and Herskovits (1936). They describe acculturation as a process by which individuals in one culture (heritage culture) take on the manifestations of another (mainstream culture), resulting in incremental and unidimensional changes to the heritage culture. According to this early model, acculturation implied that retention of the heritage culture and acquisition of the mainstream culture were cast as opposing ends of a single continuum, such that as immigrants acculturated, they lost their heritage culture and adopted the mainstream culture (Gordon, 1964). Researchers argue that earlier waves of European immigrants to the US followed this type of continuum (Schildkraut, 2007). However, this acculturation continuum was criticized for not providing a comprehensive depiction of the immigrant adaptation process and leaving important elements of the adaptation mechanisms out. In particular, this early model is criticized for being unidimensional and not accounting for the extent to which individuals retain their heritage culture while simultaneously adopting the mainstream culture.

In the early 1980s, scientists began to argue that adopting the mainstream culture did not imply relinquishing the heritage culture (Berry, 1980a, 1980b).

Berry (1984) introduces a model of acculturation that built on the earlier unidimensional model by introducing an additional dimension. Not only might immigrants take on mainstream cultural tendencies, but they might also retain their own cultural styles. This bidimensional model was divided into four ideologies that describe the processes of cultural adaptation for individuals with multiple cultural systems. Berry's framework details four ideologies that an individual may adopt when coming in contact with interacting cultures: assimilation, separation, marginalization, and integration. Assimilation proposes that individuals relinquish their ethnic identity to adapt to the norms of the mainstream culture (Berry, 1980a). In contrast, separation proposes that an individual will maintain his or her own cultural identity and reject involvement with the host country. The third ideology, marginalization, refers to situations in which an individual neither identifies with nor participates in their own culture nor the host culture. Finally, integration proposes that individuals maintain his or her own cultural identity while at the same time becoming an active participant in the host culture. Many researchers describe Berry's integration quadrant as biculturalism. Biculturalism refers to immigrants who adopt multiple cultural meaning systems (Benet-Martínez & Haritatos, 2005; Birman, 1994; LaFromboise, Coleman, & Gerton, 1993; Phinney & Devich-Navarro, 1997; Ramirez, 1984). Over time, this bicultural context may (a) produce competing cultural reference systems where individuals alternate between cultures as a function of the environment or (b) evolve and incorporate elements from both cultures creating one blended identity (Benet-Martínez & Haritatos, 2005).

Berry's acculturation ideologies have received widespread attention across the social sciences (Yoon, Langrehr, & Ong, 2011). While many to date scientists utilize this model, the four ideologies have received criticism (Alvarez, Frietze, Ramos, Field, & Zárate, 2017). In particular, the "one size fits all" approach has been questioned (Rudmin, 2003). Berry's (1980a) model of acculturation categorizes individuals into four quadrants. To do this, much of the research has utilized arbitrary cutoffs and thresholds on the associated acculturation measures. This is problematic for two reasons. First, the creation of arbitrary thresholds makes comparisons between studies difficult. This is because what is categorized as high acculturation might easily differ across studies. For example, using median splits differ across samples, making comparisons impossible (Coatsworth, Maldonado-Molina, Pantin, & Szapocznik, 2005; Giang & Wittig, 2006). Second, to assess Berry's model of acculturation without bias, one must assume all quadrants are equally observable phenomena. In practice, the reality is different and researchers have criticized the cogency of marginalization as an approach (Del Pilar & Udasco, 2004). Indeed, research has shown that the marginalization approach may be viable only for the small segment of immigrants (Berry, 2006). However, the literature argues, and to some extent shows that the likelihood that a person will develop an identity without drawing on either the heritage or mainstream culture is low.

The specificity principle of acculturation science

More recently, Bornstein (2017) proposes the Specificity Principle in Acculturation Science. The principle proposes that "specific setting conditions of specific people at specific times moderate specific domains in acculturation by specific processes" (Bornstein, 2017, p. 3). In essence, the principle calls for specificity in acculturation science and puts forth five components to guide the specificity: *setting condition*, *person*, *time*, *process*, and *domain*.

Setting conditions of acculturation include reasons for migrating, place, experience, and status. Indeed research has shown that these factors have important implications that have yet to be tied into thorough acculturation research. For example, Ogbu and Simons (1998) define two particular immigrant groups, voluntary and involuntary. Voluntary immigrants include all foreign-born people who have moved to a "host" country as a product of their own desires or motivations. Involuntary immigrants are also foreign-born people but migrated to the United States because they were displaced from their home country, feared persecution, had moved by deception or coercion, or a natural disaster. Our theories (Zárate, Reyna, & Alvarez, 2019) show that the reasons for migration have strong implications on an immigrant's process of adaptation, and none of the commonly used acculturation tools include this factor (Cuellar, Arnold, & Maldonado, 1995). Though never formally considered by acculturation scientists, the cultural inertia framework provides a unique opportunity to assess the extent to which *setting conditions* impact the process of acculturation. This is because cultural inertia describes the extent to which people accept (or reject) change when change is occurring (Quezada, Shaw, & Zárate, 2012). This framework will be discussed in detail ahead.

Bornstein's second component, *person*, refers to individual-difference characteristics such as gender, personality, and motivation. For example, greater openness is associated with greater acculturation to the mainstream culture (Mendenhall & Oddou, 1985). Traits like extraversion and agreeableness are negatively associated with an immigrants' desire to return to their heritage culture, while lower neuroticism and higher conscientiousness are associated with mainstream acculturation and maintenance (Caligiuri, 2000; Ryder, Alden, & Paulhus, 2000). The combination of traits like openness and agreeableness can promote the acculturation process, acting like a psychological propeller that once in motion, can accelerate the extent to which an individual adopts the characteristics of a new culture. In contrast, traits like neuroticism can hinder the process and function like psychological anchors, cementing individuals in a state where they will actively choose to maintain their heritage culture. Psychological anchors and propellers function similarly among a host of individual-level factors (i.e., anxiety, stress, self-esteem, and internal locus of control). Research has shown that these are linked to the acculturation process (Kosic, 2002; Valentine, 2001).

Identity is an important factor in the *person* component and is often a neglected element in acculturation science. Tajfel (1978) defines identity as "that part of an individual's self-concept which derives from knowledge of his/her membership of a social group together with the values and emotional significance attached to that membership" (p. 63). Once an identity is adopted, individuals will behave and conform to the norms of the group. For most people, this means that as a member of the group, one will behave in ways consistent with the group's norms, attitudes, beliefs, and values. When a particular identity becomes salient, individuals will adhere to prescribed norms and stereotypical behaviors associated with the group, which typically favors the ingroup as it is assumed that people like to see themselves in a positive light in relation to other groups (Tajfel & Turner, 1985).

Turner (1987) identifies three factors that contribute to the development of ingroup favoritism which we believe are important to identity. The first factor is the extent to which individuals identify with an ingroup to internalize that group membership as an aspect of their self-concept. Then, the extent to which the prevailing context provides ground for comparison between groups. Finally, the perceived relevance of the comparison group, which itself will be shaped by the relative and absolute status of the ingroup. Individuals are likely to display favoritism when an ingroup is central to their self-definition and a given comparison is meaningful or the outcome is contestable. All of these factors are essential to understanding the impact identity has on perceiving and experiencing the environment in which we live. Research shows that identity has a positive relation to well-being, and in particular, ethnic identity. Umaña-Taylor and Updegraff (2007) report that various aspects of the self (i.e., ethnic identity, cultural orientations) can protect and/or enhance the risks associated with discrimination. However, additional studies have established an indirect effect on identity and personal wellbeing. For example, high ethnic identity was reported to be a protective reactive factor that moderated the effects of discrimination on depressive symptoms among Korean Americans (Lee, 2005). These results suggest that in the face of marginalization and opposition, a strong ethnic identity helps individuals recognize positive virtues about their own ethnic groups and minimize the degrading beliefs perpetuated by society (Outten, Schmitt, Garcia, & Branscombe, 2009). Despite the ongoing and increasing research on ethnic identity, acculturation science seldom considers identity as a factor that functions as a psychological anchor or propeller in the acculturative process.

Bornstein (2017) argues that *time* is a moderator of acculturation. The Specificity Principle of Acculturation Science discusses time in the context of age, time spent in the culture of the destination, and historical period as important considerations of the concept. For example, age can impact the way in which you experience acculturation as it nearly goes without saying that the experience of a child immigrant will differ from the experiences of an adult immigrant (Carhill, Suárez-Orozco, & Páez, 2008; Jia & Aaronson, 2003). Research shows that children who migrate are often bicultural and bilingual, and experience cognitive benefits such as better phonological awareness and language competence, in comparison to monolinguals (Kovelman, Baker, & Petitto, 2008).

Furthermore, young adults who migrate to a new country tend to have the longest and most direct contact with their culture of heritage (Shuval, 1982). These two acculturation processes have strong implications on how the individual behaves in social, educational, and political spheres (Portes & Rumbaut, 2006). However, in comparison to children and adolescents, adults appear to experience the most difficulties (Schwartz, Montgomery, & Briones, 2006).

Immigrants' duration of stay in the host country can impact the acculturation process. Temporary immigrants stay in the host country temporarily and return to their heritage culture when the opportunity arises. Permanent immigrants stay in the host country indefinitely without returning to their heritage culture. Thus, immigrants who anticipate a lasting stay in a host country may exert more effort into learning the new culture and learn more about the host culture through time. For immigrants who move to a new country permanently, learning about mainstream norms, values, and beliefs may be an instrumental survival tactic, which is not often the case with temporary immigrants. Research has shown that there is cultural variation among family members based on their length of time in the host country (Mendoza, Javier, & Burgos, 2007). In addition, adults who reside in the United States for longer periods report adopting the American English language (Cabrera, Shannon, West, & Brooks-Gunn, 2006; Tamis-LeMonda, Sze, Ng, Kahana-Kalman, & Yoshikawa, 2013).

The fourth component in the Specificity Principle, *process*, refers to the progression associated with how the new culture is experienced. According to Bornstein, there are four types of processes that warrant special consideration: socialization, learning, instruction, and opportunity. Bornstein (2017) describes socialization as a necessary coping mechanism that allows individuals to learn new skills that help them function in accordance with the mainstream culture. Learning refers to the acquisition of novel behaviors and beliefs through beliefs and behaviors through observation, imitation, and reinforcement. Instruction differs from learning, as it constitutes forms of didactic acculturative transfer. For example, among adult immigrants, the workplace or community classrooms may be locations of instruction. Lastly, opportunities are affordances that impact daily life and behaviors such as access to resources and activities. Research shows that families with better access to resources are likely to invest in their children's well-being by creating opportunities that may lead to personal and professional growth (Conger & Donnellan, 2007).

The last component of Bornstein's Specificity Principle of Acculturation Science is the *domain*. This component argues acculturation is a dynamic process, such that immigrants adopt different processes which are shaped by setting, person, time, and process (Overton, 2015; Zárate et al., 2019). In general, acculturation research has differentiated between various dependent variables that acculturate differently. For example, in one study, Turkish and Moroccan immigrants in the Netherlands attributed more importance to their heritage culture the domains of home and family, but more importance to their host culture in the public domains of school and workplace (Phinney, 2006). Furthermore, this process of adaptation differs as a function of the domain, and the process itself is dynamic. Thus, increased involvement with a new culture is believed to instigate changes in immigrants that result in a better fit with the norms of the culture of the destination and reduced fit with the norms of the culture of origin. Altogether, *domain* poses that acculturation affects social, education, financial, and educational spheres differently, and this effect is dynamic and, potentially, ever changing.

The Specificity Principle of Acculturation Science provides great direction for future acculturation science for multiple reasons. First, it provides a framework that unifies acculturation research that is not solely associated with the "acculturation" term but by definition is acculturation. This is an important connection that brings together researchers from various fields and presents new methodologies that circumvent traditional acculturation scales to test acculturation theory. Second, the Specificity Principle of Acculturation Science highlights a need for careful consideration and application of acculturation theory to better understand the mechanism that impacts the processes that immigrants adopt in a host country. A benefit of specificity is that one can customize the principle to an immigrant population and discourages future research from implementing a "one size fits all" approach.

From theory to testable: A glance at acculturation and health research

The literature on acculturation is massive. Google Scholar alone provides over 541,000 articles discussing acculturation. Acculturation processes are particularly influential at the intersection of culture and health. In the health domain, researchers are interested in the impact of acculturation processes on health attitudes, health behaviors, and physiology. Many of this research focuses on Asian and Latinx issues, as they are the largest and fastest-growing immigrant populations in the United States (Lam, 2016). This section will focus on the findings of metaanalytic reviews on Asian and Latinx health behaviors as a result of acculturation.

Alcohol use

One topic that is often studied in conjunction with acculturation is alcohol use among Latinxs. The overall findings from these studies typically do not diverge from one another. Researchers often find that acculturation is positively related to alcohol use, such that the more acculturated immigrants are to US culture, the more alcohol they consume. However, what does often differ between these studies is the magnitude of this relationship. The first metaanalysis, with over 29,000 Latinx participants, conducted by Alvarez et al. (2017) found that acculturation was positively related to alcohol consumption with an overall correlation of 0.16. A second metaanalysis that focused on alcohol consumption and acculturation among Latinxs found an even smaller relationship $r=0.09$ (Lui & Zamboanga, 2018a). The general findings from both these metaanalyses may be very similar (acculturated Latinxs tend to consume more alcohol). However, it is important to note that the inability to conduct metaanalyses by ethnic-subgroup due to study constraints was evident in both of these metaanalyses. In addition, it is rarely the case that the literature differentiates between the foreign-born and native-born populations. This is a huge limitation of the field in general and will be discussed in detail ahead. Interestingly, Lui and Zamboanga (2018a) found that older studies (e.g., acculturation studies conducted in the 1990s) yielded the strongest associations.

Together, these metaanalytic reviews suggest that contrary to stereotypical perceptions of Latinxs, alcohol consumption increases as an individual increasingly acculturate to mainstream American culture. That effect, however, is very small. The correlations were 0.09 and 0.16, suggesting that acculturation is not a huge predictor of alcohol use.

The effect of acculturation and alcohol provides evidence that multiple factors function as important moderators. Alvarez et al. (2017) show that gender is an important moderator. The association was only 0.10 for Latinos and 0.18 for Latinas. These differences may indicate that the experiences of acculturation impact males and females differently. Furthermore, distinctions in the outcomes of interest produce notable different results. In addition, different acculturation measures produce different correlations between acculturation and alcohol consumption in direction and magnitude. Alvarez et al. (2017) found that the Acculturation Rating Scale for Mexican Americans (ARSMA) produced a correlation of 0.21, the ARSMA-II produced a correlation of −0.04, the Caetano acculturation scale (1987) produced a correlation of 0.14, and the Cuellar acculturation scale (1980) produced a correlation of 0.07. Given the differences in the strength of association between acculturation and alcohol use among Latinxs, one question arises from these findings: is the relationship between acculturation and alcohol use *truly* small or are researchers doing a poor job at capturing this relationship?

Cigarette use

Currently, 37.8 million Americans smoke cigarettes (Center for Disease Control and Prevention, 2018). Research on the number of immigrants who smoke is mixed, though there seems to be a consensus that smoking among immigrants is a growing problem. To identify the antecedents of smoking behaviors among immigrants, researchers have focused their attention on the relationship between acculturation and smoking (Choi, Rankin, Stewart, & Oka, 2008; Kondo, Rossi, Schwartz, Zamboanga, & Scalf, 2016). Current research suggests that acculturation may actually be a protective factor for Asian men. Acculturated Asian men are 53% less likely to engage in smoking, while acculturated Asian women are five times more likely than nonacculturated Asian women to smoke cigarettes (Choi et al., 2008). Similar results have been found for Latinas; the more acculturated Latinas are, the more they smoke cigarettes (Kondo et al., 2016). When the data is stratified by ethnic background, the relationship between acculturation and smoking varies. In comparison to Cuban and Puerto Rican women, acculturated Mexican women were significantly more likely to smoke. Further, the effect of acculturation on smoking behavior among Cuban women was null (Kondo et al., 2016).

Unlike the alcohol use metaanalyses, the metaanalysis by Choi et al. (2008) suggests that measures of acculturation may not actually lead to differences in findings, at least in regard to cigarette use. With the exception of the nativity as a proxy variable, the vast majority of scales used in this study did not result in significantly divergent findings.

Intimate partner violence

The theory of acculturation has also been extensively studied in the realm of Latinx intimate partner violence (IPV). The general prediction here is that higher acculturation to US culture leads to more reporting of IPV. However, the literature is mixed, with some studies predicting the opposite effect. Alvarez, Oviedo Ramirez, Frietze, Field, and Zárate (2018) conducted a metaanalytic review assessing the relationship between acculturation and intimate partner victimization among foreign-born and US-born Latinx adults. The metaanalysis included 27 independent effect sizes across 21 studies. Their results found that, overall, acculturation and IPV only yielded a positive correlation of 0.11. However, further analyses, revealed that the strength of the correlation differed by gender and scale. When stratified by gender, the relationship was higher for Latinx males ($r=0.26$) than females ($r=0.08$). Furthermore, when stratified by type of acculturation measure, results yielded a myriad of effect strengths that ranged from -0.003 to 0.47.

This review yielded three important findings that tie directly with previous research. First, consistent with the literature, this review uncovered that increased acculturation leads to increased intimate partner victimization. However, one must be cautious with this interpretation as the overall effect of acculturation on IPV is relatively small. Second, acculturation differentially influences male-to-female and female-to-male partner violence. This is consistent with research and promotes the argument that women and men differentially acculturate. Lastly, the strength of the correlation between acculturation and IPV differs by scale. Again, bringing to light and questioning the reliability of existing acculturation measures.

Asian vs Hispanic acculturation correlations

It is also possible that the theory of acculturation may be more applicable to some groups than others. In a recent metaanalysis, researchers investigated the link between acculturation and HIV-related sexual behaviors (Du & Li, 2015). Similar to the aforementioned findings, these findings suggest that acculturation was weakly associated with the number of contracted sexually transmitted diseases ($r=0.10$), number of sexual partners ($r=0.15$), condom use ($r=0.01$), and early sexual initiation ($r=0.13$), with no differences in magnitude when accounting for ethnicity (Asian vs Hispanic; Du & Li, 2015). Like in the aforementioned metaanalyses, the effects in this metaanalysis (Du & Li, 2015) are also particularly small. However, there were differences in the magnitude between the link of acculturation and the number of unsafe sex behaviors. Asian population had higher relationships ($r=0.25$) than Hispanics ($r=0.16$; Du & Li, 2015).

Similar results have been found in regard to enculturation, the extent to which one retains their culture of origin, and help-seeking attitudes. Asians had a stronger, negative correlation between these variables ($r=-0.14$), suggesting that as they become more acculturated to western societies, the more negative their attitudes become toward help-seeking. For Latinxs, on the other hand, enculturation and help-seeking attitudes were weakly, positively related ($r=0.02$; Sun, Hoyt, Brockber, Lam, & Tiwari, 2016). It is again important to stress that both correlations were particularly small.

Other metaanalyses on acculturation and health outcomes have resulted in similar small correlations. For example, the relationship between acculturation and depression among Asian Americans is only -0.068 (Gupta, Leong, Valentine, & Canada, 2013). Among Mexican-American women, the relationship between acculturation and depression is nonsignificant (for South Texas participants), but significant for Kansas City Mexican-American women ($r=-0.29$; Masten, Penland, & Nayani, 1994). Overall, other metaanalyses more broadly have found weak correlations between acculturation and mental health for Latinxs ($r=-0.07$) and Asians ($r=-0.11$; Yoon et al., 2013). Further, like the weak correlation ($r=0.16$) found between acculturation and alcohol use in Alvarez et al. (2017) and Lui and Zamboanga (2018b) also found that this relationship was fairly weak among Asians ($r=0.06$).

With the exception of a few findings, many of these aforementioned correlations appear to be larger for Asian populations. Thus, it can be argued that the theory of acculturation or the current measures may be more applicable to Asian populations than Latinx populations. One explanation could be that Latinxs, as a result of being a part of the second largest group in the United States (Statistical Atlas, 2015), have more space in the United States where they are allowed to maintain their ethnic identity and, as a result, experience fewer detrimental effects of acculturation.

Limitations in acculturation science

There are several factors that can impact the measured relationship between acculturation and health—most notable differences in the type of measure of acculturation, gender, and the heterogeneity among ethnic groups. Research has shown that acculturation science is uniformly applied such that factors like ethnic subgroup, gender, location, and socioeconomic status is often collapsed despite the increasing evidence that suggest these factors impact the acculturation process differently (Alvarez et al., 2017; Choi et al., 2008; Kondo et al., 2016; Lui & Zamboanga, 2018a). The section below outlines important considerations regarding acculturation measurement and operationalization.

Acculturation measuring tools

Given that acculturation science has existed for decades, it is no surprise that there are currently at least 26 measures used to assess acculturation (Wallace, Pomery, Latimer, Martinez, & Salovey, 2010). In general, acculturation scales assess the effect of acculturation perceptions of nationality, kinship, cultural processes, and perceived health beliefs (Oetzel, De Vargas, Ginossar, & Sanchez, 2007; Pérez-Escamilla & Putnik, 2007). Most scales evaluate individual's social and cultural knowledge, behaviors, and attitudes on responses to the length of time in the United States, place of birth, language and media preferences, social network composition, and subjective questions of acculturation, with the aim of quantifying an individual's degree of acculturation. These questions are typically used to evaluate the acculturation process across multiple immigrant groups, genders, and ages and lack often specificity. Acculturations scales range from 4 to 62 items and can be administered through multiple modes and in different languages. It is also the case that acculturation scales can be unidimensional or bidimensional. A unidimensional scale measures the process of acculturation on a linear continuum that ranges from total immersion in one's heritage culture to the host's culture (Lara, Gamboa, Kahramanian, Morales, & Hayes Bautista, 2005). In contrast, bidimensional scales typically measure (a) acculturation, the extent to which an individual adopts the host culture, and (b) enculturation, the extent to which they retain their heritage culture (Padilla, 1980).

In theory, the existing acculturation scales should do a fine job of capturing the theory of acculturation. However, this is not the case. Evidence shows that acculturation measures often do not agree, even among similar samples and similar outcomes. This is problematic to the field as it leads to mixed findings and inconsistent science. Though research is limited, evidence across the two metaanalyses shows that acculturation measures were strikingly inconsistent (Table 1; Alvarez et al., 2017, 2018). It is important to note that the two analyses used similar inclusion criteria. Such that (a) only studies with immigrant Latinx populations were used and (b) scientists must have measured acculturation either through a formal scale or with a language proxy.

Across both metaanalytic reviews, the most common scales were the language proxy scales, the Caetano scale, and the ARSMA scale (Alvarez et al., 2017, 2018). Across and within both health domains, the scales produced notably different patterns of results. For example, while the ARSMA had a

TABLE 1 Correlations between acculturation and health behaviors by measure.

	Acculturation and alcohol use		Acculturation and intimate partner violence	
Measures	Correlation	Number of studies	Correlation	Number of studies
Cuellar (1980)	0.07	11	–	
ARSMA	0.19*	8	0.003	5
ARSMA-II	0.11*	6	–	
Caetano (1987)	0.16*	10	0.47*	4
Language	0.23*	10	0.04	12
Others	0.19*	5	0.05	6

*Correlation is significant at $P<.01$.

correlation of 0.19 with alcohol use, the measure failed to predict intimate partner violence ($r=-0.003$). This is consistent with the pattern of associations shown in Table 1—some acculturation measures that predicted alcohol use, did not predict IPV among Latinxs and the strength of the association varied considerably within each health domain (Alvarez et al., 2017, 2018). The acculturation and alcohol use metaanalyses revealed that the strongest correlation was produced by studies that used the language proxy. The language proxy is a crude indicator of the extent to which an individual acculturates as it uses the language in which the survey was completed to designate a level of acculturation. Clearly, this is problematic because it is a limited and one-dimensional metric of the mechanism or the degree to which an individual has adopted the host culture and retained their heritage culture. Furthermore, the Cuellar (1980) scale produced the weakest correlation, which was not statistically significant. The findings in the alcohol use review produce serious questions regarding inconsistency but are heightened by the fact that the language proxies yielded a stronger and significant relationship. The acculturation and intimate partner violence review produced different findings. In this review, the Caetano (1987) scale produced the strongest relationship and the language proxy produced the weakest. The difference between these two correlations is large enough to warrant concern, given that these two measures are supposed to measure the same underlying concept and test an effect across similar samples and behaviors.

The highly inconsistent results across the two domains suggest that any particular measure of acculturation might be a poor predictor for a range of behaviors. This is consistent with the specificity hypothesis presented earlier.

Thus, we question if the measures are flawed, if the theories are flawed, or if it is simply unreasonable to expect broad measures of behavior (e.g., television watching preferences, social network choices) to predict specific forms of behavior. Furthermore, it is a call to think critically about acculturation measures and what they should predict. It may very well be the case that acculturation measures need to be domain specific, and researchers will need to analyze for important moderators to any particular effect. It may also be the case that researchers need to look beyond media consumption, for instance, and identify psychological variables that might predict the ability to adapt to new environments as the central goal of new acculturation measures.

Many of these scales have remained unchanged for decades (Wallace et al., 2010). Particularly, one can argue that the State's attitudes and behaviors toward immigrants in the 1980s and 1990s notably differed from the time this chapter was written, in 2019. Acculturation is more than one person simply adapting to a new environment. It is also how well that environment is accepting of the person attempting to acculturate. In fact, some measures of acculturation specifically include social network items in their scales. Yet, acculturation measures have not been modified or updated to account for societal turmoil that aggressively targets immigrants and, therefore, their adaptation process. While it is the case that assessing language of media consumption and social network composition are insightful given the current political context, current acculturation measures lack an evaluation of the impact negative social rhetoric can have on domain-specific acculturation. Assessing the interaction between context and acculturation can have important clinical and practical implications.

To apply or not to apply: Who acculturates and who does not?

Who should be included or excluded in an acculturation study? One theory is that children of ethnic groups born on US soil also experience a process of acculturation because of their blended identity as an American and ethnic minority. However, the theory of acculturation was developed to study how those who move from one place to another are affected by cultural change. Thus, moving is a key component of acculturation, and including ethnic minorities who have never had to migrate may contribute to weak associations in acculturation research. Nevertheless, many studies do not (or cannot) differentiate between those who are foreign born or native born (Du & Li, 2015; Lui & Zamboanga, 2018a). For example, Alvarez et al. (2017) found in their metaanalytic review, the specified sample was described as Latino or Hispanic, combining individuals from Latinx subgroups (Mexicans, Cubans, Guatemalans, Salvadorans, and Puerto Ricans). However, research has shown that group distinctions are often important. Grouping particular ethnic-group minorities together may result in misleading findings. For example and as stated earlier, acculturated Mexican women are more likely to smoke cigarettes than acculturated Puerto Rican and Cuban women. In fact, acculturation may not even play a role in smoking behavior for Cuban women (Kondo et al., 2016). In most cases, studies do not report specific effects for each subgroup; rather, the effect of acculturation on alcohol use was collapsed across all subgroups. This is problematic for the reasons mentioned above. In addition, the extent to which the acculturation process impacts first- and second-generation adults is unknown. Is the inclusion of first-, second-, third-generation minority groups appropriate in acculturation science? We argue that it is not. Studies that sample minority groups in the United States should focus on biculturalism models that investigate the possible interaction of two identities. This is because US born minorities are uniquely positioned, such that they have access to two or more cultural reference systems or cultural frame switching (Benet-Martínez, Leu, Lee, & Morris, 2002). Cultural frame switching occurs when an individual who is bicultural identifies with two cultures and alternates between two cultural interpretive frames in response to cues in the social environment, this by definition, is not acculturation.

A new lens: Cultural inertia

Cultural inertia makes specific predictions about the implications of acculturation. Cultural inertia is defined as resistance to cultural change unless the cultural change is already occurring (Zárate & Shaw, 2010; Zárate, Shaw, Marquez, & Biagas, 2012). The concept of cultural inertia parallels the understanding of inertia in physics: an object at rest remains at rest, and an object in motion remains in motion. Cultural inertia provides a new perspective to acculturation science by enhancing the understanding of the extent to which the cultural context and intergroup relations shape the immigrant experience. On the one hand, cultural inertia helps scientists understand the expectations and motivations of the majority culture. On the other, it provides a framework to understand how cultural and societal change impact the acculturative process among immigrants.

Immigrants often change to adapt to the host country's cultural norms. According to cultural inertia, immigrants cause the majority group to feel threatened because immigrants bring new cultural norms that might make the majority group change to adapt to those norms (Zárate et al., 2012). Stable or at rest groups resist movement. From the majority's perspective, immigrants who do not adopt the new culture threaten the stability of it. In a study, white Americans read an article and answered questions with differing endpoints that biased them to believe that mainstream American culture was changing or remaining stable because of an influx of immigrants (Quezada, Hitlan, Shenberger, & Zárate, 2011). The results indicated that white Americans experienced greater endorsement of antiimmigration legislation when biased to believe mainstream American culture was changing because of an influx of immigrants (Quezada et al., 2011). Furthermore, research has shown that when the majority group believes that immigrants will change the mainstream culture, they express greater realistic threat, greater symbolic threat, greater extinction threat, and anxiety for the future of their ingroup (Wohl, Branscombe, & Reysen, 2010). As a result, majority groups resist immigration if the mainstream culture is threatened and prefer assimilation processes because assimilation means other groups change and the host group remains constant (Wolsko, Park, & Judd, 2006).

Recently, cultural inertia has shifted to understand the immigrant perspective (Alvarez & Zárate, 2019). Immigrants tend to prefer multicultural approaches to cultural contact. This is because for immigrants retaining their heritage culture implies less change, whereas adopting a new culture requires more change. However, the reason for migration may be an important moderator in this relationship. Ogbu and Simons (1998) defined two particular immigrant groups, voluntary and involuntary. Voluntary immigrants include all foreign-born people who have moved to the United States as a product of their own desires or motivations. They are also often referred to as "economic seekers." Involuntary immigrants are also foreign-born people but migrated to the United States because they were displaced from their home country, feared persecution, moved due to deception or coercion, or because of a natural disaster. Verkuyten (2005) refers to voluntary and involuntary immigrants as those with the "personal choice" or "lack of choice" to migrate. Verkuyten (2004) suggests that majority members express sympathy toward involuntary immigrants and anger toward voluntary immigrants, which supports cultural inertia. When presented to the majority group, these classifications elicit distinct expectations for assimilation for the immigrant groups (Verkuyten, 2005). Conversely, cultural inertia poses that the reason for migration (voluntary or involuntary) elicits different outcomes in the degree to which the immigrant chooses to become incorporated into mainstream American culture.

It is also the case that groups in movement tend to continue in movement. Thus, for those voluntary immigrants, they choose to move and they initiated that movement—those migrants are a group in movement. Involuntary immigrants, however, did not initiate that movement, and they often hope to return to their native land. Cultural inertia constructs suggest, then, that voluntary immigrants are more likely to assimilate and acculturate to the new culture much quicker than involuntary immigrants. Current acculturation measures fail to address these motives that people might have for migrating.

Conclusion

The scientific community has used the theory of acculturation to understand a number of issues that immigrants face. Recently, research concerning the intersection of culture and health has used acculturation to explain health behaviors among ethnic minorities. While frequently used, acculturation measures typically generate weak correlations, and even those weak correlations are wildly inconsistent across domains. We assert that sampling and instrumental issues are contributing to these weak findings, and thus the theory of acculturation must be revisited and redefined.

Acculturation science is well-positioned to shift the course of multiple fields and enhance our general understanding of how migration shapes the individual and society. As the field moves forward, this chapter proposes important considerations for all future research studying immigration. First, it is important to have an in-depth understanding of samples. This goes beyond reporting demographic characteristics necessitating a deep dive into the psychological anchors and propellers that uniquely shape one's everyday experiences and subsequently behavior. In particular, we posit that the acculturation process is highly influenced by identity—mainstream and ethnic. Social psychological research provides strong evidence for this notion (Marcia, Waterman, Matteson, Archer, & Orlofsky, 1993). As such, it might be most beneficial to move forward by integrating both acculturation and identity research in innovative ways that provide both new theoretical paths and insightful practical implications. Second, we detail the extent to which variation in measurement has led to inconsistent findings within and between health domains, highlighting a need to reconceptualize current acculturation instruments. However, it is most important to ask if it is feasible to test the acculturation theory with only one instrument. We believe that is it not. This is because if we truly adopt a specificity approach coupled with the cultural inertia framework, acculturation theory becomes an entire mechanism, where researchers must test specific, varied components.

As globalization increases cultural contact among nations, acculturation science is the foundation to understand individual behavior and intergroup relations. It also serves as a springboard for a new way of immigration research that integrates social psychological processes to increase the affinity of the field's understanding of acculturation as a mechanism that shapes individuals and societies. Furthermore, the application of the cultural inertia model makes a viable contribution to the literature as it provides a novel framework to understand group interactions and individual differences with direct applicability to the real world. As the US' population grows, its demographics are becoming increasingly diverse. This demographic shift is shaping a new chapter in American history to the extent that demographic diversity is reaching every state of the nation. As the landscape of the American population continues to change, it is important for scientists to remain at the forefront of research that seeks to understand how these changes will impact everyone's future.

References

Alvarez, M. J., Frietze, G., Ramos, C., Field, C., & Zárate, M. A. (2017). A quantitative analysis of Latino acculturation and alcohol use: Myth versus reality. *Alcoholism: Clinical and Experimental Research*, *41*, 1246–1256.

Alvarez, M. J., Oviedo Ramirez, S., Frietze, G., Field, C., & Zárate, M. A. (2018). A meta-analysis of Latinx acculturation and intimate partner violence. *Trauma, Violence & Abuse*, *41*, 1246–1256.

Alvarez, M. J., & Zárate, M. A. (2019). *Understanding immigration: A look into migrants' attitudes*. [Unpublished raw data].

Benet-Martínez, V., & Haritatos, J. (2005). Bicultural identity integration (BII): Components and psychosocial antecedents. *Journal of Personality, 73*, 1015–1050.

Benet-Martínez, V., Leu, J., Lee, F., & Morris, M. (2002). Negotiating biculturalism: Cultural frame switching in biculturals with oppositional versus compatible cultural identities. *Journal of Cross-Cultural Psychology, 33*, 492–516.

Berry, J. W. (1980a). Acculturation as varieties of adaptation. In A. Padilla (Ed.), *Acculturation: Theory, models and some new findings*. Boulder: Westview Press.

Berry, J. W. (1980b). Social and cultural change. In H. C. Triandis & R. Brislin (Eds.), *Handbook of cross-cultural psychology*. Boston: Allyn & Bacon.

Berry, J. W. (1984). Cultural relations in plural societies: Alternatives to segregation and their sociopsycological implications. In N. Miller & M. B. Brewer (Eds.), *Groups in contact: The psychology of desegregation* (pp. 11–27). New York: Academic Press.

Berry, J. W. (2006). Mutual attitudes among immigrants and ethnocultural groups in Canada. *International Journal of Intercultural Relations, 30*, 719–734.

Birman, D. (1994). Acculturation and human diversity in a multicultural society. In E. J. Trickett, R. J. Watts, & D. Birman (Eds.), *Human diversity: Perspective on people in context* (pp. 261–284). San Francisco: Jossey-Bass.

Bornstein, M. H. (Ed.), (2010). *Handbook of cultural developmental science*. New York: Psychology Press.

Bornstein, M. H. (2017). The specificity principle in acculturation science. *Perspectives on Psychological Science, 12*, 3–45.

Cabrera, N. J., Shannon, J. D., West, J., & Brooks-Gunn, J. (2006). Parental interactions with Latino infants: Variation by country of origin and English proficiency. *Child Development, 77*, 1190–1207.

Caetano, R. (1987). Acculturation and drinking patterns among US Hispanics. *British Journal of Addiction, 82*, 789–799.

Caligiuri, P. M. (2000). Selecting expatriates for personality characteristics: A moderating effect of personality on the relationship between host national contact and cross-cultural adjustment. *MIR: Management International Review, 40*, 61–80.

Carhill, A., Suárez-Orozco, C., & Páez, M. (2008). Explaining English language proficiency among adolescent immigrant students. *American Educational Research Journal, 45*, 1155–1179.

Center for Disease Control and Prevention. (2018, February 18). *Current cigarette smoking among adults in the United States* Retrieved from: https://www.cdc.gov/tobacco/data_statistics/fact_sheets/adult_data/cig_smoking/index.htm.

Choi, S., Rankin, S., Stewart, A., & Oka, R. (2008). Effects of acculturation on smoking behavior in Asian Americans: A meta-analysis. *Journal of Cardiovascular Nursing, 23*, 67–73.

Coatsworth, J. D., Maldonado-Molina, M., Pantin, H., & Szapocznik, J. (2005). A person-centered and ecological investigation of acculturation strategies in Hispanic immigrant youth. *Journal of Community Psychology, 33*, 157–174.

Conger, R. D., & Donnellan, M. B. (2007). An interactionist perspective on the socioeconomic context of human development. *Annual Review of Psychology, 58*, 175–199.

Cuellar, I. (1980). An acculturation scale for Mexican American normal and clinical populations. *Hispanic Journal of Behavioral Sciences, 2*, 199–217.

Cuellar, I., Arnold, B., & Maldonado, R. (1995). Acculturation rating scale for Mexican Americans-II: A revision of the original ARSMA scale. *Hispanic Journal of Behavioral Sciences, 17*, 275–304.

Del Pilar, J. P., & Udasco, J. O. (2004). Deculturation: Its lack of validity. *Cultural Diversity & Ethnic Minority Psychology, 10*, 169–176.

Du, H., & Li, X. (2015). Acculturation and HIV-related sexual behaviours among international migrants: A systemic review and meta-analysis. *Health Psychology Review*, *9*, 103–122.

Florida, R. (2004). America's looming creativity crisis. *Harvard Business Review*. Retrieved from https://hbr.org/2004/10/americas-looming-creativity-crisis.

Giang, M. T., & Wittig, M. A. (2006). Implications of adolescents' acculturation strategies for personal and collective self-esteem. *Cultural Diversity and Ethnic Minority Psychology*, *12*, 725.

Gordon, M. M. (1964). *Assimilation in American life: The role of race, religion, and national origins*. New York: Oxford University Press on Demand.

Gupta, A., Leong, F., Valentine, J. C., & Canada, D. D. (2013). A meta-analytic study: The relationship between acculturation and depression among Asian Americans. *American Journal of Orthopsychiatry*, *83*(2), 372–385.

Halloran, M. J., & Kashima, E. (2006). Culture, social identity, and the individual. In T. Postmes & J. Jetten (Eds.), *Individuality and the group: Advances in social identity*. London: Sage.

Jia, G., & Aaronson, D. (2003). A longitudinal study of Chinese children and adolescents learning English in the United States. *Applied PsychoLinguistics*, *24*, 131–161.

Joint Economic Committee. (2016). *The 2016 joint economic report*. Washington: U.S. Government printing office.

Kondo, K. K., Rossi, J. S., Schwartz, S. J., Zamboanga, B. L., & Scalf, C. D. (2016). Acculturation and cigarette smoking in Hispanic women: A meta-analysis. *Journal of Ethnicity in Substance Abuse*, *15*, 46–72.

Kosic, A. (2002). Acculturation attitudes, need for cognitive closure, and adaptation of immigrants. *The Journal of Social Psychology*, *142*, 179–201.

Kovelman, I., Baker, S. A., & Petitto, L. A. (2008). Bilingual and monolingual brains compared: A functional magnetic resonance imaging investigation of syntactic processing and a possible "neural signature" of bilingualism. *Journal of Cognitive Neuroscience*, *20*, 153–169.

LaFromboise, T., Coleman, H. L., & Gerton, J. (1993). Psychological impact of biculturalism: Evidence and theory. *Psychological Bulletin*, *114*, 395–412.

Lam, C. (2016). Asians remain fastest-growing U.S. group as pacific islanders, mixed-race numbers grow: Census. *NBC News*, (June 23). Retrieved from https://www.nbcnews.com/news/asian-america/asians-remain-fastest-growing-us-group-pacific-islanders-mixed-race-n597711.

Lara, M., Gamboa, C., Kahramanian, M. I., Morales, L. S., & Hayes Bautista, D. E. (2005). Acculturation and Latino health in the United States: A review of the literature and its sociopolitical context. *Annual Review of Public Health*, *26*, 367–397.

Lee, R. M. (2005). Resilience against discrimination: ethnic identity and other-group orientation as protective factors for Korean Americans. *Journal of Counseling Psychology*, *52*(1), 36.

Lui, P. P., & Zamboanga, B. L. (2018a). A critical review and meta-analysis of the associations between acculturation and alcohol use outcomes among Hispanic Americans. *Alcoholism: Clinical and Experimental Research*, *42*, 1841–1862.

Lui, P. P., & Zamboanga, B. L. (2018b). Acculturation and alcohol use among Asian Americans: A meta-analytic review. *Psychology of Addictive Behaviors*, *32*, 173–186.

Marcia, J. E., Waterman, A. S., Matteson, D. R., Archer, S. L., & Orlofsky, J. L. (1993). *Ego identity: A handbook for psychosocial research*. New York: Springer.

Masten, W. G., Penland, E. A., & Nayani, E. J. (1994). Depression and acculturation in Mexican-American women. *Psychological Reports*, *75*, 1499–1503.

McCann, A. (2019). Economic impact of immigration by state. *Wallethub*, (January 29). Retrieved from https://wallethub.com/edu/economic-impact-of-immigration-by-state/32248/.

Mendenhall, M., & Oddou, G. (1985). The dimensions of expatriate acculturation: A review. *Academy of Management Review*, *10*, 39–47.

Mendoza, F. S., Javier, J. R., & Burgos, A. E. (2007). Health of children in immigrant families. In J. E. Lansford, K. Deater-Deckard, & M. H. Bornstein (Eds.), *Immigrant families in contemporary society*. New York: Guilford Press.

New American Economy. (2017). *How Hispanics contribute to the U.S. economy*. New American Economy. Retrieved from http://research.newamericaneconomy.org/wp-content/uploads/sites/2/2017/12/Hispanic_V5.pdf.

Oetzel, J., De Vargas, F., Ginossar, T., & Sanchez, C. (2007). Hispanic women's preferences for breast health information: Subjective cultural influences on source, message, and channel. *Health Communication*, *21*, 223–233.

Ogbu, J. U., & Simons, H. D. (1998). Voluntary and involuntary minorities: A cultural-ecological theory of school performance with some implications for education. *Anthropology & Education Quarterly*, *29*, 155–188.

Outten, H. R., Schmitt, M. T., Garcia, D. M., & Branscombe, N. R. (2009). Coping options: Missing links between minority group identification and psychological well-being. *Applied Psychology*, *58*, 146–170.

Overton, W. F. (2015). Process and relational developmental systems. In W. F. Overton & P. C. Molenaar (Eds.), *Handbook of child psychology and developmental science*. Hoboken, NJ: Wiley.

Padilla, A. M. (1980). *Acculturation: Theory, models, and some new findings*. Boulder, CO: Westview.

Pérez-Escamilla, R., & Putnik, P. (2007). The role of acculturation in nutrition, lifestyle, and incidence of type 2 diabetes among Latinos. *The Journal of Nutrition*, *137*, 860–870.

Phinney, J. S. (2006). Acculturation is not an independent variable: Approaches to studying acculturation as a complex process. In M. H. Bornstein & M. H. L. Cote (Eds.), *Acculturation and parent child relationships. Measurement and development* (pp. 79–95). Mahwah, NJ: Erlbaum.

Phinney, J., & Devich-Navarro, M. (1997). Variations in bicultural identification among African American and Mexican American adolescents. *Journal of Research on Adolescence*, *7*, 3–32.

Pokhrel, P., Herzog, T. A., Sun, P., Rohrbach, L. A., & Sussman, S. (2013). Acculturation, social self-control, and substance use among Hispanic adolescents. *Psychology of Addictive Behaviors*, *27*, 674.

Portes, A., & Rumbaut, R. G. (2006). *Immigrant America: A portrait*. University of California Press.

Quezada, S. A., Hitlan, R., Shenberger, J., & Zárate, M. A. (2011). *Reactions to immigration in the United States*. . [Unpublished raw data].

Quezada, S. A., Shaw, M. P., & Zárate, M. A. (2012). The relationship between ethnic identity and reactions to cultural change. *Social Psychology*, *43*, 243–251.

Ramirez, M. (1984). Assessing and understanding biculturalism-multiculturalism in Mexican-American adults. In J. Martinez & R. Mendoza (Eds.), *Chicano psychology* (pp. 77–94). Orlando, FL: Academic.

Redfield, R., Linton, R., & Herskovits, M. (1936). Memorandum on the study of acculturation. *American Anthropologist*, *38*, 149–152.

Rudmin, F. W. (2003). Critical history of the acculturation psychology of assimilation, separation, integration, and marginalization. *Review of General Psychology*, *7*, 3–37.

Ryder, A., Alden, L., & Paulhus, D. (2000). Is acculturation unidimensional or bidimensional? A head-to-head comparison in the prediction of personality, self-identity, and adjustment. *Journal of Personality and Social Psychology*, *79*, 49–65.

Schildkraut, D. J. (2007). Defining American identity in the twenty-first century: How much "there" is there? *The Journal of Politics*, *69*(3), 597–615.

Schwartz, S. J., Montgomery, M. J., & Briones, E. (2006). The role of identity in acculturation among immigrant people: Theoretical propositions, empirical questions, and applied recommendations. *Human Development*, *49*, 1–30.

Shore, B. (2002). Taking culture seriously. *Human Development, 45*, 226–228.

Shuval, J. T. (1982). Migration and stress. In L. Goldberger & S. Breznitz (Eds.), *Handbook of stress: Theoretical and clinical aspects*. New York: Free Press.

Statistical Atlas. (2015, April 28). *Race and ethnicity in the United States*. Retrieved from https://statisticalatlas.com/United-States/Race-and-Ethnicity.

Sun, S., Hoyt, W. T., Brockber, D., Lam, J., & Tiwari, D. (2016). Acculturation and enculturation as predictors of psychological Help-Seeking Attitudes (HSAs) among racial and ethnic minorities: A meta-analytic investigation. *Journal of Counseling Psychology, 63*, 617–632.

Tajfel, H. E. (1978). *Differentiation between social groups: Studies in the social psychology of intergroup relations*. London: Academic Press.

Tajfel, H., & Turner, J. C. (1985). The social identity theory of intergroup behavior. In S. Worchel & W. G. Austin (Eds.), *Psychology of intergroup relations*. (2nd ed., pp. 7–24). Chicago: Nelson-Hall.

Tamis-LeMonda, C. S., Sze, I. N. L., Ng, F. F. Y., Kahana-Kalman, R., & Yoshikawa, H. (2013). Maternal teaching during play with four-year-olds: Variation by ethnicity and family resources. *Merrill-Palmer Quarterly, 59*, 361–398.

Triandis, H. C. (1995). *Individualism and collectivism*. Boulder, CO: Westview Press.

Turner, J. (1987). *Rediscovering the social group: A self-categorization theory*. Oxford: Blackwell.

U.S. Census Bureau. (2012). *Projections of the population by sex, race, and Hispanic origin for the United States: 2015 to 2060*. Retrieved from http://www.census.gov/population/projections/data/national/2012/summarytables.html.

Umaña-Taylor, A. J., & Updegraff, K. A. (2007). Latino adolescents' mental health: Exploring the interrelations among discrimination, ethnic identity, cultural orientation, self-esteem, and depressive symptoms. *Journal of Adolescence, 30*, 549–567.

Valentine, S. (2001). Self-esteem, cultural identity, and generation status as determinants of Hispanic acculturation. *Hispanic Journal of Behavioral Sciences, 23*, 459–468.

Verkuyten, M. (2004). Emotional reactions to and support for immigrant policies: Attributed responsibilities to categories of asylum seekers. *Social Justice Research, 17*, 293–314.

Verkuyten, M. (2005). Immigration discourses and their impact on multiculturalism: A discursive and experimental study. *British Journal of Social Psychology, 44*, 223–240.

Wallace, P. M., Pomery, E. A., Latimer, A. E., Martinez, J. L., & Salovey, P. (2010). A review of acculturation measures and their utility in studies promoting Latino health. *Hispanic Journal of Behavioral Sciences, 32*, 37–54.

Wohl, M. J., Branscombe, N. R., & Reysen, S. (2010). Perceiving your group's future to be in jeopardy: Extinction threat induces collective angst and the desire to strengthen the ingroup. *Personality and Social Psychology Bulletin, 36*, 898–910.

Wolsko, C., Park, B., & Judd, C. M. (2006). Considering the tower of babel: Correlates of assimilation and multiculturalism among ethnic minority and majority groups in the United States. *Social Justice Research, 19*, 277–306.

Yoon, E., Chang, C., Kim, S., Clawson, A., Cleary, E., Hansen, M., et al. (2013). A meta-analysis of acculturation/enculturation and mental health. *Journal of Counseling Psychology, 60*, 15–30.

Yoon, E., Langrehr, K., & Ong, L. Z. (2011). Content analysis of acculturation research in counseling and counseling psychology: A 22-year review. *Journal of Counseling Psychology, 58*, 83.

Zárate, M. A., Reyna, C., & Alvarez, M. J. (2019). Cultural inertia, identity, and intergroup dynamics in a changing context. *Advances in Experimental Social Psychology, 59*, 175–204.

Zárate, M. A., & Shaw, M. P. (2010). The role of cultural inertia in reactions to immigration on the US/Mexico border. *Journal of Social Issues, 66*, 45–57.

Zárate, M. A., Shaw, M., Marquez, J., & Biagas, D. (2012). Cultural inertia: The effects of cultural change on intergroup relations and the self-concept. *Journal of Experimental Social Psychology*, *48*, 634–645.

Further reading

Berry, J. W. (1997). Immigration, acculturation, and adaptation. *Applied Psychology An International Review*, *46*, 5–68.

Section B

Mental health

Chapter 5

A gendered look at work-family conflict among diverse US immigrants

Lizette Ojeda, Cristal Lopez and Abigail Sharer
Texas A&M University, College Station, TX, United States

Work is a central activity that holds a fundamental role in an individual's life as it ensures a means of survival via wages, social connectedness, and self-determination (Blustein, Kenny, Di Fabio, & Guichard, 2019). While traditional US culture is individualistic, with an individual expected to care for themselves and is seen as responsible for their path in life, many immigrants come from communities that are collectivistic in which they value the greater good over individual needs and do not see caring for others as unwarranted. This core cultural difference between individualistic US work culture and collectivistic immigrant communities, along with the gendered expression of work and family roles, has the potential to cause conflict with work and family domains.

The traditional US corporate culture is distinct from that of the rest of the world. It has a reputation of adhering to the "good ol' boys" network, and the "pull yourself up by the bootstraps" mentality. There is a strong individualistic message that calls for "each man for his own," which conflicts with the more collectivistic orientation of African, Asian, and Latino immigrants. There is a hidden undertone that at the end of the day, it is not what you know or who you know, but rather who knows you *and* what they know about you, that determines career success. This calls for immigrants to engage in self-promotion and networking strategies that might go against their cultural values of unity and based on a Japanese proverb, not be "the nail that stands out." This is further complicated by gender role expectations in an immigrant's culture that might call for women to be self-sacrificing, nurturing, and meek (Chuang & Tamis-LeMonda, 2013).

Unspoken approaches to work in the US can make it difficult for immigrants to integrate themselves into the US work culture on top of navigating a host of issues that come with the immigrant experience, such as the immigration process in and of itself, acculturative stress, and family separation issues

Mental and Behavioral Health of Immigrants in the United States
https://doi.org/10.1016/B978-0-12-816117-3.00005-1

(Balidemaj & Small, 2019). As such, the purpose of this chapter is to shed light on the challenges that African, Asian, and Latino US immigrants face as they navigate demands between work and family through a gendered cultural lens.

Immigrants at work in the US

In 2018, the total US workforce was comprised of 17.4% immigrants, with 47.7% comprised of Latino, 25% Asian, and 9.5% Black immigrants (US Bureau of Labor Statistics, 2019). Immigrant men (77.9%) were more likely to be employed than US-born men (67.3%), whereas immigrant women (54.3%) were somewhat less likely to work outside the home than US-born women (57.6%). A greater gap exists when women have children under the age of 18, with immigrant mothers (61%) being less likely to work outside the home than US-born mothers (74%). In regards to employment settings, immigrants were more likely than US-born workers to work in service occupations (23.3% vs 15.9%) and less likely to work in management, professional, and related occupations (32.7% vs 41.6%). Wage gaps exist for immigrants and even more so by gender. Immigrant men earned 80.9% of what US-born men were paid while the gap for immigrant women is slightly lower at 83.7% of their US-born female counterparts' earnings. Interestingly, Latino immigrants made 83.8% of what US-born Latinos earned, while non-Hispanic Black immigrants earned about the same as Black Americans at 100.3%, whereas Asian immigrants earned more than Asian Americans at 106%. When education levels were at or above a bachelor's degree, immigrants made 104% of what US-born college-educated workers earned.

In light of these statistics, it is not uncommon for immigrants to be stereotyped as overwhelmingly occupying labor-intensive, under-the-table pay types of jobs. However, immigrants do hold space in corporate America though they are often confined to entry-level jobs, making their presence and influence rare at the executive leadership level (US Bureau of Labor Statistics, 2019). Whether engaged in blue-collar or white-collar work, immigrants experience several challenges that vary based on factors such as work authorization, educational background, and English-language proficiency.

Work authorization

Many immigrants venture to the US in search of improved livelihood for themselves and their family and/or better work opportunities (Bautista, Bressler, & Bosworth, 2019). Varying constraints placed by their authorization to work in the US can lead to stress about job security and financial stability (Held, Cuellar, & Cook Heffron, 2018). For instance, holding an undocumented status poses a different set of challenges in the workforce than for documented immigrants, leading to a sense of having less certainty about their future on a regular day-to-day basis. For instance, even the threat of ICE raiding their employment sites may be sufficient to cause serious distress (Hamann & Reeves, 2012). Undocumented immigrants still have some protections in the US such as health and safety standards, prohibition of sexual harassment, and limited wage/hour protections (Cook, Gleeson, Griffith, & Kahn, 2018) though they may not be aware of the full extent of their rights.

Although immigrants with a valid visa do not have the same stressors of nonauthorized workers when it comes to documented immigration issues, if one's company sponsored their visa, this may be enough for the individual to feel indebted to their workplace. They may believe that it is because of their employer that they are able to work toward the proverbial "American Dream." Some immigrant groups may be more inclined to experience this due to cultural norms. For example, the traditional Asian cultural value of filial piety may foster a sense of loyalty or indebtedness when helped to succeed (Bedford & Yeh, 2019). Further, immigrant women may be less likely to speak up and assert themselves at work if doing so violates gender role expectations. Together, cultural norms can foster the coercion that immigrants may feel as they seek to remain loyal to their employers and have more tolerance toward excessive job expectations or work-related stress that affects their family life.

Gaps in achievement, opportunity, and pay

Education levels among immigrants and the perceived level of prestige of education obtained can impact the way their skill value is assessed by colleagues. Overall, educational attainment among US immigrants is low (US Bureau of Labor Statistics, 2019). Nonetheless, college-educated immigrants are still more likely to have lower wages if higher education was obtained through a non-Western institution (Lancee & Bol, 2017). Further, immigrants may face the issue of nontransferable skills if they have certain standardized licensing or skills in their country of origin that are not recognized in the US. Aside from missed job opportunities and a hit to one's career advancement, denial of skills or credentials can compromise self-esteem and self-efficacy (Titzmann & Jugert, 2017). Mental health can take a further hit with the compounding effects of other variables such as acculturative stress, documentation status, language barriers, and education. These consequences may then start a ripple effect that can impact more than just the individual but the workplace as a whole. For example, an individual with lower self-efficacy may be more inclined to remain silent in work meetings in which their expertise can be utilized. They may feel devalued and begin to view their skillset or credentials as subpar. They may even need to complete further certification requirements to qualify for certain roles, requiring them to test their knowledge through unfamiliar US testing standards. Should they be unable to successfully demonstrate competence during the credentialing process, the companies miss out on the opportunity of having diverse cultural skills and ideas and in turn society as a whole is also deprived of these skills.

The achievement gap in terms of education level and opportunity gap based on underuse of transferable skills can contribute to the pay gap for immigrants and even more so for foreign-born women (US Bureau of Labor Statistics, 2019). The Institute for Women's Policy Research (2018) stated that females of all racial and ethnic groups earned less than white males. Latinos had the lowest wages compared to their Black, White, and Asian peers. Furthermore, Latinas had the lowest earned wages and Asian men had the highest. The financial hardships and burden that some immigrants have to financially support families in their country of origin may add significant stress.

Linguistics

Linguistic barriers may require immigrants to put in additional effort into work-related duties if they are concerned about their English language comprehension skills, which in turn can create more workplace stress. Language barriers may also pose misunderstandings between employees. For example, individuals from different cultures have certain proverbs that may not translate into a different language well. This may trigger anxiety for the individual if they have to "read between the lines" and remain hyperalert to cross-cultural exchanges. Other components of linguistics that are associated with proverbs may be an interpretation of humor, which can be perceived differently or as inappropriate in the workplace (Robert, 2017). Further, immigrants with a strong accent may be vulnerable to stereotype threat, which can negatively impact well-being by creating additional stress (Thoman, Smith, Brown, Chase, & Lee, 2013). It is not uncommon for immigrants with "ethnic-sounding" names that are perceived as difficult to pronounce to change their name altogether into a common English-sounding name to help them fit in (Zhao & Biernat, 2019). Fear of mispronouncing technical terms or not being familiar with a term at all in English may hold immigrants back from facing possible embarrassment among their colleagues.

Cultural considerations for diverse immigrants

Many immigrate to the US in search of upward mobility but find themselves at the bottom of a corporate chasm, their education and skills disregarded if not earned from US or western schools. This can particularly threaten masculinity through having to accept a low-paying job to keep a family afloat, not maintaining previous prestige, needing additional training, or even having one's abilities questioned. In fact, many countries also have entrenched values that define gender roles, with an overall theme that women are held to a specific dominant narrative of being caretakers, in some cases being forced to forego an education to birth and care for children at relatively young ages. Family overall is of exceptional importance; collectivistic values center the identity of groups over individuals, especially in families as ancestors pass down traditions, rituals, and customs held sacred for decades (Taras et al., 2014).

Immigrants not only may experience difficulty fitting into the workplace culture but also with their US-born counterparts. They might feel pressure to integrate the norms, customs, behaviors, and mannerisms of their US-born counterparts. For instance, the experience of African immigrants and African Americans in the US is completely different but similar physical features might cause people to put them into the same cultural box. There may also be internalized antiimmigrant sentiments from the US-born ethnic minorities toward their immigrant counterparts. They may feel threatened by their success and internalize the "they are taking our jobs" mentality. For immigrant workers with limited social or familial support, to not be accepted by their US-born counterparts would make it more difficult to integrate themselves at work and have a sense of belonging.

It bears mentioning that lumping together dozens of countries under the shared moniker of "immigrant" is problematic. For instance, Africa is a continent, not a country, in which within-group differences are greater than those between groups, such as differences in religion/spiritual beliefs, language, and colonization. As countries that have been overwhelmingly subject to western influences and ideals, trying to define an entire continent in broad brushstrokes is reminiscent of a colonist mentality. With that said, it is beyond the scope of this chapter to go in-depth on the wide diversity that exists among collectivistic immigrant groups. To that end, certain important considerations are discussed as they relate to or are traditionally central to the lives of immigrants from Africa, Asia, and Latin America.

African immigrants

Some countries in Africa have named English as an official language (e.g., South Africa, Zambia, and Kenya) and other countries have French, Portuguese, or Arabic as their official tongues. While slavery was rampant in many African countries, particularly on the west coast, not all countries faced the same cruelty; some nations like Uganda were largely self-ruled while others like Kenya were British colonies (Kamya, 2005). Unfortunately, historical and ongoing combat, even genocide, are reasons why some Africans immigrate to the US, often suffer from posttraumatic stress and other lasting generational traumas. Even African immigrants coming to the US today may seek out African American neighborhoods, and communities, only to discover the depths of segregation lurking in the shadows of a supposedly more conscious country. With a lack of experience with systematic and structural racism that is perpetuated in the US, both consciously and unconsciously, Africans can find themselves at odds with the US population at large, including African Americans, with whom they may not share many experiences.

Asian immigrants

Much like the African continent, the Asian community is more diverse than is often credited. Asia includes countries like China, India, much of the Middle

East, and many islands like the Philippines, Sri Lanka, and Papua New Guinea. Living a life in accordance with filial piety, which one "saves face," makes one a good child, a good subject, and good in whatever role one takes on—including the role at work (Bedford & Yeh, 2019). Individual accomplishments may help one gain notoriety, but the most important thing for an individual to maintain is their face, or how others see the individual in the context of their family. Conflicts can arise between an individual and their family if they want to pursue occupations that are not stereotypically well-regarded or those that are not traditionally "for" their gender. Further, Chinese men have reported more work-family conflict than Chinese women, attributed to men chasing success and security as their wives sought to keep the family stable and supported (Yang, Liu, Liu, Zhang, & Duan, 2017). Filial piety motivates people to be respectful of family hierarchy and duties in the private sphere, and loyal to the ruler, peaceful, industrious in the public sphere. A child who has learnt to be filial through proper upbringing (or, one may say, through indoctrination), must "glorify" his parents; therefore, he must be a virtuous and successful member of society. These high expectations can contribute to the "model minority myth," which is the stereotype that Asians are good at math and science (Leong & Tang, 2016). This perception may contribute to higher pay for people of Asian descent but it comes with added pressure to perform and maintain a "saved face."

Latino/a/x immigrants

A collectivistic value known as "allocentrism" calls for individuals to focus more on their group or others around them than on themselves, bears similarities to the aforementioned importance placed by both African and Asian cultures on the family and collectivistic values. *Familismo* is another value of utmost importance in Latinx culture. The term denotes a strong emphasis on one's entire family and on belonging, no matter how extended they may be, and even includes those close to a family who are not biologically related. Other central values include hierarchies (jerarquísmo), respect toward elders and authority (respeto), belief that what happens to them was intended to happen (fatalismo), politeness (personalismo), and kindness (simpatía) even in the face of stress (Castillo & Cano, 2007). Embedded within Latinx culture are the notions of machismo, the traditional male gender role defined by aggressive self-reliance, but this limited view of Latino masculinity can serve to pathologize them. In fact, Latino male roles also include a more positive side known as *caballerismo*, which includes chivalry and working for the greater good (Ojeda & Organista, 2015). The traditional female role known as *marianismo* calls for women to emulate the Virgin Mary, be pure, and self-sacrificing (Castillo & Cano, 2007).

The work-family interface among diverse US immigrants

More often than not, the hierarchical structure of many corporate organizations has a White able-bodied cisgender heterosexual man at the top, with true diversity being found at lower ranks. In fact, children as young as 3 years old already have gender-specific ideas on what professions are available to them, ideas that are only reinforced and strengthened as they learn and grow into adulthood and experience the workplace.

Storti (1999) proposes four broad and dynamic "building blocks" of culture that can help to explain cross-cultural work-family conflict: (a) individualistic or collectivistic self-concept, (b) universalistic or particularistic societal responsibility, (c) monochronic or polychronic time orientation, and (d) internal or external locus of control. An understanding of various worldviews can aid both employees and employers by offering a better understanding of where individuals of different identities and backgrounds may fall on the same construct. This can help reduce miscommunication, misunderstandings, and frustration when trying to work together as people who come from different worldviews. For instance, the US as an individualistic culture may conflict with the more collectivistic worldview of immigrants, in which they see themselves as *part* of something (e.g., company and family) rather than separate from it. Such views can impact how they carry out this value and how it is perceived by employers. Further, the US is primarily a universalistic culture in which it is expected that everyone should follow the same rules and regulations. Such rigidness can make it difficult for immigrant workers to follow the same expectations at work if they have restrictions imposed on them as workers or also have to navigate responsibilities back home. This can cause a misperception of the immigrant worker as nonabiding to company policies or asking for special considerations.

Time in the US is traditionally monochronic and is seen as limited, a resource so scarce the world seems to move at a frightening speed. It is seen as disrespectful and inconsiderate to be late or to go past the expected time reserved for meetings. For an individual from Latin America, time is polychronic, meaning time is much less scarce; it is normal for folks to arrive late if it is due to wrapping up a prior matter that took longer than anticipated. In fact, it may be perceived as rude to cut someone off even if it means running late for their next meeting. In contrast, corporate culture values efficiency and timeliness over relationships. Culture and corporate America are like oil and water—it is rare in the business world for anyone, regardless of the identities they may hold, to arrive late to a meeting, to dress in colorful clothing, even to not tout their own accomplishments as they seek to climb higher in their organization's hierarchy. The degree to which immigrant employees learn about and successfully navigate these often unwritten rules has a great impact on their experience at work—and how well they are able to do their job.

It is difficult to try to separate the demands of one's professional and personal life in a clear cut way. This is especially difficult when the personal expands into the familial in which an individual is responsible for others in their personal life as caregivers for young children, aging parents, or ill partners. With modernization, women's movement, and increased cost of living, gone are the days when women stay at home while men work as the sole breadwinner. Unlike in the US, many collectivistic countries, do not expect women to work outside the home, where in the US it is oftentimes an economic necessity. This has implications for the adjustment of immigrants of color to the US work-life culture and has the potential to cause confusion about norms, conflict with values, and various work-life-family stressors that can negatively affect their well-being as workers, family caregivers, and human beings as a whole.

Work-family conflict

With the advancement of technology, it has become easier to expect people to be more easily accessible, readily available, and quickly responsive to work-related matters outside the ever-expanding 9-to-5 traditional work hours, and late-night requests, it becomes difficult to keep work at work. It leaves little time to be present for quality family activities let alone personal time to unwind from the day's labor.

Within the family, members may feel obliged to support relatives still in their home country, placing an even greater financial burden on their shoulders. These same relatives may have misconceptions that their family in the US has accrued great wealth and ask them for resources or even to help them visit or immigrate themselves. Many East Asian cultures see caring for one's parents as they age as nonnegotiable, a means of returning the care provided when they were young, a feat more readily accomplished by those who are successful and have the financial capital to do so. Among Latinos, it is not uncommon for greetings to include inquiries about one's family, not just the individual they are interacting with. For example, one might ask "How is your family?" instead of just "How are you?" This cultural difference in social etic can lead to misinterpretations about the interaction in which a Latino immigrant might perceive not being asked about their family as "cold" or "uncaring," whereas the person interacting with them might perceive the same inquiry as "intrusive."

Work-family stress

There are three categories of stress related to work and family conflict: time-, strain-, and behavior-conflict (Shockley, Shen, DeNunzio, Arvan, & Knudsen, 2017). Time-based conflict occurs when the amount of time one spends in one domain affects the time spent in the other, for example, missing bedtime due to having to spend more time at the office to complete projects. This could also result in having to take time off from work to attend to a child's needs such as school events and sickness, as well as visit family overseas. Strain-based conflict occurs when one's internal resources are exhausted and therefore affect the other domain. This could result in decreased tolerance for people's mistakes and irritability with family or coworkers. Behavior-based conflict occurs when the actions one takes in one role negatively affect that of the other domain. For instance, if one is expected by the family to travel to their home country whenever there is a special family event, they might need to decrease the physical presence they have at work, which might cause their employer to question their work ethic or dedication to the company. In examining gender differences, men are more likely to resent work than women, whereas women are more likely to experience family task-related stressors than men. Furthermore, men tend to report more work resentments than women.

When positive or negative experiences in one role spillover and affect that of the other role, spillover has occurred (Westman, 2006). It can include the level of satisfaction or dissatisfaction experienced with either the work or life domain. For instance, the experience of fatigue due to overwhelming home responsibilities, such as caretaking needs, or family matters overseas can bring on fatigue at work and potentially result in increased chances of making mistakes when energy reserves have been depleted. It can also cause decreased engagement if one is too tired to get involved above and beyond managing their task at hand. All of this can affect their overall work performance. On the positive side, if a worker experiences a sense of belonging within the company, it may help compensate for homesickness because they are getting their needs for community met at work. This, in turn, increases engagement at work because they feel welcomed and valued as a contributor to the greater good of the company. It is easier for men than women to compartmentalize thoughts, feelings, and behaviors between work and home, which could help protect against negative spillover. However, if experiences are at an extreme, they may still spillover to the other domain (Kinnunen, Feldt, Mauno, & Rantanen, 2010). To further light flame to the fire, the crossover can occur in which the stress experienced by one individual crosses over onto another, such as a spouse, child, or coworker. As can be imagined, spillover and crossover if not handled appropriately have the potential to affect an entire company and family system.

Research on parent-child attachment among children who attend childcare vs home family care is mixed (Shirvanian & Michael, 2017). Nonetheless, in the US, it is not typical to be raised at home by several family members who are available as is more so the case in other countries. As such, immigrants may experience mistrust in having a stranger care for their child, making it difficult for immigrant parents to choose between career and their kids, or they may have difficulty focusing at work if they are preoccupied over their child's safety while in the hands of nonfamily members.

When it comes to reuniting with family back home, overseas vacations and family emergencies are restricted with the typical 2-week vacation allotted, especially when long-distance travel time and jet lag cut into the time off. Furthermore, immigrants may have to choose between reserving their limited vacation days for potential family emergencies and taking a chance of actually enjoying a vacation for the purpose it is supposed to serve.

Society still expects women to be primary caregivers. This assumption can have an impact on a mother's earning potential and professional advancement and being perceived as less committed to their career and therefore the company (Halbesleben, Harvey, & Bolino, 2009). Women are more likely to carry the responsibility of handling daytime caregiving needs, such as taking off from work on short notice when a family member falls sick. Handle health-care appointments during working hours. Women spend significantly more time engaging in family-related activities than men. At the end of the day, research shows that family boundaries are more likely to be violated than work boundaries, in that workers are less likely to intentionally allow family demands to interfere with work (Shockley et al., 2017).

Coping with work-family conflict

It is virtually impossible to attain the proverbial "best of both worlds" in an equally balanced way as a working parent in the fast-paced pull yourself up by your own bootstraps US corporate culture. Being stretched in either direction often leaves working parents feeling like they have to sacrifice one for the other. They can experience relationship issues at work and at home when members on either side complain about being undervalued or not considered. They may question the individual's commitment to the company or family, often leaving the individual to put their own well-being last, if at all. This, in turn, creates a self-fulfilling prophecy because they are now completely depleted of any energy reserves to contribute in a meaningful and engaging way to their profession or relatives.

One way immigrants may attempt to manage work-family dissatisfaction is through compensation in which one attempts to compensate for unmet needs in one domain by the other (Halbesleben et al., 2009). Compensation can cause one to decrease the significance they previously placed on the dissatisfying domain, which can result in decreased actions to do their best in that domain. For instance, if one is experiencing substantial family stress, one might poor themselves deeper into their work if they perceive it as a favorable environment more so than their home environment. On the flip side, if one feels underappreciated and overwhelmed at work, one might start to focus more on family life where they feel supported and accepted. Relatedly, enrichment aims to help one's positive experiences in one role enrich that of the other role (Masuda, McNall, Allen, & Nicklin, 2012). Work-family facilitation is encouraged. If employers trust their employees to get the job done right while giving them the flexibility to take care of their home needs in a responsible way, they will likely be more engaged in work because they are being taken into consideration and allowed to not have to sacrifice family for work.

An additional way to manage work-family demands is to engage in segmentation in which one intentionally creates a boundary between their work and home life (Halbesleben et al., 2009). This can be difficult to maintain if role responsibilities in each domain are high and the person perceives that they are unable to set clear boundaries for the demands they are made. Things like leaving work at work and not doing personal-related activities during working hours. This is not practical given school events and doctor appointments are conducted during regular business hours. This makes it a slippery slope for work and family needs to affect each other. An opposite approach to segmentation would be integration in which one does not attempt to keep work and home life separate but rather integrate them into their life and adjust with the ebbs and flow of each demand when called for. For instance, one might do a "split shift" in which they take a longer lunch break to exercise or engage with family and make up work that has been paused at night after one's children fall asleep.

One's ability to cope with work-family conflict depends on the number of internal and external resources they have available. Internal resources include thought processes, problem-solving abilities, emotional regulation, and time management skills. External resources can include financial and social support, as well as job rank and stability, which can vary for immigrants who are on a work visa or are US residents. The more threats to their resources they perceive, the more likely they are to experience stress within the domain it affects. The Conservation of Resources model (Halbesleben et al., 2009) suggests that if one perceives themselves to be depleted of reserves that are essential to fulfill their role duties at work or at home, they are more likely to experience stress. How the individual interprets stress and its consequences matter. Some may fear that not being able to keep up at work will put them at risk of losing everything they have sacrificed and built in the US at the cost of leaving their home country and family. Others may fear losing their job, putting their visa sponsorship at risk as it is a work benefit that is not easy to come by. If the person interprets a situation as threatening to their professional or personal life, then stress levels will increase.

While some levels of stress are helpful to keep people "on their toes," an excess amount can trigger a worse outcome depending on how an individual decides to cope with stress (Biggs, Brough, & Drummond, 2017), for instance, pretending that the problem does not exist or is not that big of a deal can cause the issue to become even bigger than if it were faced and actively addressed. Such denial renders the person helpless to do anything about it. Perhaps they think the outcome is out of their control and is in the destiny of God or their employer, which coincides with the cultural value of fatalism among Latino immigrants. To cope with the perceived lack of control, they may ignore facing the circumstance to preserve their ego. Others might make light of the situation or use humor to cope with it. Others may cope by suppressing thoughts and feelings about the situation and not voicing their concerns to their boss for a number of reasons, such as cultural values that do not condone questioning authority. Others may vent about the stress they are dealing with but not actively do anything about it. They might not have family support if they are not accompanied by family members in the US. Further, family members in their home country might not understand the complexities of working in the US. They might have a distorted perception of what it means to live in the US as the place of "opportunity" and assume that the person has "made it" and can now provide for family back home. This can cause stress for the worker because they feel pulled to provide for their family, give back to their community, and show gratitude that they have made it in the US. If one experiences a family emergency that requires their physical presence or financial contribution, this can put them in a bind to have to pick between their work, their own responsibilities at home, and that of their family in their home country.

Misunderstandings between an employer, the individual, and their family can cause turmoil between the things and people that matter most to immigrants. Things like regret for not being able to be present with family back home should it be a life-threatening circumstance and resentment from family for not being there, to begin with. Given family is at the core of immigrants' values, this can negatively affect their well-being and, in turn, bring them to work when not at their best. They may harbor resentment and frustration toward their job for putting them in the position to sacrifice their family and may show up in decreased performance either consciously or subconsciously. This decreases their chances of career advancement, promotions, performance reviews, and can even put their position at risk. Decreased engagement, states of flow, and altruistic efforts. They can start to see their job as just a paycheck rather than their calling.

Work-family conflict and mental health

Conflict experienced between work and family life can negatively impact outcomes related to their vocational, familial, and personal lives. They may feel less satisfied with their job, family, or life in general. They may be less engaged at work or with family and friends. They might push themselves beyond their limit to increase harmony between work and family life that they take a hit to their own well-being, triggering mental and physical health problems. If work and family conflicts, they might be less engaged, be perceived as not dedicated to their career, or passed up for promotions. Stress due to work-family conflict can be further compounded by the immigration and cultural integration process (Balidemaj & Small, 2019). Taken together, these hardships and traumatic experiences create adverse outcomes for US immigrants. In turn, these adverse outcomes can spill over and directly impact their work life in various ways. For some immigrants, this may create a decrease in success and motivation.

One ongoing psychological pattern that individuals experience when they believe that their accomplishments arose from external factors (e.g., luck, charm, etc.) rather than internal factors (e.g., talent) is known as the impostor phenomenon or impostorism (Crawford, Shanine, Whitman, & Kacmar, 2016). Individuals who experience the impostorism worry that others will find out that they are incompetent and unworthy. They fear being evaluated, not being able to continue their successes, and that they might not be as capable as others. Research shows that workers who experience impostor feelings are more likely to decrease efforts in career planning, career striving, and motivation to be leaders (Neureiter & Traut-Mattausch, 2016). As minorities, immigrants may be more susceptible to impostorism if they experience added stressors such as discrimination, stereotype threats, beliefs that they are in certain spots due to affirmative action, distressing environment, feelings of isolation, and prejudice (Cokley et al., 2017). Thus, not only may immigrants feel like a fraud but also a fraud in an unfamiliar environment to which they do not belong culturally. Given the current political climate and negative perception of immigrants in the US, it is not uncommon for many of these similar stressors to be experienced.

For some US immigrants, feeling like a "perpetual foreigner" refers to any ethnic minority individual is perceived as "other" or not American by the White-dominated majority group regardless of whether that individual is native-born or naturalized in the US (Huynh, Devos, & Smalarz, 2011). Despite the individual's level of acculturation or assimilation to the host culture, others will still perceive them to be perpetual foreigners based on phenotypic characteristics. It is not uncommon for the individual to be constantly questioned by others about their origins (e.g., the "where are you from" question). This experience has been shown to have negative effects on the individual's well-being by way of ethnic discrimination (Armenta et al., 2013). Furthermore, labels such as "alien, foreigner, noncitizens" (Rucker, Murphy, & Quintanilla, 2019) can be internalized by US immigrants to deepen the impostor experience of not belonging. It is possible that the added stress of impostorism at work can spill over to cause stress at home depending on frequency, intensity, and severity (Crawford et al., 2016). However, to date, there is no known research that has looked at this relationship.

Due to the conditions and hardships that are experienced by US immigrants, they may be susceptible to burnout. Burnout includes emotional exhaustion, cynicism/disengagement, and decreased personal sense of accomplishment, which in turn can lead to decreased work ethic, motivation, and capacity for work-related engagement (Yang et al., 2017). Although to our knowledge, burnout within vocational settings among US immigrants specifically has not been examined, there has been some work done on the international level to support this idea. One study that did not measure burnout directly, measured similar variables such as job dissatisfaction and psychological well-being among Filipino immigrants in the US and found that job dissatisfaction had significant implications for psychological well-being in this population (de Castro, Gee, & Takeuchi, 2008). Furthermore, these analyses controlled for many sociodemographic variables (e.g., age, income, job category, etc.) and results were consistent thus, further supporting the idea that immigrants suffering from job dissatisfaction may be more susceptible to symptoms of burnout.

Implications for practice and recommendations

Mental health practitioners, career counselors, and human resource managers have the power and therefore the potential to help immigrants address work-family conflict so they can be at their best at work and at home without sacrificing either domain. Such professionals are called to first and foremost recognize that there are many within-group differences among immigrants and that the intersecting differences that arise due to factors such as gender norms, cultural values, and histories. For example, an African immigrant from Ghana will likely have vast differences from an immigrant from Kenya. At the same time, there are commonalities that unite many cultures such as filial piety among Asian immigrants despite differences in language. At the same time, immigrants from collectivistic cultures as a whole tend to express family values in a vastly different way than the more individualistic US culture. It is also important to understand the systematic oppression faced by many immigrants, especially by those with other intersecting minoritized identities.

History and politics also impact immigrants; between events in their country of origin and in the US. It is vital to not make assumptions based on their demographic information, initial presentation, language skills or accent, or any other surface-level factors. It is also vital to understand the cultural expectations surrounding many, for example, if they have grown up believing in filial piety and are struggling to care for their elders who may be overseas. Some cultures prize eye contact, while others see it as disrespectful, especially toward authority. For some, a handshake is an inappropriate greeting while for others a kiss on the cheek is normal. As such, it is the responsibility of professionals to be familiar with the experiences and histories of immigrants while also recognizing that there are great variations in adherence to certain cultural values or the degree to which certain cultural factors pose a challenge within the work-life interface. In essence, be informed, but do not make assumptions. Show the individual that you have a vested interest in helping them navigate their work-family needs by asking them how they might be supported. At the same time, take the initiative to provide culturally informed solutions and assistance, as it may be seen as violating a hierarchy or disrespectful for immigrants from collectivistic cultures to "impose" their needs in a way that gets them "special treatment."

Mental health professionals and career counselors should recognize that results on assessments might be biased or pathologize immigrants when cultural factors are not considered when interpreting test results. It is important to recognize the meaning that is placed on work and recognize cultural values within the context of work and family. For instance, it is assumed that work is to be enjoyed in the US but that is not always the case in other countries. Immigrants may view work as a means of survival rather than a means of personal fulfillment because it goes beyond them. The work they do might be perceived as an expression of the sacrifices made by their home community and family that should not be taken for granted. This places a burden on them to perform and to have a legacy in the name of their family because they are the one that "made it."

Within the work setting, human resource professionals are challenged with establishing communication between a workplace and its workers. As such, they are in a position of power to convey metamessages regarding the nature of an organization and what explicit and implicit values are being introduced. Human resource departments should promote and support diversity training as an ongoing initiative. It is not sufficient to see diversity workshops as a "one and done" type of exercise; diversity training is not a checkbox that can be completed every calendar year and not thought about again until 365 days later, rather it must be an ongoing effort, included in daily conversation, operations, and initiatives. It will take time through a process of change to fight potential stereotyping and archaic notions, such as picturing the entire continent of Africa as a monolith of primitive towns without electricity, technology, or even knowledge of the outside world. This is not to say that coming from a poorer area or country are less valid; rather it speaks to the importance of not making assumptions simply upon meeting a person and letting them tell their own story. African, Latinx, and Asian individuals may be coming from centuries of historical, potentially even present-day, trauma. It is not up to the individual in question to inform others of the entire history of their country, its conflicts, or the ways in which European nations have stripped resource-rich countries of their autonomy by destroying democratic leadership, instilling corruption, and squandering natural resources and reserves.

Although corporate America is a busy environment, diversity programs and training should still be prioritized for the sake of longevity of the company and its employees. Diversity initiatives impact the success of an entire company and allow for a more holistic view of employees as multifaceted individuals who bring a great deal to the conference table. Individuals should not shy away from practices and programs that promote diversity in the workplace, but instead, strive to create a culture that showcases strengths. The workplace should not be a melting pot or a place where there is a collective culture that is formed as an amalgamation of the narratives and experiences most represented at a company.

Companies in various parts of the world fail to provide support and services for their female employees, especially mothers who have recently given birth. For some, help from family, friends, or other caretakers is a viable option to displace responsibility, but for others it is not a part of their reality. By providing designated nursing rooms for breastfeeding mothers can help send a message that their family matters. Further, conflict between work and family life can also be potentially decreased by providing nap rooms and exercise facilities to improve energy and performance, a flexible schedule to take care of family needs during the day, work from home options when a child is sick, and incentives that include performance-based bonus vacation days that can come in handy for overseas travel. Installation of gender-neutral restrooms can help convey that inclusivity is part of the company culture. One no-cost recommendation is to put gender pronouns and name pronunciation in email signatures so that workers can feel more comfortable with how they want to be referred to and how they want their name to be pronounced in a non-Americanized way. Similarly, the use of more inclusive language such as "Latinx" helps to challenge and dismantle the gender binary as a system of oppression, and makes no assumptions of gender identity, further allowing employers and employees to communicate a desire to understand and support each other (Adames, Chavez-Dueñas, Sharma, & La Roche, 2018). These types of recommendations can help immigrant workers feel not just included but valued as well.

In conclusion, this chapter has covered conditions experienced by immigrants in the US. For many, there is an overwhelming feeling of not being included nor valued not only in their new country but at work, too. The understudied and recently emerging focus on burnout within vocational settings may apply to immigrant populations as they experience compounding conditions that other groups may not while they navigate their work and family demands. More research is needed to understand the complexities of the compounding effects of psychological, vocational, and familial needs of African, Asian, and Latino immigrants in the United States.

References

Adames, H. Y., Chavez-Dueñas, N. Y., Sharma, S., & La Roche, M. J. (2018). Intersectionality in psychotherapy: The experiences of an AfroLatinx queer immigrant. *Psychotherapy*, *55*(1), 73–79.

Armenta, B. E., Lee, R. M., Pituc, S. T., Jung, K.-R., Park, I. J. K., Soto, J. A., … Schwartz, S. J. (2013). Where are you from? A validation of the Foreigner Objectification Scale and the psychological correlates of foreigner objectification among Asian Americans and Latinos. *Cultural Diversity and Ethnic Minority Psychology*, *19*(2), 131–142.

Balidemaj, A., & Small, M. (2019). The effects of ethnic identity and acculturation in mental health of immigrants: A literature review. *International Journal of Social Psychiatry*, *65*(7–8), 643–655.

Bautista, J., Bressler, K., & Bosworth, N. (2019). Immigration detention: Perspectives from Maine law students working on the ground at the Laredo Detention Center in Texas. *Maine Law Review*, *71*(1), 2–35.

Bedford, O., & Yeh, K.-H. (2019). The history and the future of the psychology of filial piety: Chinese norms to contextualized personality construct. *Frontiers in Psychology*, *10*, 100.

Biggs, A., Brough, P., & Drummond, S. (2017). Lazarus and Folkman's psychological stress and coping theory. In C. L. Cooper & J. Quick (Eds.), *The Wiley handbook of stress and health: A guide to research and practice* (pp. 341–364). London, UK: John Wiley & Sons.

Blustein, D. L., Kenny, M. E., Di Fabio, A., & Guichard, J. (2019). Expanding the impact of the psychology of working: Engaging psychology in the struggle for decent work and human rights. *Journal of Career Assessment*, *27*(1), 3–28.

Castillo, L., & Cano, M.Á. (2007). Mexican American Psychology: Theory and clinical application. In C. Negy (Ed.), *Cross-cultural psychotherapy: Toward a critical understanding of diverse client populations* (2nd ed., pp. 85–102). Reno, NV: Bent Tree Press, Inc..

Chuang, S., & Tamis-LeMonda, C. (2013). *Current perspectives on gender roles and relationships in immigrant families*. In *Gender roles in immigrant families*. (pp. 1–5). New York, NY: Springer.

Cokley, K., Smith, L., Bernard, D., Hurst, A., Jackson, S., Stone, S., & Roberts, D. (2017). Impostor feelings as a moderator and mediator of the relationship between perceived discrimination and mental health among racial/ethnic minority college students. *Journal of Counseling Psychology*, *64*(2), 141–154.

Cook, M. L., Gleeson, S., Griffith, K. L., & Kahn, L. M. (2018). Introduction to a special issue on the impact of immigrant legalization initiatives: International perspectives on immigration and the world of work. *ILR Review*, *71*(4), 807–822.

Crawford, W. S., Shanine, K. K., Whitman, M. V., & Kacmar, K. M. (2016). Examining the impostor phenomenon and work-family conflict. *Journal of Managerial Psychology*, *31*(2), 375–390.

de Castro, A. B., Gee, G. C., & Takeuchi, D. (2008). Relationship between job dissatisfaction and physical and psychological health among Filipino immigrants. *AAOHN Journal*, *56*(1), 33–40.

Halbesleben, J. R. B., Harvey, J., & Bolino, M. C. (2009). Too engaged? A conservation of resources view of the relationship between work engagement and work interference with family. *Journal of Applied Psychology*, *94*, 1452–1465.

Hamann, E. T., & Reeves, J. (2012). ICE raids, children, media, and making sense of Latino newcomers in flyover country. *Anthropology & Education Quarterly*, *43*(1), 24–40.

Held, M. L., Cuellar, M. J., & Cook Heffron, L. (2018). A study of social work students' knowledge and perceptions of stages of Latino immigration. *Journal of Social Work Education*, *54*(1), 61–78.

Huynh, Q.-L., Devos, T., & Smalarz, L. (2011). Perpetual foreigner in one's own land: Potential implications for identity and psychological adjustment. *Journal of Social & Clinical Psychology*, *30*(2), 133–162.

Institute for Women's Policy Research. (2018). *The gender wage gap: 2018 earnings differences by race and ethnicity*. Retrieved 6 August 2019 from https://iwpr.org/publications/gender-wage-gap-2018/.

Kamya, H. (2005). African immigrant families. In M. McGoldrick, J. Giordano, & N. Garcia-Preto (Eds.), *Ethnicity and family therapy* (pp. 101–116). New York: Guilford Press.

Kinnunen, U., Feldt, T., Mauno, S., & Rantanen, J. (2010). Interface between work and family: A longitudinal individual and crossover perspective. *Journal of Occupational and Organizational Psychology*, *83*, 119–137.

Lancee, B., & Bol, T. (2017). The transferability of skills and degrees: Why the place of education affects immigrant earnings. *Social Forces*, *96*(2), 691.

Leong, F. T. L., & Tang, M. (2016). Career barriers for Chinese immigrants in the United States. *Career Development Quarterly*, *64*(3), 259–271.

Masuda, A. D., McNall, L. A., Allen, T. D., & Nicklin, J. M. (2012). Examining the constructs of work-to-family enrichment and positive spillover. *Journal of Vocational Behavior*, *80*, 197–210.

Neureiter, M., & Traut-Mattausch, E. (2016). An inner barrier to career development: Preconditions of the impostor phenomenon and consequences for career development. *Frontiers in Psychology*, *7*, 48.

Ojeda, L., & Organista, K. C. (2015). Latino American men. In Y. J. Wong & S. R. Wester (Eds.), *APA handbook of the psychology of men and masculinities*. Washington, DC: American Psychological Association.

Robert, C. (2017). Humor at work. Often experienced, seldom studied. In C. Robert (Ed.), *The psychology of humor at work: A psychological perspective* (pp. 1–9). New York, NY: Routledge.

Rucker, J. M., Murphy, M. C., & Quintanilla, V. D. (2019). The immigrant labeling effect: The role of immigrant group labels in prejudice against noncitizens. *Group Processes & Intergroup Relations*, *22*(8), 1139–1160.

Shirvanian, N., & Michael, T. (2017). Implementation of attachment theory into early childhood settings. *International Education Journal: Comparative Perspectives*, *16*(2), 97–115.

Shockley, K. M., Shen, W., DeNunzio, M. M., Arvan, M. L., & Knudsen, E. A. (2017). Disentangling the relationship between gender and work–family conflict: An integration of theoretical perspectives using meta-analytic methods. *Journal of Applied Psychology*, *102*(12), 1601–1635.

Storti, C. (1999). *Figuring foreigners out*. Yarmouth, ME: Intercultural Press.

Taras, V., Sarala, R., Muchinsky, P., Kemmelmeier, M., Singelis, T. M., Avsec, A., … Sinclair, H. C. (2014). Opposite ends of the same stick? Multi-method test of the dimensionality of individualism and collectivism. *Journal of Cross-Cultural Psychology*, *45*(2), 213–245.

Thoman, D. B., Smith, J. L., Brown, E. R., Chase, J., & Lee, J. Y. K. (2013). Beyond performance: A motivational experiences model of stereotype threat. *Educational Psychology Review*, *25*, 211–243.

Titzmann, P. F., & Jugert, P. (2017). Transition to a new country: Acculturative and developmental predictors for changes in self-efficacy among adolescent immigrants. *Journal of Youth and Adolescence*, *46*(10), 2143–2156.

US Bureau of Labor Statistics. (2019). *Labor force characteristics of foreign-born workers summary*. Retrieved 15 April 2019 from https://www.bls.gov/news.release/pdf/forbrn.pdf.

Westman, M. (2006). Crossover of stress and strain in the work-family context. In: F. Jones, R. J. Burke, & M. Westman (Eds.), *Work-life balance: A psychological perspective* (pp. 163–184). Psychology Press.

Yang, S., Liu, D., Liu, H., Zhang, J., & Duan, Z. (2017). Relationship of work-family conflict, self-reported social support and job satisfaction to burnout syndrome among medical workers in Southwest China: a cross-sectional study. *PLoS ONE*, *12*(2), e0171679.

Zhao, X., & Biernat, M. (2019). Your name is your lifesaver: Anglicization of names and moral dilemmas in a trilogy of transportation accidents. *Social Psychological and Personality Science*, *10*(8), 1011–1018.

Chapter 6

Being a Latina/o immigrant parent in the United States: Links with parents' and adolescents' mental health and health risk behaviors

Elma I. Lorenzo-Blanco and Seth J. Schwartz
Department of Human Development and Family Sciences, University of Texas at Austin, Austin, TX, United States; Department of Public Health Sciences, University of Miami, Miami, FL, United States

The Hispanic population in the United States

The US Hispanic population has increased exponentially in the past 50 years. In 1970, less than 5% of the US population was Hispanic (US Census Bureau, 2012). In 2019, nearly 60 million Hispanics resided in the United States, representing 18% of the US population (Flores, Lopez, & Krogstad, 2019). This growth has occurred both through immigration and to fertility—currently, approximately one-third of US Hispanics are foreign born and two-thirds are US born (Flores, 2017). By 2050, Census projections suggest that 25%–30% of the US population will be Hispanic (Krogstad, 2014).

The Hispanic population has become increasingly diverse in recent years. Whereas Mexicans have traditionally represented the largest Hispanic group in the United States, their immigration has slowed since the Great Recession of 2008–2009 (Portes & Rumbaut, 2014). On the other hand, other Hispanic groups have been arriving in greater numbers—including Guatemalans, Salvadorans, Colombians, and Dominicans. The crisis in Venezuela has sent nearly half a million people to the United States (see US Citizenship and Immigration Services, 2019, for an example of 1 month's asylum workload). Nearly 150,000 Puerto Ricans moved to the US mainland in the year following Hurricane Maria (Flores & Krogstad, 2019). The undocumented immigrant population—with recent arrivals comprised largely of Central Americans—may increase by several hundred thousand in 2019 alone (Chishti, Pierce, & Telus, 2019).

Mental and Behavioral Health of Immigrants in the United States
https://doi.org/10.1016/B978-0-12-816117-3.00006-3

This growth, however, has occurred fairly unevenly across US regions, states, and cities. The Southwestern states have the largest Hispanic populations by proportion (e.g., 55% of New Mexico residents are Hispanic; and New York, California, Florida, and New Jersey house the majority of foreign-born Hispanics in the United States (Flores, 2017). Cities such as Miami, Los Angeles, New York, Houston, and Chicago are home to large Spanish-speaking enclaves where residents—especially adults who did not attend school in the United States—can go about their daily lives without learning or using much English (Schwartz, Pantin, Sullivan, Prado, & Szapocznik, 2006).

Reactions to this growth in the US Hispanic population have ranged from extremely positive and supportive to extremely negative and threatened. Liberal commentators have celebrated the increasing diversity of the United States, whereas conservative commentators have labeled mass Hispanic immigration—especially undocumented immigration—as an invasion. For example, Macias (2000) referred to large-scale Hispanic immigration as "the flowering of America," whereas Buchanan (2007) referred to large-scale Hispanic immigration as "a Third World invasion." Huntington (2004) framed Hispanic population growth, and especially the emergence of large Spanish-speaking enclaves, as a challenge to the Anglo-Protestant heritage of the United States and to the status of English as the country's dominant language. Buchanan (2011a, 2011b) went as far as to claim that Hispanic immigrants were "invading" the US Southwest as part of an organized Mexican plan to reconquer the territory that the US took from Mexico following the Mexican American War and the Treaty of Guadalupe Hidalgo in the 19th century.

Generally speaking, mass immigration activates threat and defense dynamics among many destination-society individuals. In the 19th and early 20th centuries, mass Italian and Jewish immigration to the Northeastern and Midwestern United States was met with derisive comments, such as calling the immigrants "human garbage" (Sterba, 2003), as well as with restrictive immigration legislation in 1924 that effectively ended this wave of immigration (Gjelten, 2015). Coenders, Lubbers, Scheepers, and Verkuyten (2008) reviewed Dutch responses to mass Muslim migration and found that attitudes were least favorable during the heaviest migration flows. Woods and Arthur (2017) argue that the election of Donald Trump as US president, and his advocacy for "tough" immigration enforcement policies, represent an attempt by certain segments of the US population to end mass Hispanic immigration. Restrictive immigration policies represent a form of defense against the perceived threats posed by mass immigration—especially mass immigration of people perceived as being different from the "mainstream" population (e.g., Hogan & Haltinner, 2015).

Chavez (2013) reviews empirical research debunking most of these negative and "threatened" reactions among some conservative commentators. For example, loyalty to the United States is quite high among Hispanic immigrants (Schildkraut, 2014), challenging the idea that their arrival is part of a subversive plan to harm the country. Further, the vast majority of Hispanic children (including those born outside the United States) master and prefer English (Tran, 2010). Interviews with undocumented immigrants indicate that escaping untenable living conditions (e.g., war, gang violence, extreme poverty, natural disasters)—not "invading" the United States—was their primary motivation for crossing the border illegally (Sladkova, 2007).

Notwithstanding this evidence against the threatened positions adopted by some US residents, a key principle is that threat is in the eye of the beholder. In other words, although many Venezuelan and Central American immigrants view themselves as running for their lives, some Americans view them as invaders. Integrated threat theory (Stephan, Ybarra, & Bachman, 1999) enumerates three primary reasons why ingroup members might find outgroups to be threatening or potentially harmful—realistic threat, symbolic threat, and stereotyping. *Realistic threats* involve perceived harms that outgroup members pose to the ingroup's physical, financial, or other tangible resources. For example, one commonly held assumption in many immigration contexts is that migrants take jobs away from native-born citizens (Chomsky, 2007). *Symbolic threats* involve perceived harm to intangible assets possessed by the ingroup, such as its national identity. Right-wing, nationalist political parties, and movements in the United States, Australia, Austria, Italy, Hungary, Poland, Brazil, and elsewhere have won elections, at least in part, by demonizing immigrants as "invaders" who will "ruin our culture" if the invasion is not stopped (Wodak & Krzyżanowski, 2017). Velasco González, Verkuyten, Weesie, and Poppe (2008) examined Dutch attitudes toward Muslim migrants and found that symbolic threats, but not realistic threats, predicted endorsement of discrimination against Muslims. *Stereotypes* are portrayals of the "typical" outgroup member and are usually negative and demeaning. For example, Mexican and Central American immigrants in the United States are often typecast as invaders who live off of the US government (Chavez, 2013).

Mass Hispanic immigration activates all three threat processes in some Americans. Working-class White and Black Americans may perceive large-scale immigration of low-skilled workers as a realistic threat to their earning potential. Immigration research based on integrated threat theory has found that immigrant groups that share a common unifying characteristic (such as a language or religion that is different from that endorsed by the majority of people within the country's dominant ethnic group) are viewed as especially threatening (Hartman, Newman, & Bell, 2014). Individuals from migrant groups that are viewed as threatening—whether because of their large numbers or because of a common outgroup characteristic (such as language or religion)—are most likely to be received and treated poorly in the destination society. Often, symbolic threats result in these migrants and groups being excluded from the shared national ingroup, and nations or regions may enact policies to limit the presence or impact of "threatening" migrant groups.

These policies include the "English only" laws enacted in various states, California's Proposition 187 that would have denied education and medical care to the children of undocumented immigrants, and the 2009 Arizona "racial profiling" law allowing police to detain anyone who they believe may be in the United States illegally (see Selden, Pace, & Nunn-Gilman, 2011, for an example). English-only laws are intended to remove the Spanish language from public places—though these laws clearly will not prevent Hispanics from speaking their ethnic language in private spaces. "Tough" immigration laws are intended to discourage illegal immigration, though there is no evidence that these laws serve their intended purpose. Indeed, immigration appears to be governed by "push" and "pull" factors (e.g., poverty and war in the sending country, peace, and prosperity in the destination country)—such that, in extreme cases, individuals will risk their lives to enter the destination country (Sabates-Wheeler, Sabates, & Castaldo, 2008). The Arizona law facilitated the harassment of indigenous-looking individuals, who may be viewed by some Americans as posing symbolic threats to the European heritage of the United States. Simply put, these policies are designed to reduce threats to the English-speaking, European-descent majority group in the United States (Jardina, 2019).

At the same time, Hispanic immigrants *may be unintentionally discouraged from becoming American*. In a series of experimental studies, Devos and Banaji (2005) found that US participants—both Whites and ethnic minorities—more readily identified Whites as American and non-White groups as foreigners. Foreigner objectification syndrome (Lee, Lee, & Tran, 2017) refers to a phenomenon where visible-minority individuals (primarily Hispanic and Asian) are regarded as foreigners even if they speak perfect English and are well versed in the US culture. Individuals may be repeatedly asked where they are from or spoken to very slowly or loudly—insinuating that the person is not American. Further, visible-minority individuals who attempt to "pass as White American" are *more* likely to be rejected and discriminated against than are visible-minority individuals who remain separated from the White American mainstream (Staerklé, Sidanius, Green, & Molina, 2010). Self-verification theory (North & Swann, 2009) holds that one's claim to membership in a social group requires validation from other group members before it can be considered secure. As a result, individuals who identify as American, but who are not accepted as such, may be emotionally hurt or scarred as a result.

In essence, then, many Hispanic immigrants are demonized for remaining separate from the US mainstream—but they may also be rejected if they attempt to integrate into the US mainstream. Although laws and policies designed to reduce perceived threats posed by Hispanic immigration may be comforting for those individuals who feel threatened, they are in fact quite hurtful to immigrants. These policies denigrate Hispanic immigrants' linguistic and cultural heritage—which paradoxically undermines their ability and desire to integrate into the US "mainstream" (Rumbaut, 2008). Simply put, people are unlikely to identify with a group that rejects them, that rejects their culture, and regards them as a threat. Those who *do* identify as Americans may experience pushback insinuating that they are not really American.

These negative intergroup interactions may lead to cultural stress among Hispanic immigrant families. Theories of dehumanization (e.g., Moshman, 2011) hold that once individuals have been grouped into "us" (ingroup) versus "them" (outgroup), ingroup members can discriminate against, exclude, and even physically harm outgroup members as a way of defending themselves and their ingroup against the threats posed by the outgroup. For example, the Southern Poverty Law Center (2009) and Piedrabuena (2018) provide first-hand accounts of Hispanic immigrants' experiences in Suffolk County, New York, where an Ecuadorean day laborer was murdered in 2009 by a group of white men because he was undocumented—and where Hispanic residents are often denigrated for speaking Spanish in public places. In her article, Piedrabuena notes that beatings of Hispanic day laborers are not uncommon in eastern Long Island. Countless other examples can be found in other parts of the United States. Quite likely, these incidents reflect the dehumanization and exclusion of Hispanic residents because their presence is perceived as "threatening." The pushback against immigrants may lead to discrimination and a negative context of reception, where immigrants perceive themselves as being marginalized and excluded. Perceived threats posed by large immigrant *groups* may lead to defensive policies that exert deleterious effects on *individuals* and *families*. In all, these dynamics contribute to the cultural stress experience of Hispanic families, which can influence the mental and behavioral of parents and youth (Lorenzo-Blanco, Meca, et al., 2016; Schwartz, Unger, Des Rosiers et al., 2014; Schwartz, Unger, Lorenzo-Blanco, et al., 2014; Yoshikawa, 2011).

Cultural stress among Hispanic parents in the United States

Parental stress has been described as a normative experience for parents that requires parents to balance the demands of their role as a parent (e.g., providing shelter and food) with their access to available resources (e.g., employment and financial resources) (Deater-Deckard, 2008). Stress and coping theories (Folkman, Lazarus, Gruen, & DeLongis, 1986) suggest that parental stress arises when there is a mismatch between the demands placed on parents and their available resources to manage these demands. Many studies have documented the negative effects of parental stressors on the development of adolescents from diverse backgrounds (Kim, Schwartz, Perreira, & Juang, 2018; Perreira, Chapman, & Stein, 2006; Tran, 2014). According to the Family Stress Model (FSM), parental stressors may influence adolescents' mental and behavioral health by compromising parents' mental and behavioral health, which in turn, may compromise their parenting and marital relationship (Conger, Conger, & Martin, 2010).

Many parents experience parental stressors (Deater-Deckard, 2008). Yet, as mentioned above, Hispanic immigrant parents in the United States can experience additional cultural stressors related to having to navigate multiple cultural contexts and to belonging to an ethnic-minority and stigmatized group (Conger et al., 2012; Tran, 2014; White, Roosa, Weaver, & Nair, 2009), increasing their overall stress level. In the literature, *cultural stress* has been conceptualized as a constellation of interrelated but distinct factors that can contribute to the stress experience of Hispanic immigrant families. Some cultural stressors include perceived discrimination, a negative context of reception, and acculturative/bicultural stress (Cano et al., 2015; Lorenzo-Blanco, Meca, et al., 2016). *Perceived discrimination* refers to Hispanic parents' experiences of being treated unfairly or differentially due to their ethnicity, immigration status, and/or skin color, such as being teased or ostracized for being a Hispanic immigrant or for having an accent when speaking English (Pérez, Fortuna, & Alegria, 2008). A *negative context of reception* refers to Hispanic immigrant parents' perceptions of not feeling welcomed in their US receiving contexts such as not having access to good employment, schools, health care, and safe neighborhoods (Schwartz, Unger, Des Rosiers, et al., 2014). *Acculturative/bicultural stress* includes the pressure of having to learn a new language; maintain one's native language; balance differing cultural values and ways of behaving; teach ones' children the native language and Hispanic cultural values and ways of behaving (Torres, Driscoll, & Voell, 2012).

Related to the above experiences of discrimination, a negative context of reception, and acculturative/bicultural stress, Cervantes, Padilla, and Salgado de Snyder (1991) have identified additional cultural stressors recent Hispanic immigrant parents can experience when navigating the US cultural context. These cultural stressors include marital stress, parenting stress, occupational and economic stress, immigration stress, and cultural/family conflict stress (Cavazos-Rehg, Zayas, Walker, & Fisher, 2006; Cervantes et al., 1991). While many parents/couples experience *marital stress* (Cavazos-Rehg et al., 2006; Cervantes et al., 1991), Hispanic immigrant parents/couples can experience additional marital stressors related to the immigration/adaptation process. For example, parents/couples may argue about which language to speak at home and whether to raise children the Hispanic or the American way. Also, in some families, one parent/couple may acculturate to US culture faster than the other parent/couple, which can create differences in values and behaviors, resulting in cultural conflict within the marital relationship/family.

One form of *parenting stress* Hispanic parents can experience is *acculturation-gap stress*, which can occur when children adopt US American culture faster than their parents, resulting in differences between children's and parents' values, expectations, and behaviors. These differences, in turn, can result in parent-child conflict and distanced parent-child relationships (Cavazos-Rehg et al., 2006; Cervantes et al., 1991). Hispanic parents can also experience stress related to mismatches in acculturation patterns and/or cultural values between parents and their children (Lui, 2015). Similar to acculturation gaps between parents and children, acculturation mismatch can result in intergenerational cultural conflict, contributing to parents' stress experience.

Another parenting stressor for Hispanic parents can include parents' concern and worry about their children experiencing discrimination and/or parents' worry about their children receiving substandard education given that Hispanic immigrant families often reside in poor neighborhoods (Alegría, Green, McLaughlin, & Loder, 2015; Landale, McHale, & Booth, 2010; Suárez-Orozco, Yoshikawa, & Tseng, 2015). Schools in these neighborhoods tend to lack adequate resources, impacting Hispanic parents' and youths' experiences at school.

Occupational and *economic stress* for Hispanic parents includes their perceptions of being expected to work harder due to their ethnicity and/or for being an immigrant. It can also include parents having to work multiple jobs or having to accept work far away from family to be able to provide for their families. Another occupational stressor includes parents' experiences with the wage gap and promotion discrimination that may prevent Hispanic parents from getting raises and promotions at work (Cavazos-Rehg et al., 2006; Cervantes et al., 1991).

Immigration stress for Hispanic immigrant parents has been described as parents' fear of experiencing deportation or about family members and friends experiencing deportation and separation (Cavazos-Rehg et al., 2006; Cervantes et al., 1991). Immigration stress can also entail for parents and children to have limited contact with family or friends due to parents' or childrens' immigration status, which can result in feeling isolated and disconnected. Another cultural stressor identified by Cervantes et al. (1991) includes *cultural/family conflict* which involves differences in values and customs between family members, resulting in arguments and conflicts among family members. As described later and consistent with the FSM, these additional parent cultural stressors may negatively affect the emotional and behavioral health of parents and adolescents by compromising the overall functioning of the family (Conger et al., 2010, 2012).

Barriers Hispanic immigrant parents face when navigating US social institutions

In addition to above cultural stressors, Hispanic immigrant parents can face personal, community, and system-level barriers in accessing and navigating social institutions such as schools; government agencies (e.g., department of motor vehicles); health and mental health services; and other public programs that provide economic, housing, school, mental, and physical health support (Crosnoe et al., 2012; Perreira et al., 2012; Yoshikawa, Weiland, Ulvestad, Perreira, & Crosnoe, 2014). These barriers can contribute to the stress experience of Hispanic parents and families, thereby impacting adolescents' and parents' mental and behavioral health (Yoshikawa, 2011). These barriers can further prevent parents from accessing resources that could reduce families' economic hardship, improve parents' and adolescents' mental and behavioral health, and contribute to students' success and stability in school, as well as to families' stability at work and home. The Immigrant to Health and Human Services Project (Crosnoe et al., 2012;

Perreira et al., 2012; Yoshikawa et al., 2014), for example, has identified several barriers that parents and families can face when accessing public services and programs that can provide economic and health support to families. Other studies have identified similar barriers for Hispanic families when accessing mental health services (Alegría et al., 2015; Lorenzo-Blanco, Torres, & Smithwick, 2016; Ramirez, Gallion, Aguilar, & Dembeck, 2017). These barriers generally fall within four larger categories including (a) complex application processes and eligibility rules; (b) administrative burdens and errors; (c) language, literacy, and cultural barriers; and (d) transportation and other logistical challenges.

The complexity of application processes and eligibility rules can create barriers for Hispanic immigrant families, as some parents may not be familiar with government and public programs (including programs offered at school and workplaces) and they may not understand how to benefit from these programs or how to navigate the enrollment/application process (e.g., how to show proof of residence). Moreover, because some Hispanic immigrant parents may arrive in the United States with limited education, language, and computer literacy, they may have difficulty filling out application forms which can be lengthy, complicated, and difficult to navigate (even when forms are available in the parents' native language). Another barrier related to the complexity of the application process and eligibility rules can include rapid and frequent changes in application processes and administrators'/staffs' ability to keep up with changes to effectively guide Hispanic parents. Also, Hispanic immigrant parents may face barriers when having to provide documentation to complete applications or when accessing programs. For example, because Hispanic immigrant parents often work irregular or nontraditional jobs (e.g., day laborers, farm laborers, subcontractors, etc.), they may not be able to show proof of income. Similarly, because some Hispanic immigrant families may share housing with other families and they may not appear on leases or utility bills, parents can face difficulty in showing proof of residence which can complicate enrollment/application processes. Also, questions regarding parents' or family members' social security numbers and legal status can discourage parents and families to take advantage of public programs as parents and/or other family members may not have the required documentation (Crosnoe et al., 2012; Lorenzo-Blanco, Torres, et al., 2016; Perreira et al., 2012; Yoshikawa et al., 2014). These barriers may create stress for parents and families and contribute to their cultural stress experience (Yoshikawa, 2011).

Administrative errors or burdens that can present barriers for Hispanic immigrant parents in accessing schools and other government and nongovernment programs can include administrators/staff difficulty in reviewing documents from Latin American countries. For example, some administrative staff may have difficulty with using and understanding Latin American conventions for names and dates, which can result in data errors, mismatching of records and applications, and delay in successfully processing paperwork. Moreover, some administrators/agency staff may not have the training and skills needed to form trusting relationships with Hispanic immigrant parents and families, keeping parents and families away from accessing and participating in public events/programs. Similarly, some of the cultural stressors reviewed above (e.g., perceived discrimination, negative context of reception, immigration stress) may occur while immigrant parents navigate schools, government agencies, and other public programs (Falicov, 2014; Gassman-Pines, 2015; Gold, 2017) suggesting that administrators/agency staff may not be aware of ways they may be alienating Hispanic parents and families from services and programs they need. These experiences, in turn, may contribute to the cultural stress experience of Hispanic immigrant families.

Hispanic immigrant parents and families can also face language and cultural barriers when navigating US institutions or agencies (Perreira et al., 2012; Yoshikawa et al., 2014). Many Hispanic immigrant parents do not speak English or do not speak it proficiently, and they may not have yet acquired cultural knowledge of how US institutions operate. Although many schools and other agencies make application forms available in Spanish, parents and families often still have to navigate English dominant schools and agency buildings that may lack bilingual staff; bilingual signage to help them navigate buildings; and bilingual internet portals. Moreover, application forms can be lengthy and complicated and may be difficult to understand even for educated English speakers, making the application process even more difficult for Hispanic parents with limited English language and literacy skills. Moreover, because many schools and other public agencies/programs lack bilingual and bicultural staff, many immigrant parents rely on untrained interpreters such as friends, relatives, or children which can pose stress to and suboptimal conditions for Hispanic parents, families, and service providers, creating additional stressors for parents and families (Lorenzo-Blanco, Torres, et al., 2016; Perreira et al., 2012; Yoshikawa et al., 2014). There are also some cultural barriers that may inhibit Hispanic parents' interactions with schools and other public agencies, including differences in cultural beliefs and practices between parents' and the institutions where parents are navigating (Falicov, 2014; Perreira et al., 2012; Suárez-Orozco, Suárez-Orozco, & Todorova, 2009). For example, in some Latin American countries, parents are not expected to actively participate in their children's schooling, and doing so could be interpreted as lacking respect for teachers and school administrators (Falicov, 2014; Suárez-Orozco et al., 2009). As such, Hispanic immigrant parents may not participate in school events or reach out to teachers to help their children succeed. Similarly, many Hispanic immigrant parents value hard work, family support, and self-reliance and may find it difficult and stressful to seek help from public programs and government agencies (Perreira et al., 2012). Moreover, Hispanic immigrant families may feel discomfort with navigating Western medical systems for physical and mental health conditions. Their beliefs about physical and mental health may be incongruent with medical belief systems (Alegría et al., 2015; Perreira et al., 2012), thereby preventing parents and families from seeking help for physical and mental health concerns.

Lastly, Hispanic immigrant parents can face transportation and logistical barriers when accessing schools and other public programs or agencies (Lorenzo-Blanco, Torres, et al., 2016; Perreira et al., 2012). For example, not all Hispanic immigrant parents have cars or driver's licenses; and public transportation may not be a viable option, especially for families living in rural or urban areas with poorly developed public transportation infrastructure. Without dependable transportation and/or training in how to navigate transportation systems, Hispanic immigrant parents may be less able to control their schedules and access or participate in public programs and agencies. Another logistical barrier Hispanic immigrant parents may face involves being able to visit public agencies or participate in school events during working hours, given that many Hispanic immigrants have irregular job schedules and may not have the necessary benefits that allow them to leave their work to take care of family matters (Falicov, 2014; Perreira et al., 2012).

In sum, recent Hispanic immigrant parents and families can encounter numerous barriers in navigating US institutions (e.g., schools). While these barriers have not traditionally been conceptualized as cultural stressors, they can constitute a form of stress and contribute to the cultural stress experience of Hispanic immigrant parents and families, impacting their own and their youths' mental and behavioral health.

Linking Hispanic parents' experiences in the United States with parent and youth mental and behavioral health

Ecodevelopmental theories of development-in-context (e.g., Pantin, Schwartz, Sullivan, Coatsworth, & Szapocznik, 2003; Szapocznik & Coatsworth, 1999) suggest that youth outcomes are directly embedded within multiple social ecologies, including the family system, neighborhood contexts, immigration policies, broader economic forces, and other macrosystemic influences. Within the Hispanic family, closeness to parents is among the strongest predictors of positive youth outcomes and the strongest protective forces against health risk behaviors (e.g., Lorenzo-Blanco et al., 2019). Hispanic parents not only engage in "typical" parenting tasks such as involvement with children, monitoring and shaping behavior, and administering positive discipline, but many Hispanic parents also choose to socialize their children toward their cultural heritage (e.g., Umaña-Taylor, Bhanot, & Shin, 2006). Parents may do this both because of a desire to transmit their heritage language, symbols, and values, as well as to counter the strong assimilationist pressures in the United States (Lutz, 2008). Indeed, Portes and Rumbaut (2014) document that, among Hispanic youth in the United States, Spanish language use declines precipitously between first- and second-generation individuals—and by the third-generation, Spanish is generally lost.

Research indicates that retaining heritage practices, values, and identifications is beneficial for Hispanic youth mental and behavioral health.

Spanish-language use tends to protect against internalizing problems and suicidality (Zayas, 2011), against aggressive and delinquent behavior (Smokowski & Bacallao, 2006), and against sexual risk-taking (Schwartz, Unger, Lorenzo-Blanco, et al., 2014). Traditional Hispanic values, such as familism (valuing the needs of family members over one's own needs), simpatía (being kind and non-confrontational with others), and respeto (showing respect to others), have been shown to protect against internalizing symptoms (Telzer, Tsai, Gonzales, & Fuligni, 2015) and against marijuana use (Ramirez et al., 2004). Telzer et al. found that family obligations may be less protective against internalizing symptoms when the obligation is to a family member who is in crisis.

Immigration rhetoric, policy, and effects on Hispanic families

The larger sociocultural environment also exerts strong impacts on adjustment outcomes among Hispanic families. For example, even for those families who are in the United States legally, the current US climate regarding undocumented immigration and asylum seeking is likely to exert harmful effects (Nguyen & Kebede, 2017). Indeed, exposure to news about the Trump administration's immigration policies, including rescinding Deferred Action for Childhood Arrivals and Temporary Protected Status, has been shown to cause distress among Hispanic parents (Roche, Vaquera, White, & Rivera, 2018). Many Hispanic adolescents and adults worry about themselves, family members, or friends being detained and deported (Quiroga, Medina, & Glick, 2014). In particular, Hispanic people who are undocumented (or know someone who is undocumented), were born outside the US mainland, and/or prefer to speak Spanish may be most likely to experience distress when reminded about the Trump administration's immigration policies (Callister, Galbraith, & Galbraith, 2019). On the other hand, Hispanics who prefer English—and especially those who voted for Trump and/or consider themselves politically conservative—are far less likely to be bothered by the administration's policies on immigration.

Harsh immigration policies also affect Hispanic youth *through* parental stress. Chavez, Lopez, Englebrecht, and Viramontez Anguiano (2012) interviewed immigrant families in Indiana and found that many parents had less patience with their children because of worries about detention or deportation. Further, when undocumented parents are deported, their US-born children must either remain in the United States as orphans or leave with their parents as exiles (Zayas, 2015). Both options are traumatic for youth: Zayas provides a number of case studies of children and adolescents whose parents were deported, and the effect that parental deportation exerts on children's lives. Guadalupe Garcia de Rayos, an undocumented Mexican mother, had been living in Phoenix, Arizona, with her husband and US-born teenage children when she was deported in February 2017—less than a month after Trump's inauguration (Gonzalez, 2018). She is barred from entering the United States and is able to speak with her husband and children only through video chat. Rojas-Flores, Clements, Koo, and

London (2017) found that, according to self, parent, and teacher reports, such forced separation from parents is associated with symptoms of depression, anxiety, posttraumatic stress, and disruptive behavior.

Although many conservative commentators (e.g., Buchanan, 2011a, 2011b) demonize undocumented immigrants as a monolithic "threat" to the United States, in reality, the picture is far more complex. Whereas the stereotypical portrayal of undocumented families involves parents sneaking illegally across the Mexican border in the middle of the night with children in tow, many Hispanic families are "mixed status"—that is, some family members are in the United States legally whereas others are undocumented (Golash-Boza, 2012). Further, there are multiple ways to be undocumented. One can cross the border illegally, overstay a visa, refuse to leave the country following a denied asylum request, or turn 18 before one's parents have become naturalized US citizens. In fact, visa overstays—not illegal border crossers—represent the majority of undocumented immigrants (Gonzales, 2019).

Parent-adolescent acculturation discrepancies

Aside from the main effects of family and wider ecosystemic processes, *discrepancies* between parent and adolescent acculturation profiles may also be predictive of adolescent outcomes. Based on their clinical work with Hispanic behavior-problem youth, Szapocznik and Kurtines (1993) introduced the "acculturation discrepancy hypothesis." This hypothesis proposed that, in immigrant families, youth adapt to the destination culture far more quickly and completely than their parents do. As a result, a cultural disconnect emerges in the family, whereby youth are more "Americanized" whereas parents are more traditional. These discrepancies, the hypothesis proposes, then serve to compromise family functioning—which in turn leads to problematic adolescent outcomes such as delinquency, drug, and alcohol use, and sexual risk-taking.

Subsequent iterations of the parent-adolescent acculturation discrepancy hypothesis have been more nuanced. Because acculturation consists of both heritage-culture retention and destination-culture acquisition, discrepancies can emerge in either or both of these dimensions (Telzer, 2010). Telzer argues that discrepancies in US-culture acquisition are largely benign and may even be beneficial to families. The concept of cultural brokering, whereby children and adolescents help their parents to open bank accounts, communicate with doctors, and purchase cars and homes, rests on the assumption that youth are more familiar and comfortable with US culture than their parents are (see Weisskirch, 2017, for a collection of reviews). The more pernicious discrepancies are likely to be those where youth relinquish their cultural heritage whereas parents remain loyal to that heritage. For example, because language is a marker and transmitter of cultural heritage (Kang, 2006), youth who are unable to unwilling to communicate in Spanish with their families may be viewed as disrespectful and disloyal (Smokowski & Bacallao, 2011).

Although earlier, cross-sectional tests of the acculturation discrepancy hypothesis were inconclusive, more recent longitudinal tests have supported Telzer's (2010) predictions. Unger, Ritt-Olson, Soto, and Baezconde-Garbanati (2009) found that discrepancies between adolescents' behavioral acculturation and how they believed their parents expected them to acculturate predicted reduced levels of adolescent-reported family cohesion, which in turn predicted cigarette and marijuana use. In a recent meta-analysis on acculturation mismatch, intergenerational cultural conflict, and mental health outcomes among Asian and Hispanic families, Lui (2015) found that acculturation mismatch in terms of acculturation patterns and/or cultural values between parents and their children was positively associated with intergenerational cultural conflict, which in turn was positively associated with internalizing problems, but not externalizing problems. Gonzales et al. (2018) found, among Mexican American families in Arizona, mother-adolescent and father-adolescent gaps in heritage values predicted family conflict and youth internalizing and externalizing problems—but only in cases where adolescents' heritage values declined over time and parents' heritage values remained consistent. Schwartz et al. (2016) found that parent-adolescent discrepancies in heritage-cultural practices (e.g., speaking Spanish), values (e.g., familism), and identifications (e.g., taking pride in being from one's country of origin) were significantly and negatively predictive of family functioning (parental involvement, positive parenting, and parent-adolescent communication). In turn, compromised family functioning was predictive of depressive symptoms, delinquency, and binge drinking, and negatively predictive of self-esteem, optimism, and prosocial behavior. Supporting Telzer's (2010) argument, discrepancies in individualist (US) values and in identification with the United States were *positively* predictive of family functioning and indirectly predictive of youth outcomes. What can be surmised here is that, when youth begin to relinquish their heritage values, *or* when parents increase in heritage-culture orientations but youth do not, family functioning may be impaired.

What is less well known, however, is what larger forces may be *responsible* for parent-adolescent acculturation discrepancies. Gonzales et al. (2018) found a number of different types of discrepancies, only some of which posed risks for family functioning and youth outcomes. The majority of families in the recent-immigrant sample of Schwartz et al. (2016) were not characterized by parent-adolescent acculturation discrepancies. Macrosocial forces such as immigration policies and rhetoric are likely constant across families (although US states differ in terms of the extent to which they support or oppose such policies and rhetoric; Young & Wallace, 2019). Other factors, such as association with Americanized peers and pressure to become a monolingual English speaker may be more likely to create cultural discrepancies within the family. It is essential to conduct research to identify such predictors so that acculturation discrepancies within the family can be prevented or ameliorated.

Recommendations for future research

Research on cultural stressors in the lives of Hispanic immigrant parents and families have employed survey and qualitative research methods with Hispanic parents, youth, and families to better understand their cultural stress experiences (Cano et al., 2015; Leon, 2014; Perreira et al., 2006). Data from these studies have informed interventions to improve the emotional and behavioral health of youth by teaching parents how to support their youth; how to strengthen their relationships with their youth; how to advocate for their youth; and how to navigate US social institutions (Cervantes, Goldbach, & Santos, 2011; Coatsworth, Pantin, & Szapocznik, 2002; Martinez, Eddy, & McClure, 2014; Martinez & Eddy, 2005). These intervention efforts are timely and needed. However, these intervention efforts put the sole burden of dealing with cultural stressors and navigating barriers on Hispanic parents and families. However, because cultural stressors and barriers Hispanic parents and families face are embedded in social institutions and systems, such as schools, over which Hispanic immigrant parents have little personnel control, we propose that additional efforts are needed that also target social institutions and their organizational structures (e.g., policies). Yet, few studies have examined how social institutions and their organizational structures and policies contribute to the cultural stress experience of Hispanic parents and families. We propose that future research needs to examine how social institutions impact the day-to-day experiences of Hispanic parents and families. Also, because we could not identify any efforts or strategies that target social institutions and their organizational structures to promote the mental and behavioral health of Hispanic parents, youth, and families, we further propose that research needs to investigate how organizational structures and policies may be altered to reduce barriers and cultural stressors for Hispanic immigrant parents and families; and to mitigate the impact of cultural stressors and barriers on the well-being of parents and their families. This may be done by making social institutions, their policies, and their processes the focus of research on the mental and behavioral health of Hispanic parents, youth, and families.

Although numerous studies have documented the various cultural stressors and barriers Hispanic immigrant parents and families can face, we know almost nothing regarding how parents and families manage these stressors and barriers. Many parents and youth experience cultural stressors and may face barriers in accessing and navigating US institutions, yet, not all parents and youth experience emotional and behavioral health problems. Understanding how parents and families successfully manage cultural stressors and barriers can provide important information about how to create community-informed programs to support recent immigrant Hispanic parents and their families (Ford-Paz, Reinhard, Kuebbeler, Contreras, & Sánchez, 2015; Jason, Keys, Suarez-Balcazar, Taylor, & Davis, 2004; Romero, 2016). As such, we propose that research is needed that documents strategies that parents and families are utilizing to manage the cultural stressors and barriers they face. In addition, we propose that research is needed that documents the kind of support and resources Hispanic immigrant parents, youth, and families would like to further develop so that efforts can address the needs of parents and families. This information could be used to develop community-informed strategies to support Hispanic immigrant parents and families, thereby reducing barriers and cultural stressors and mitigating their negative effects (Ford-Paz et al., 2015; Ramirez et al., 2017).

Studies have also documented barriers Hispanic immigrant parents can face when navigating social institutions such as social institutions such as schools, government agencies, health and mental health services (Crosnoe et al., 2012; Perreira et al., 2012; Yoshikawa et al., 2014); however, much of what we know comes from interviews and surveys with individuals working at these institutions. Thus, we know less about how parents and families experience social institutions. We propose that research on barriers among Hispanic families could also benefit from incorporating the perspectives of parents and families and examine how recent immigrant parents and families experience the organizational structures and policies of social institutions they navigate. Understanding the perspectives of Hispanic stakeholders and individuals working in social institutions can inform more comprehensive strategies to reduce barriers and cultural stressors and to mitigate their negative effects on the mental and behavioral health of immigrant parents and their families.

References

Alegría, M., Green, J. G., McLaughlin, K., & Loder, S. (2015). *Disparities in child and adolescent mental health and mental health services in the US*. New York: William T. Grant Foundation.

Buchanan, P. J. (2007). *State of emergency: The Third World invasion and conquest of America*. New York: St. Martin's Press.

Buchanan, P. J. (2011a). *State of emergency: The Third World invasion and conquest of America*. New York: St. Martin's Press.

Buchanan, P. J. (2011b). *Suicide of a superpower*. New York: St. Martin's Press.

Callister, A. H., Galbraith, Q., & Galbraith, S. (2019). Immigration, deportation, and discrimination: Hispanic political opinion since the election of Donald Trump. *Hispanic Journal of Behavioral Sciences*, *41*, 166–184.

Cano, M.Á., Schwartz, S. J., Castillo, L. G., Romero, A. J., Huang, S., Lorenzo-Blanco, E. I., … Baezconde-Garbanati, L. (2015). Depressive symptoms and externalizing behaviors among Hispanic immigrant adolescents: Examining longitudinal effects of cultural stress. *Journal of Adolescence*, *42*, 31–39.

Cavazos-Rehg, P. A., Zayas, L. H., Walker, M. S., & Fisher, E. B. (2006). Evaluating an abbreviated version of the Hispanic stress inventory for immigrants. *Hispanic Journal of Behavioral Sciences*, *28*(4), 498–515.

Cervantes, R., Goldbach, J., & Santos, S. M. (2011). Familia adelante: A multi-risk prevention intervention for Latino families. *Journal of Primary Prevention*, *32*(3–4), 225–234.

Cervantes, R. C., Padilla, A. M., & Salgado de Snyder, N. (1991). The Hispanic stress inventory: A culturally relevant approach to psychosocial assessment. *Psychological Assessment: A Journal of Consulting and Clinical Psychology*, *3*(3), 438.

Chavez, L. R. (2013). *The Latino threat*. Berkeley: University of California Press.

Chavez, J. M., Lopez, A., Englebrecht, C. L., & Viramontez Anguiano, R. P. (2012). *Sufren los niños*: Exploring the impact of unauthorized immigration status on children's well-being. *Family Court Review, 50*, 638–649.

Chishti, M., Pierce, S., & Telus, H. (2019). Spike in unaccompanied child arrivals at U.S.-Mexico border proves enduring challenge; citizenship question on 2020 census in doubt. *Migration Policy Institute*. Retrieved from https://www.migrationpolicy.org/article/spike-unaccompanied-child-arrivals-proves-enduring-challenge.

Chomsky, A. (2007). *They take our jobs!: And 20 other myths about immigration*. Boston: Beacon Press.

Coatsworth, J. D., Pantin, H., & Szapocznik, J. (2002). Familias Unidas: A family-centered ecodevelopmental intervention to reduce risk for problem behavior among Hispanic adolescents. *Clinical Child and Family Psychology Review, 5*(2), 113–132.

Coenders, M., Lubbers, M., Scheepers, P., & Verkuyten, M. (2008). More than two decades of changing ethnic attitudes in the Netherlands. *Journal of Social Issues, 64*, 269–285.

Conger, R. D., Conger, K. J., & Martin, M. J. (2010). Socioeconomic status, family processes, and individual development. *Journal of Marriage and Family, 72*(3), 685–704.

Conger, R. D., Song, H., Stockdale, G. D., Ferrer, E., Widaman, K. F., & Cauce, A. M. (2012). Resilience and vulnerability of Mexican origin youth and their families: A test of a culturally informed model of family economic stress. In P. K. Kerig, M. S. Schulz, S. T. Hauser, P. K. Kerig, M. S. Schulz, & S. T. Hauser (Eds.), *Adolescence and beyond: Family processes and development* (pp. 268–286). New York, NY: Oxford University Press.

Crosnoe, R., Pedroza, J., Purtell, K., Fortuny, K., Perreira, K., Ulvestad, K., ... Chaudry, A. (2012). *Promising practices for increasing immigrants' access to health and human services*. Washington, DC: Office of the Assistant Secretary for Planning and Evaluation (ASPE), US Department of Health and Human Services.

Deater-Deckard, K. (2008). *Parenting stress*. Yale University Press.

Devos, T., & Banaji, M. R. (2005). American = White? *Journal of Personality and Social Psychology, 88*, 447–466.

Falicov, C. J. (2014). *Latino families in therapy* (2nd ed.). New York: Guilford Press.

Flores, A. (2017). *How the US Hispanic population is changing*. Retrieved from https://www.pewresearch.org/fact-tank/2017/09/18/how-the-u-s-hispanic-population-is-changing/.

Flores, A., & Krogstad, J. M. (2019). *Puerto Rico's population declined sharply after Hurricanes Maria and Irma* Retrieved from https://www.pewresearch.org/fact-tank/2019/07/26/puerto-rico-population-2018/.

Flores, A., Lopez, M. H., & Krogstad, J. M. (2019). *US Hispanic population reached a new high in 2018, but growth has slowed*. Retrieved from https://www.pewresearch.org/fact-tank/2019/07/08/u-s-hispanic-population-reached-new-high-in-2018-but-growth-has-slowed/.

Folkman, S., Lazarus, R. S., Gruen, R. J., & DeLongis, A. (1986). Appraisal, coping, health status, and psychological symptoms. *Journal of Personality and Social Psychology, 50*(3), 571.

Ford-Paz, R. E., Reinhard, C., Kuebbeler, A., Contreras, R., & Sánchez, B. (2015). Culturally tailored depression/suicide prevention in Latino youth: community perspectives. *Journal of Behavioral Health Services & Research, 42*(4), 519–533.

Gassman-Pines, A. (2015). Effects of Mexican immigrant parents' daily workplace discrimination on child behavior and family functioning. *Child Development*, (4), 1175–1190.

Gjelten, T. (2015). *Nation of nations: A great American immigration story*. New York: Simon and Schuster.

Golash-Boza, T. M. (2012). *Immigration nation: Raids, detentions, and deportations in post-9/11 America*. New York: Routledge.

Gold, L. A. (2017). *"They don't say it up front": Immigrant-origin high school students' experiences of disrespect and racial microaggressions by teachers: A project based upon a group research investigation* [Theses and Dissertations]. Smith College.

Gonzales, R. (2019). *For 7th consecutive year, visa overstays exceeded illegal border crossings.* National Public Radio. Retrieved from https://www.npr.org/2019/01/16/686056668/for-seventh-consecutive-year-visa-overstays-exceeded-illegal-border-crossings.

Gonzales, N. A., Knight, G. P., Gunn, H. J., Tein, J.-Y., Tanaka, R., & White, R. M. B. (2018). Intergenerational gaps in Mexican American values trajectories: Associations with parent–adolescent conflict and adolescent psychopathology. *Development and Psychopathology, 30*, 1611–1627.

Gonzalez, D. (2018). *Deported mom makes new life in Mexico but misses kids "dearly".* Arizona Republic. Retrieved from https://www.azcentral.com/story/news/politics/immigration/2018/02/09/deported-arizona-mom-guadalupe-garcia-de-rayos-1-year-later-life-mexico/308079002/.

Hartman, T. K., Newman, B. K., & Bell, C. S. (2014). Decoding prejudice toward Hispanics: Group cues and public reactions to threatening immigrant behavior. *Political Behavior, 36*, 143–163.

Hogan, J., & Haltinner, K. (2015). Floods, invaders, and parasites: Immigration threat narratives and right-wing populism in the USA, UK and Australia. *Journal of Intercultural Studies, 36*, 520–543.

Huntington, S. P. (2004). *Who are we? The challenge to America's national identity.* New York: Simon and Schuster.

Jardina, A. (2019). *White identity politics.* New York: Cambridge University Press.

Jason, L. A., Keys, C. B., Suarez-Balcazar, Y. E., Taylor, R. R., & Davis, M. I. (2004). *Participatory community research: Theories and methods in action*. American Psychological Association.

Kang, S. M. (2006). Measurement of acculturation, scale formats, and language competence: Their implications for adjustment. *Journal of Cross-Cultural Psychology, 37*, 669–693.

Kim, S. Y., Schwartz, S. J., Perreira, K. M., & Juang, L. P. (2018). Culture's influence on stressors, parental socialization, and developmental processes in the mental health of children of immigrants. *Annual Review of Clinical Psychology, 14*, 343–370.

Krogstad, J. M. (2014). *With fewer new arrivals, Census lowers Hispanic population projections.* Retrieved from https://www.pewresearch.org/fact-tank/2014/12/16/with-fewer-new-arrivals-census-lowers-hispanic-population-projections-2/.

Landale, N., McHale, S., & Booth, A. (2010). *Growing up Hispanic: Health and development of children of immigrants.* Urban Institute Press.

Lee, J. P., Lee, R. M., & Tran, A.G.G.T. (2017). Theory and measurement of foreigner objectification. In S. J. Schwartz & J. B. Unger (Eds.), *Oxford handbook of acculturation and health* (pp. 157–174). New York: Oxford University Press.

Leon, A. L. (2014). Immigration and stress: The relationship between parents' acculturative stress and young children's anxiety symptoms. *Inquiries Journal, 6*(03). Retrieved from http://www.inquiriesjournal.com/a?id=861.

Lorenzo-Blanco, E. I., Meca, A., Piña-Watson, B., Zamboanga, B. L., Szapocznik, J., Cano, M. A., … Schwartz, S. J. (2019). Longitudinal trajectories of family functioning among recent immigrant Latino families: Links with cultural stress, emotional well-being, and behavioral health. *Child Development, 90*, 506–523.

Lorenzo-Blanco, E. I., Meca, A., Unger, J. B., Romero, A., Gonzales-Backen, M., Piña-Watson, B., … Soto, D. W. (2016). Latino parent acculturation stress: Longitudinal effects on family functioning and youth emotional and behavioral health. *Journal of Family Psychology, 30*(8), 966.

Lorenzo-Blanco, E. I., Torres, M. E., & Smithwick, J. (2016). *Latino/a Mental Health in South Carolina: An assessment of mental health needs, existing resources, and current challenges*.

Lui, P. P. (2015). Intergenerational conflict, mental health, and educational outcomes among Asian and Latino/a Americans: Qualitative and meta-analytic review. *Psychological Bulletin, 141*, 404–446.

Lutz, A. (2008). Spanish maintenance among English-speaking Latino youth: The role of individual and social characteristics. *Social Forces, 84*, 1417–1433.

Macias, R. F. (2000). The flowering of America: Linguistic diversity in the United States. In S. McKay & S. Wong (Eds.), *New immigrants in the United States: Readings for second language educators* (pp. 11–57). Cambridge: Cambridge University Press.

Martinez, C. R., Jr, & Eddy, J. M. (2005). Effects of culturally adapted parent management training on Latino youth behavioral health outcomes. *Journal of Consulting and Clinical Psychology, 73*, 841.

Martinez, C., Jr., Eddy, J., & McClure, H. (2014). Nuestras Familias: Replicating the effects of a preventive intervention to promote strong Latino families. *Family Relations, 55*(3), 306–317.

Moshman, D. (2011). Identity, genocide, and group violence. In S. J. Schwartz, K. Luyckx, & V. L. Vignoles (Eds.), *Handbook of identity theory and research* (pp. 881–896). New York: Springer.

Nguyen, C., & Kebede, M. (2017). Immigrant students in the Trump era: What we know and do not know. *Educational Policy, 31*, 716–742.

North, R. J., Swann, W. B., Jr. (2009). Self-verification 360: Illuminating the light and dark sides. *Self and Identity, 8*, 131–146.

Pantin, H., Schwartz, S. J., Sullivan, S., Coatsworth, J. D., & Szapocznik, J. (2003). Preventing substance abuse in Hispanic immigrant adolescents: An ecodevelopmental, parent-centered approach. *Hispanic Journal of Behavioral Sciences, 25*, 469–500.

Pérez, D. J., Fortuna, L., & Alegria, M. (2008). Prevalence and correlates of everyday discrimination among US Latinos. *Journal of Community Psychology, 36*(4), 421–433.

Perreira, K. M., Chapman, M. V., & Stein, G. L. (2006). Becoming an American parent: Overcoming challenges and finding strength in a new immigrant Latino community. *Journal of Family Issues, 27*(10), 1383–1414.

Perreira, K. M., Crosnoe, R., Fortuny, K., Pedroza, J., Ulvestad, K., Weiland, C., … Chaudry, A. (2012). *Barriers to immigrants' access to health and human services programs*. ASPE Issue Brief Washington, DC: Office of the Assistant Secretary for Planning and Evaluation.

Piedrabuena, M. (2018). *Here's what it feels like to be Latino on Long Island right now*. Retrieved from https://riverheadlocal.com/2018/08/26/heres-what-it-feels-like-to-be-latino-on-long-island-right-now/.

Portes, A., & Rumbaut, R. G. (2014). *Immigrant America: A portrait* (3rd ed.). Berkeley: University of California Press.

Quiroga, S. S., Medina, D. M., & Glick, J. (2014). In the belly of the beast: Effects of anti-immigration policy on Latino community members. *American Behavioral Scientist, 58*, 1723–1742.

Ramirez, J. R., Crano, W. D., Quist, R., Burgoon, M., Alvaro, E. M., & Grandpre, J. (2004). Acculturation, familism, parental monitoring, and knowledge as predictors of marijuana and inhalant use in adolescents. *Psychology of Addictive Behaviors, 18*, 3–11.

Ramirez, A., Gallion, K., Aguilar, R., & Dembeck, E. (2017). *Mental health and Latino kids: A research review* (pp. 1–22). Salud America.

Roche, K. M., Vaquera, E., White, R. M., & Rivera, M. I. (2018). Impacts of immigration actions and news and the psychological distress of US Latino parents raising adolescents. *Journal of Adolescent Health, 62*, 525–531.

Rojas-Flores, L., Clements, M. L., Koo, J. K., & London, J. (2017). Trauma and psychological distress in Latino citizen children following parental detention and deportation. *Psychological Trauma: Theory, Research, Practice, and Policy*, *9*, 352–361.

Romero, A. (2016). *Youth-community partnerships for adolescent alcohol prevention: "We can't do it alone"*. In *Youth-community partnerships for adolescent alcohol prevention* (pp. 1 -17). Springer.

Rumbaut, R. G. (2008). Reaping what you sow: Immigration, youth, and reactive ethnicity. *Applied Developmental Science*, *12*, 108–111.

Sabates-Wheeler, R., Sabates, R., & Castaldo, A. (2008). Tackling poverty-migration linkages: Evidence from Ghana and Egypt. *Social Indicators Research*, *87*, 307–328.

Schildkraut, D. J. (2014). Boundaries of AmericanIdentity: Evolving understandings of "us". *Annual Review of Political Science*, *17*, 1–20.

Schwartz, S. J., Pantin, H., Sullivan, S., Prado, G., & Szapocznik, J. (2006). Nativity and years in the receiving culture as markers of acculturation in ethnic enclaves. *Journal of Cross-Cultural Psychology*, *37*, 345–353.

Schwartz, S. J., Unger, J. B., Baezconde-Garbanati, L., Zamboanga, B. L., Córdova, D., Lorenzo-Blanco, E. I., … Szapocznik, J. (2016). Testing the parent-adolescent acculturation discrepancy hypothesis: A five-wave longitudinal study. *Journal of Research on Adolescence*, *26*, 567–586.

Schwartz, S. J., Unger, J. B., Des Rosiers, S. E., Lorenzo-Blanco, E. I., Zamboanga, B. L., Huang, S., … Szapocznik, J. (2014). Domains of acculturation and their effects on substance use and sexual behavior in Hispanic recent immigrant adolescents. *Prevention Science*, *15*, 385–396.

Schwartz, S. J., Unger, J. B., Lorenzo-Blanco, E. I., Des Rosiers, S. E., Villamar, J. A., Soto, D. W., … Szapocznik, J. (2014). Perceived context of reception among recent Hispanic immigrants: Conceptualization, instrument development, and preliminary validation. *Cultural Diversity and Ethnic Minority Psychology*, *20*(1), 1.

Selden, D. A., Pace, J. A., & Nunn-Gilman, H. (2011). Placing S.B. 1070 and racial profiling into context, and what S.B. 1070 reveals about the legislative process in Arizona. *Immigration and Nationality Review*, *27*, 27.

Sladkova, J. (2007). Expectations and motivations of Hondurans migrating to the United States. *Journal of Community and Applied Social Psychology*, *17*, 187–202.

Smokowski, P. R., & Bacallao, M. L. (2006). Acculturation and aggression in Latino adolescents: a structural model focusing on cultural risk factors and assets. *Journal of Abnormal Child Psychology*, *34*, 657–671.

Smokowski, P. R., & Bacallao, M. L. (2011). *Becoming bicultural: Risk, resilience, and Latino youth*. New York: New York University Press.

Southern Poverty Law Center. (2009). *Climate of fear: Latino immigrants in Suffolk County, New York*. Retrieved from https://www.splcenter.org/20090831/climate-fear-latino-immigrants-suffolk-county-ny.

Staerklé, C., Sidanius, J., Green, E. G. T., & Molina, L. E. (2010). Ethnic minority-majority asymmetry in national attitudes around the world: A multilevel analysis. *Political Psychology*, *31*, 491–519.

Stephan, W. G., Ybarra, O., & Bachman, G. (1999). Prejudice toward immigrants: An integrated threat theory. *Journal of Applied Social Psychology*, *29*, 2221–2237.

Sterba, C. M. (2003). *Good Americans: Italian and Jewish immigrants during the First World War*. New York: Oxford University Press.

Suárez-Orozco, C., Suárez-Orozco, M. M., & Todorova, I. (2009). *Learning a new land*. Harvard University Press.

Suárez-Orozco, C., Yoshikawa, H., & Tseng, V. (2015). *Intersecting inequalities: Research to reduce inequality for immigrant-origin children and youth*. William T. Grant Foundation.

Szapocznik, J., & Coatsworth, J. D. (1999). An ecodevelopmental framework for organizing the influences on drug abuse: A developmental model of risk and protection. In *Drug abuse: Origins & interventions*. American Psychological Association. (pp. 331–366).

Szapocznik, J., & Kurtines, W. M. (1993). Family psychology and cultural diversity: Opportunities for theory, research, and application. *American Psychologist*, *48*, 400–407.

Telzer, E. H. (2010). Expanding the acculturation gap-distress model: An integrative review of research. *Human Development*, *53*, 313–340.

Telzer, E. H., Tsai, K. M., Gonzales, N. A., & Fuligni, A. J. (2015). Mexican American adolescents' family obligation values and behaviors: Links to internalizing symptoms across time and context. *Developmental Psychology*, *51*, 75–86.

Torres, L., Driscoll, M. W., & Voell, M. (2012). Discrimination, acculturation, acculturative stress, and Latino psychological distress: A moderated mediational model. *Cultural Diversity and Ethnic Minority Psychology*, *18*(1), 17.

Tran, V. C. (2010). English gain versus Spanish loss? Language assimilation among second-generation Latinos in young adulthood. *Social Forces*, *89*, 257–284.

Tran, A. G. (2014). Family contexts: Parental experiences of discrimination and child mental health. *American Journal of Community Psychology*, *53*(1–2), 37–46.

Umaña-Taylor, A. J., Bhanot, R., & Shin, N. (2006). Ethnic identity formation during adolescence: The critical role of families. *Journal of Family Issues*, *27*, 390–414.

Unger, J. B., Ritt-Olson, A., Soto, D. W., & Baezconde-Garbanati, L. (2009). Parent–child acculturation discrepancies as a risk factor for substance use among Hispanic adolescents in Southern California. *Journal of Immigrant and Minority Health*, *11*(3), 149–157.

US Census Bureau. (2012). *A look at the 1940 Census*. Retrieved from https://www.census.gov/newsroom/cspan/1940census/CSPAN_1940slides.pdf.

US Citizenship and Immigration Services. (2019). *Asylum office workload, January 2019*. Retrieved from https://www.uscis.gov/sites/default/files/USCIS/Outreach/Notes%20from%20Previous%20Engagements/PED_AffirmativeAsylumStatisticsJan2019.pdf.

Velasco González, K., Verkuyten, M., Weesie, J., & Poppe, E. (2008). Prejudice towards Muslims in The Netherlands: Testing integrated threat theory. *British Journal of Social Psychology*, *47*, 667–685.

Weisskirch, R. S. (Ed.), (2017). *Language brokering in immigrant families: Theories and concepts*. New York: Routledge.

White, R. M., Roosa, M. W., Weaver, S. R., & Nair, R. L. (2009). Cultural and contextual influences on parenting in Mexican American families. *Journal of Marriage and Family*, *71*(1), 61–79.

Wodak, R., & Krzyżanowski, M. (2017). Contesting politics & discourse: Beyond 'Orbanism' and 'Trumpism'. *Journal of Language and Politics*, *16*, 471–484.

Woods, J., & Arthur, C. D. (2017). *Debating immigration in the age of terrorism, polarization, and Trump*. New York: Lexington Books.

Yoshikawa, H. (2011). *Immigrants raising citizens: Undocumented parents and their children*. Russell Sage Foundation.

Yoshikawa, H., Weiland, C., Ulvestad, K., Perreira, K. M., & Crosnoe, R. (2014). *Improving access of low-income immigrant families to health and human services*. Washington, DC: Urban Institute.

Young, M.-E.D.T., & Wallace, S. P. (2019). Included, but deportable: A new public health approach to policies that criminalize and integrate immigrants. *American Journal of Public Health*, *109*, 1171–1176.

Zayas, L. H. (2011). *Latinas attempting suicide: When cultures, families, and daughters collide*. New York: Oxford University Press.

Zayas, L. H. (2015). *Forgotten citizens: Deportation, children, and the making of American exiles and orphans*. New York: Oxford University Press.

Further reading

Lorenzo-Blanco, E. I., Meca, A., Unger, J. B., Romero, A., Szapocznik, J., Piña-Watson, B., … Des Rosiers, S. E. (2017). Longitudinal effects of Latino parent cultural stress, depressive symptoms, and family functioning on youth emotional well-being and health risk behaviors. *Family Process*, *56*(4), 981–996.

Martinez, C. R., Jr., DeGarmo, D. S., & Eddy, J. M. (2004). Promoting academic success among Latino youths. *Hispanic Journal of Behavioral Sciences*, *26*(2), 128–151.

Schwartz, S. J., Unger, J. B., Baezconde-Garbanati, L., Zamboanga, B. L., Lorenzo-Blanco, E. I., Des Rosiers, S. E., … Córdova, D. (2015). Trajectories of cultural stressors and effects on mental health and substance use among Hispanic immigrant adolescents. *Journal of Adolescent Health*, *56*(4), 433–439.

Suárez-Orozco, C., & Suárez-Orozco, M. M. (2014). Structuring opportunity for immigration origin children. In *Bread and brain, education and poverty, Vatican City*.

Chapter 7

Contextual stressors and the role of religion and spirituality in the mental health of Latino/a immigrant parents and youth

Rosario Ceballo, Francheska Alers-Rojas, Jessica P. Montoro and Andrea S. Mora
University of Michigan, Ann Arbor, MI, United States

Latino/as are the fastest-growing and largest ethnic minority group in the United States, now representing 18% of the total US population. Only one-third of the 58.9 million Latino/as currently living in the US were born in a foreign country (U.S. Census Bureau, 2018). Latino/a immigrants are defined as individuals who have moved across national borders, away from their country of origin. In this chapter, we use Suárez-Orozco, Motti-Stefanidi, Marks, and Katsiaficas (2018) definitions for immigrant youth. Whereas first-generation immigrant youth are those who were born outside of the United States, second-generation immigrant youth were born in the United States and have at least one foreign-born parent. Historically, three primary reasons for Latino/as' immigration to the United States have remained consistent over time: (1) to seek economic opportunities and employment, (2) to improve the educational opportunities for their children and future generations, and (3) to flee political and criminal violence in their home countries (Alcántara, Chen, & Alegria, 2014; Perreira, Chapman, & Stein, 2006).

Over the past 50 years, patterns of migration among Latino/as have dramatically changed the demographics of the United States. Before 1970, Latino/as were ethnically less diverse and geographically concentrated in the Southwest, Northeast, and the Miami Metropolitan area (Massey, Durand, & Pren, 2016). New patterns of migration, starting in the 1970s, brought Latino/as from different countries and into new regions. Although outside the scope of this chapter, these new patterns emerged, in part, due to the US interventionist policies that created political, economic, and social turmoil in Latin America and the Caribbean (Massey et al., 2016). Between 1970 and 2010, 11.7 million Latin

Mental and Behavioral Health of Immigrants in the United States
https://doi.org/10.1016/B978-0-12-816117-3.00007-5

Americans legally migrated to the United States. At the same time, the undocumented Latino/a population increased to around 8.8 million (Massey et al., 2016). The majority of Latin American migrants do not enter the United States illegally; rather, they arrive with legal visas and overstay their departure date (Passel & Cohn, 2019). Others have temporary permission but could be subject to deportation, including people from three Latin American nations with former Temporary Protected Status (Nicaragua, El Salvador, and Honduras), beneficiaries of Deferred Action for Childhood Arrivals (DACA), and asylum seekers (Passel & Cohn, 2019). Finally, Puerto Rican migrants who come to the US mainland are US citizens.

Issues affecting Latino/a immigrants' mental health will understandably vary before migration, during the process of migration itself, and postmigration. Even though Latino/a immigrant youth and parents are susceptible to experiences of trauma throughout their lives, a preponderance of research has focused on postmigration experiences. Before migration, low family income and less educational attainment in Latino/a immigrants' home countries are linked to higher rates of depressive symptoms (Ornelas & Perreira, 2011). Moreover, premigration traumatic experiences (e.g., criminal victimization, physical or sexual abuse, wars, and natural disasters) are not uncommon for Latino/a immigrants (Li, 2016). For children and adults, traumatic events related to the migration process itself are associated with a host of psychological difficulties, including symptoms of anxiety, depression, externalizing behaviors, and post-traumatic stress disorder (PTSD) (Caballero et al., 2017; Perreira & Ornelas, 2013; Torres & Wallace, 2013). Moreover, Ornelas and Perreira (2011) found that the impact of premigration and migration-related stressors on depressive symptomatology persisted for years after Latino/a immigrant parents were settled in the United States.

Following migration, different patterns of mental health issues emerge among Latino/as. Specifically, scholars have reported evidence of an "immigrant paradox" whereby foreign-born, Latino/a immigrants experience lower rates of mental health problems and psychiatric disorders when compared to US-born Latino/as of later generations and non-Latino/a White individuals (Grant et al., 2004; Ornelas & Perreira, 2011). Since higher lifetime rates of psychiatric disorders are thought to coincide with various aspects of a US lifestyle, it is not surprising that Latino/a immigrants who are born in or who spend more time in the United States will be subjected to greater mental health risks. Nonetheless, caution is warranted in viewing the immigrant paradox as a phenomenon applicable to all Latino/as across all types of psychiatric disorders. Indeed, Alegria et al. (2008) found that while the immigrant paradox held for Mexicans with regard to anxiety, mood, and substance disorders, it was only apparent among other Latino/as for substance disorders, and no evidence of the immigrant paradox was found among Puerto Ricans. Thus, the picture of Latino/a immigrant mental health is likely to be more complex than the immigrant paradox may lead us to believe. On the whole, it is important to remember that Latino/as consist of a highly heterogenous group of people, representing a host of different subethnicities, premigration histories, and so forth. Latino/as can be of any race, sexual identity, socioeconomic status, and any of over 30 different ethnic identities. This diversity also accounts for different experiences based on Latino/as' intersectional identities. For example, in one study, 53% of Latino/as with darker skin reported that they were subjected to slurs or jokes compared to 34% of those with lighter skin (Gonzalez-Barrera, 2019).

Despite the protection conferred by the immigrant paradox, many Latino/a immigrants in the United States encounter significant challenges, including acculturative stress, community violence, educational barriers, financial stressors, language barriers, limited access to health care, migration-related traumas, as well as racism and discrimination; furthermore, all of these challenges present a threat to Latino/a immigrants' mental health (Arbona et al., 2010; Cobb, Meca, Xie, Schwartz, & Moise, 2017; Siemons, Raymond-Flesh, Auerswald, & Brindis, 2017). Anxiety and major depression are the most prevalent mental health disorders reported among Latino/a youth; moreover, Latino/a adolescents report higher rates of suicide attempts when compared to African American and non-Latino/a White youth (Caballero et al., 2017; Lee & Liechty, 2015). However, compared to non-Latino Whites, Latino/a immigrants are less likely to seek mental health-care services for depression (Tyson, Arriola, & Corvin, 2016).

In this chapter, we provide a review of the literature addressing the mental health of Latino/a immigrant youth and parents. In doing so, we rely upon the integrative risk and resilience model proposed by Suárez-Orozco et al. (2018). Their model integrates several theoretical frameworks, including Bronfenbrenner's ecological model, García Coll and colleagues' integrative model for the study of developmental competencies in minority children, and Masten's developmental framework of risk and resilience. We will first review various challenges in the political and social contexts of reception (e.g., attitudes toward immigrants) and in the microsystem (e.g., neighborhood and school climates) that influence the mental health of both Latino/a immigrant youth and parents. Next, we focus on one of the specific intersecting social positions identified by Suárez-Orozco and colleagues, namely religion and spirituality. We examine religiosity and spirituality as sources of strength and resilience for Latino/a immigrant youth and parents. Finally, we conclude with a discussion of the mechanisms by which religiosity and spirituality may influence the psychological functioning and well-being of Latino/a immigrant families.

Challenges affecting the mental health of Latino/a immigrant youth and parents

Sociopolitical climate

Recent restrictive immigration policies and enforcement strategies have heightened stress and fear among undocumented immigrants and their families

(Lopez et al., 2017). Discussions of stronger border security and mass deportations, an attempt to end the Deferred Action for Childhood Arrivals (DACA) program, and the end of the Temporary Protected Status (TPS) program are only some examples of restrictive immigration policies. Focus groups with Latino/a adults have revealed that anti-immigrant sentiment contributes to parents' feelings of worthlessness, increased fear, and experiences with discrimination (Gurrola & Ayón, 2018). Further, Latino/a parents expressed that their fears of discrimination have led them to avoid public spaces and have only increased feelings of isolation (Gurrola & Ayón, 2018). Such anti-immigrant and anti-Latino rhetoric can also lead to psychological distress among Latino immigrant communities (Roche, Vaquera, White, & Rivera, 2018).

The current sociopolitical climate is clouded with xenophobic and discriminatory policies that reinforce structural racism and amplify mental health disparities in the United States (Morey, 2018). Hatzenbuehler et al. (2017) explored the links between state policies specific to immigration, agricultural worker protections, as well as language and mental health outcomes among Latino/a adults. As expected, a greater number of poor mental health days were reported by Latino/a adults residing in states with more restrictive state policies. Similar associations between policies and Latino/a mental health are found in other studies. For example, Lopez et al. (2017) reported decreases in Latino/a adults' health following an immigration raid. Brabeck and Xu (2010) found that Latino/a immigrant parents who were more legally vulnerable (e.g., were undocumented, had current deportation orders, had been previously detained by immigration authorities, and had a family member currently in detention or previously deported) reported a more negative impact on familial well-being following a family member's deportation/detention.

Recently implemented policies have resulted in similarly detrimental mental health outcomes among Latino/a immigrant youth. First- and second-generation Latino/a immigrant youth reported feeling afraid and/or anxious, expressed anger, and reported contempt and/or disgust when describing their views on immigration-related topics (Wray-Lake et al., 2018). Children of deported and/or detained parents were significantly more likely to exhibit externalizing behaviors, including aggressive and avoidant behavior, and were also more likely to report more internalizing symptoms, such as higher levels of anxiety, depressive, and PTSD symptoms, compared to children whose families remained intact (Rojas-Flores, Clements, Hwang Koo, & London, 2017). In a recent study, undocumented Latino/a parents conveyed more messages of mistrust to their children, which in turn, were associated with increased depressive symptoms among adolescents (Cross et al., 2020). In focus groups and interviews with both undocumented children and children of undocumented parents, over half of the participants scored within borderline or clinical ranges on scales of anxiety, depressive symptoms, externalizing behaviors, and somatic complaints (Delva et al., 2013). Taken together, restrictive immigration policies and anti-immigrant rhetoric contribute to a hostile, discriminatory environment, which is highly detrimental to the health and well-being of Latino/a immigrant youth and families (Androff, Ayón, Becerra, & Gurrola, 2011; Ayón, 2016; Hatzenbuehler et al., 2017).

Discrimination

A prevalent anti-immigrant and xenophobic rhetoric in the United States have made discrimination a more salient contextual stressor for Latino/a immigrant families (Ayón, Valencia-Garcia, & Kim, 2017; Hooghe & Dassonneville, 2018). Ethnic or racial discrimination is defined as unfair, differential treatment based on a person's race or ethnicity (García Coll et al., 1996). Characteristics such as language proficiency, phenotypic features like skin color, and documentation status have all been associated with increased perceived discrimination and in turn, poorer psychological well-being (Córdova Jr & Cervantes, 2010; Finch, Kolody, & Vega, 2000). Multiple meta-analyses and studies have examined the detrimental effect of perceived discrimination on psychological well-being (Pascoe & Smart Richman, 2009; Schmitt, Branscombe, Postmes, & Garcia, 2014; Williams, Neighbors, & Jackson, 2003) and the link between discrimination and poor mental health among Latino/as has been well established (Ayón, Marsiglia, & Bermudez-Parsai, 2010; Flores et al., 2008). Examples of ethnic or racial discrimination experienced by Latino/a immigrants include racial profiling (Giles, Linz, Bonilla, & Gomez, 2012), various types of microagressions (Huynh, 2012), foreigner objectification (Juang et al., 2016), and stereotyping (Guyll, Madon, Prieto, & Scherr, 2010). Focus groups revealed that discrimination, at both the institutional and individual level, was a daily stressor for first-generation Latino/a immigrant adults (Ayón & Becerra, 2013).

Mirroring the reports of Latino/a immigrant adults, Latino/a youth who perceive more discrimination also report heightened anxiety, greater depressive symptoms, increased psychological distress, more externalizing behaviors, and lower self-efficacy, as well as lower self-esteem (Benner et al., 2018; Delgado, Updegraff, Roosa, & Umaña-Taylor, 2011; Fisher, Wallace, & Fenton, 2000; Greene, Way, & Pahl, 2006; Juang et al., 2016; Stein, Gonzalez, Cupito, Kiang, & Supple, 2015; Umaña-Taylor & Updegraff, 2007; Zeiders, Umaña-Taylor, & Derlan, 2013). Cano et al. (2015) found that discrimination experiences upon arrival to the United States and throughout a 5-year period influenced aggression, optimism, and self-esteem levels among Latino/a immigrant adolescents. School is one context in which Latino/a youth may experience discrimination from peers, teachers, and school administrators. As examples of school-based discrimination, Benner and Graham (2011) found that Latino/a adolescents reported that they were placed in lower-ability groups, disciplined unfairly, and graded more harshly because of their ethnicity. Among a sample of ethnically diverse adolescents, Latino/as reported that their ethnicity influenced how they were disciplined at school and treated in public spaces (Fisher et al., 2000).

Financial stress and economic inequality

A wealth of data demonstrates an association between living in poverty and heightened risks for mental health problems among parents and youth (Purtell & Gershoff, 2016; Reiss, 2013). Among Latino/as in the United States, 18.3% lived below the poverty line in 2017 (U.S. Census Bureau, 2018). Upon arrival in the United States, many Latino/a immigrants and their families encounter racial and ethnic stratification, economic disparities, and financial disadvantages (Campbell & Kaufman, 2006; Catanzarite & Aguilera, 2002; Painter, Holmes, & Bateman, 2015). As a result of these systems of inequality, immigrant workers are often compensated with lower wages, are overworked and underpaid by employers, forced to take more physically strenuous jobs, and discriminated in workplace settings (Peri & Sparber, 2009). Discrimination, limited social networks, and stigmatized legal status amplified feelings of social isolation and psychological distress among Latino/a immigrant day laborers (Negi, 2013). Moreover, undocumented immigrant workers are especially vulnerable to workplace exploitation (Miller, 2007). More specifically, among Latino/a immigrant populations, economic inequality and financial stressors have been linked to poor psychological well-being such as heightened anxiety, depressive symptoms, and externalizing behaviors (Dennis, Parke, Coltrane, Blacher, & Borthwick-Duffy, 2003; Mendoza, Dmitrieva, Perreira, Hurwich-Reiss, & Watamura, 2017; Suárez-Morales & Lopez, 2009).

Latino/a immigrant families often live in segregated ethnic neighborhoods with high rates of poverty, violence, and overcrowded housing conditions, all of which have negative mental health implications (Osypuk, Bates, & Acevedo-Garcia, 2010; Reiss, 2013; Yoshikawa & Kalil, 2011). In a longitudinal study with over 70,000 families, findings revealed that compared to native whites, Mexican and Central American immigrant families were more likely to live in crowded homes within densely populated cities and reported greater concern about environmental and neighborhood conditions (Hall & Greenman, 2013). Further evidence reveals that Latina mothers who report community violence exposure also report greater rates of anxiety, depression, and PTSD symptoms, which in turn, can contribute to behavioral problems in their children (Aisenberg, 2001).

Poor, urban neighborhoods also place Latino/a immigrant youth at increased risk of exposure to violence and crime (Gudiño, Nadeem, Kataoka, & Lau, 2011). Exposure to community violence includes instances of personal victimization, such as being personally threatened with serious physical harm, as well as witnessing acts of violence, such as seeing someone get shot with a gun (Aisenberg & Herrenkohl, 2008; Cooley-Strickland et al., 2009). In one study, Latino/a immigrant youth reported similarly high rates of exposure to violence compared to nonimmigrant Latino/a youth, but Latino/a immigrant youth reported exposure to more severe forms of violence, including weapon-related violence exposure (Gudiño et al., 2011). A wealth of literature documents a strong association between exposure to community violence and reports of anxiety, delinquency, depressive symptoms, PTSD symptoms, school disengagement, and substance abuse among youth (Cooley-Quille, Boyd, Frantz, & Walsh, 2001; Cooley-Strickland et al., 2009; Denson, Marshall, Schell, & Jaycox, 2007; Jocson, Alers-Rojas, Ceballo, & Arkin, 2018; Kennedy & Ceballo, 2014; Lynch, 2003). In sum, many Latino/a immigrant youth and parents experience economic insecurity, poverty, inadequate housing, and violence in their neighborhoods, factors that impact the psychological well-being of all family members.

Acculturative stress

Latino/a immigrants must simultaneously navigate their culture-of-origin and their new host culture, a process that can result in numerous experiences of *acculturative stress* within Latino/a immigrant families (Suárez-Orozco & Carhill, 2008). Acculturative stress arises from intercultural contact that is brought on by postimmigration factors such as difficulties assimilating to the beliefs, values, and norms of a dominant culture, and the frustration of limitations imposed by language barriers (Berry, 1997). Studies have found that acculturative stress serves as a strong predictor of depressive symptoms and suicidal ideation among Latino/a immigrants (Hovey, 2000; Hovey & King, 1996). Further, acculturation gaps and conflicts may arise when Latino/a youth and parents become culturally involved in their new "American" culture at different rates (Dennis, Basañez, & Farahmand, 2010; Smokowski, Rose, & Bacallao, 2008; Telzer, 2010). For instance, while children and youth navigate their new culture through daily experiences in the American school system, parents may have fewer opportunities to engage with US culture (Telzer, 2010). As a result, children and youth are often exposed to more individualistic American values (Kwak, 2003), and parents may shame their children for speaking more English than Spanish or may insist upon culturally based family obligations. Parent-child discrepancies in attitudes about family obligations can amplify Latino/a youth's stress (Stein et al., 2015), and such intergenerational discrepancies may result in parent-youth conflicts (Lau et al., 2005). Parent-child acculturation gaps have been linked to greater depressive symptoms, increased family conflict, and overall poor adjustment among racial/ethnic minority youth (Céspedes & Huey Jr, 2008; Hwang & Wood, 2009; Lau et al., 2005).

Religion and spirituality among Latino/a immigrant families

Religiosity and spirituality are notoriously hard to define because they are multilevel, multidimensional, and intertwined constructs (Pargament, Mahoney, Exline, Jones, & Shafranske, 2013). In general, religiosity refers to beliefs, practices, and values within an established community of faith or specific religious ideology, while spirituality refers to beliefs, activities, relationships, or experiences having to do with the sacred that may include God, higher powers, or the divine (Loewenthal, 2012). Traditionally, Latino/as have primarily identified as Roman Catholics, but more recently the number of evangelical Protestants and unaffiliated Latino/as has increased (Pew Research Center, 2014). Age differences also interact with religious affiliation. A Pew Research Center (2014) study found that among Latino/as between the ages of 18–29 years, identification as Catholic decreased from 60% in 2010 to 45% in 2013. In fact, immigrant Latino/as are more likely to identify as Catholic (60%) when compared to their US-born counterparts (48%) and less likely to identify as religiously unaffiliated (15% vs. 23%). Further, about 65% of Latino Catholics were born outside of the United States (Pew Research Center, 2014). For some Latino/as, religious affiliations are integrated with spiritual practices (e.g., curanderismo, espiritismo, Mesa Blanca, and santería) carried out in lieu of or in conjunction with Catholicism and Protestantism (Koss-Chioino, 2013).

It is widely accepted that religion and spirituality are important aspects of Latino/a culture and a shared Latino/a identity (Calzada, Fernandez, & Cortes, 2010; Comas-Díaz, 2006; Koss-Chioino, 2013). Among a sample of Dominican and Mexican mothers, religiosity was identified as one of the most important values to pass from one generation to the next via Latino/a family and community practices (Calzada et al., 2010). It is common, for example, for many Latino/a children, even from a very young age, to ask for blessings (*bendición*) and to receive God's blessing (*Dios te bendiga*) from parents, grandparents, and other extended family (Koss-Chioino, 2013). It is also not uncommon for small stores (*botánicas*) in Latino communities to sell iconic statues, prints, healing herbs, oils, candles, perfumed alcohols, and prayer sheets, as well as for the owner to give advice (Koss-Chioino, 2013). In short, many Latino/a immigrant families practice religiosity and spirituality in public and private spheres and transmit religious beliefs and practices across generations.

Religiosity, spirituality, and mental health among Latino/a adults

For Latino/a immigrant parents who must navigate various contextual stressors, religiosity and spirituality may serve as sources of faith-based strength and resilience; further, religious coping and spirituality may foster Latino/a parents' mental health in a number of ways (Cadge & Ecklund, 2007; Calvillo & Bailey, 2015). Prayer, church attendance, involvement in religious or spiritual communities, and religious coping are all types of religious and spiritual expressions that may contribute to positive mental and physical health among Latino/a adults (Abraído-Lanza, Vásquez, & Echeverría, 2004; Garcia, Ellison, Sunil, & Hill, 2013; Negi, 2013; Reyes-Ortiz, Rodriguez, & Markides, 2009). Interestingly, older Latino/a immigrants attend more religious services and engage in more private prayer than their US-born counterparts (Aranda, 2008). Among Latino/a immigrants above the age of 50, religious involvement, such as attending worship-related services, was negatively associated with depressive symptoms. More specifically, participants who attended religious services were 24% less likely to be diagnosed with depression (Aranda, 2008). In another study with 868 Mexican immigrant and Mexican American participants, immigrants reported greater religious attendance and those who attended more religious services had lower lifetime rates of anxiety, depressive disorder, and substance use (Moreno & Cardemil, 2018). Among another sample of predominantly Central American immigrant elders, believing in a higher power impacted their attitudes toward aging, success, and well-being (Beyene, Becker, & Mayen, 2002). Faith in God, expressing gratitude toward God and believing in God's will all facilitated elders' coping with daily stressors, provided faith-based strength, and eased their concerns regarding their own mortality.

When challenging and traumatic events are followed by an increase in spiritual growth and positive virtues, it is often described as stress-related growth or post-traumatic growth (Ai & Park, 2005). It is important to note that such positive life changes, in the aftermath of trauma, do not negate the emotional difficulties encountered. In fact, despite the accumulation of positive outcomes for religiosity, spirituality, and religious coping, there are nonetheless also findings of little or negative effects of religiosity on Latina/os' mental health and psychological functioning (Dunn & O'Brien, 2009). For some, experiencing challenging and traumatic events can lead to the disavowal of religious beliefs and a loss of faith, whether lasting for an initial, short period or having a longer duration (Ai & Park, 2005). Immigrants who were highly involved in their country-of-origin religious organizations may experience a sense of loss after migration, especially among undocumented migrants (Sanchez, Dillon, Ruffin, & de la Rosa, 2012). Higher levels of negative religious coping (e.g., seeing stressful events as punishment from a higher power) have also been linked to more alcohol use among recent Latina/o immigrants with high levels of acculturative stress (Sanchez et al., 2012). Involvement in formal religious institutions, on the other hand, has been associated with more negative attitudes toward seeking professional mental health services, especially among Latino men (Moreno, Nelson, & Cardemil, 2017).

Religious communities may provide Latino/a immigrants with tangible resources as well as social and emotional support. Qualitative findings from a mixed-method study by Negi (2013) revealed that religiosity, church attendance, and religious involvement helped foster a sense of spiritual social support among Latino/a day laborers. Moreover, participants reported that religious communities lessened their feelings of isolation and improved their overall mental health (Negi, 2013). Religious spaces can also function as places of refuge as well as places for faith-based companionship and celebration. Irazábal and Dyrness (2010) observed the ways in which Latino/a immigrants navigated religious spaces in Southern California. Religious spaces such as churches served as physical locations, where Latino/a immigrants could openly discuss restrictive anti-immigrant policies, express frustrations with national and local politics, and participate in both religious and civic engagement with others who share similar values (Djupe & Neiheisel, 2012; Irazábal & Dyrness, 2010). This was particularly true for undocumented Latino/a immigrants who embody stigmatized identities as unauthorized foreigners on a daily basis (Irazábal & Dyrness, 2010). In response to anti-immigrant state sanctioned policies and practices, some churches and places of worship have become physical sanctuaries, protecting undocumented migrants from detention and deportation (Burke, 2019). Some undocumented migrants have spent months, even years, in these places to avoid being separated from their families. Congregation members have become activists, advocating in different ways for undocumented migrants and the estimated 50 people currently living in sanctuary churches around the country (Timpane & Delp, 2019).

Latino/a immigrants who frequent religious spaces reported feeling a sense of empowerment and a greater sense of well-being (Irazábal & Dyrness, 2010). Religious festivities, such as *Dia de Los Muertos*, *Posadas*, and *Virgen de Guadalupe,* are some examples of celebrations that foster a sense of community, cultural pride, and strong ethnic identity, all of which have been associated with positive psychological well-being (Gómez-Barris & Irazabal, 2009; Phinney, Horenczyk, Liebkind, & Vedder, 2001; Rivas-Drake et al., 2014). Finally, among Latino/a immigrant couples, religious beliefs and spirituality are linked to better relationship quality (Austin & Falconier, 2013; Ellison, Burdette, & Wilcox, 2010). For example, when each partner expressed high levels of spirituality, they reported fewer aggressive behaviors and in turn, reported more common dyadic coping as a couple (Austin & Falconier, 2013).

Religiosity, spirituality, and psychological well-being among Latino/a youth

In keeping with the literature on religiosity and spirituality among Latino/a immigrant adults and parents, studies also support a positive impact of religiosity and spirituality on Latino/a youth's mental health. In general, religiosity is an important part of the lives of many American children and adolescents, with a large proportion of youth participating in some form of public (e.g., attendance at religious services) or private (e.g., praying) religious activity (Salas-Wright, Vaughn, Hodge, & Perron, 2012). When compared to non-Latino/a White youth, there is evidence that Latino/a immigrant adolescents in the United States report even higher levels of religiosity (Lopez, Huynh, & Fuligni, 2011). Moreover, religion is identified as a salient factor in the lives of many immigrant youth in the United States (Abo-Zena & Barry, 2013; Suárez-Orozco, Singh, Abo-Zena, Du, & Roeser, 2011). Suárez-Orozco et al. (2011) illustrate how religiosity and spirituality provide some immigrant youth with an ever-present moral compass, a sense of protection, and a higher power to call upon in times of crisis. All of these personal belief systems are rooted in the familial and cultural transmission of religious values. Importantly, research indicates that greater endorsement of religiosity and spirituality among adolescents is associated with numerous indicators of positive mental health, such as fewer symptoms of anxiety, delinquency, depression, substance use, and suicidality (Dew et al., 2008; Nonnemaker, McNeely, & Blum, 2003; Petts, 2014; Salas-Wright et al., 2012; Yonker, Schnabelrauch, & DeHaan, 2012).

Martinez (2017) relied on general strain theory to investigate the role of religiosity in buffering the effects of societal strain and negative psychological emotions (e.g., anger, anxiety, and depression) with a sample of 2258 Latino/a US-born and foreign-born adolescents (24% were foreign-born). Nationally representative, longitudinal survey data from the first two waves (1994–95) of the Add Health study were used with exposure to community violence and experiences of health or emotional problems assessed as measures of strain. The findings demonstrated that higher rates of personal religiosity at Wave 1 reduced the likelihood of engaging in delinquent behaviors at Wave 2 for foreign-born, Latino/a adolescents. In addition, among foreign-born adolescents, personal religiosity buffered the relation between exposure to violence and excessive alcohol use. Finally, regardless of immigrant status, personal religiosity also buffered the effects of depression/anxiety on alcohol use such that Latino/a youth with higher levels of personal religiosity were less likely to cope with depression/anxiety by using alcohol compared to depressed/anxious Latino/a youth with low levels of personal religiosity.

Martinez's (2017) findings are consistent with those reported by Jocson et al. (2018) who found that spirituality, compared to other measures of religiosity, demonstrated the strongest protective effects for Latino/a youth exposed to community violence. More specifically, spirituality—a private and personal set of beliefs—protected Latino/a youth from the deleterious effects of community violence on symptoms of depression and post-traumatic stress disorder. Thus, researchers have found evidence that religiosity and spirituality serve as protective factors for Latino/a youth exposed to contextual stressors, with some indication that these buffering relations are even stronger for Latino/a immigrant youth.

Despite the many benefits reported for religiosity and spirituality, Latino/a immigrant youth are not all equally likely to experience such positive effects. Lesbian, gay, bisexual, and transgender (LGBT) youth, in particular, are vulnerable to internalized rejecting or disapproving messages about their sexual identities given the homonegative and homophobic positions many religions endorse (Page, Lindahl, & Malik, 2013). When parents adhere to these religious positions, LGBT youth may hide their sexual identity or stop practicing their parents' religion which, in turn, may increase family conflict and lead to negative mental health outcomes among youth.

Religion and spirituality: Identifying mechanisms of influence

We now turn to a discussion of the mechanisms by which religiosity and spirituality may serve Latino/a immigrant youth and parents as sources of strength and resilience. Here, we rely on Jocson et al.'s (2018) categorization of religious and spiritual factors as fitting into different ecological levels: namely, individual, family, and community levels. Spirituality and private dimensions of religious beliefs and faith operate primarily at the individual level. For Latino/a immigrant children and parents, religious beliefs and spirituality may provide a sense of purpose, direction, and meaning in life. When faced with difficult, unpredictable, and challenging life events or societal stressors, having a personal sense of faith and moral grounding can provide an important sense of self-reliance and self-worth. A spiritual inner anchor may bestow stability and coherence amidst fragmenting traumatic events (Jocson et al., 2018). Given the centrality of identity development during adolescence, it stands to reason that developing a religious identity and belief system can be particularly salient for Latino/a immigrant teenagers. In other words, embracing a religious identity may be especially important when youth are in the throes of establishing their own identities and seeking purpose in life (Abo-Zena & Barry, 2013).

At the family level, various aspects of religious participation and involvement may occur within a family context, like church attendance and the celebration of religious holidays. For Latino/a parents, teaching children about religious values and faith is seen as an important part of their parental responsibilities and the generational transmission of shared values (Calzada et al., 2010). Not surprisingly, many behaviors and other activities associated with religious faith are performed in home-based settings, such as daily prayers, offering blessings, and listening to or watching church services on the radio or television. In this sense, the protective benefits of religiosity may be rooted in the strength of family cohesion, familial support and closeness, or parent-child relational bonds—all are primary examples of *familismo*, a commonly held, Latino/a cultural value stressing the importance of family relationships (Calzada et al., 2010).

At the community level, attendance at religious services and participation in religious events may foster a sense of belonging and connection to community. For both parents and youth, religious communities may provide access to a network of supportive people, practical educational and financial information, and tangible resources or opportunities. Latino/a immigrant youth reveal that religious communities bolster their prosocial behavior, as opposed to engagement in risky behaviors, and provide valuable social support (Abo-Zena & Barry, 2013). At times, the support structures provided to youth are quite formal as seen in faith-based youth programs. In addition to a sense of belonging and community, religious settings may provide Latino/a immigrant families with a sense of safety and security that is directly attached to a physical space and location.

Religious institutions may offer refuge and safety from acculturative stressors, discrimination, stigmatization, and the like. Many Latino/a immigrants turn to religious institutions as a way to connect with other Latino/as, to be in a place where Spanish is spoken, to maintain their ethnic identity, and to receive material assistance and counseling without fear of detention or deportation

(Koss-Chioino, 2013). Mora (2013) posits that churches offer small group settings, like prayer groups, that provide internal settings for connection and support, while also providing links to external organizations that offer opportunities for civic engagement. Further, as highlighted by Abo-Zena and Barry (2013), religious settings may provide immigrant Latino/a youth with a bridge between cultural priorities from one's family and country of origin to those in their new US context. Hence, religious organizations may simultaneously meet a number of critical needs for Latino/a immigrant youth and parents. Although we have placed various dimensions of religiosity and spirituality into neatly ordered ecological categories, it is important to emphasize that the benefits provided within different ecological levels are not mutually exclusive. For example, it may be the spiritual component of engaging in private, reflective prayer that most supports a Puerto Rican adolescent who is attending a religious service with her family, even as she also benefits from the sense of shared connection to her parents during the weekly routine of attending religious services.

In conclusion, we agree with Suárez-Orozco et al. (2011) that the role of religion in the lives of immigrant youth and parents remains relatively understudied and is in need of greater scholarly attention. The lack of consistency and variability in the measurement of religiosity and spirituality make it difficult to both identify the key underlying components and to generalize findings across studies. More research is needed that examines the causal pathways by which religiosity is protective or not protective. For instance, researchers should examine when, how, and what specific dimensions of religiosity and spirituality are protective (Pargament et al., 2013). The answers to these questions will help us construct more effective points of intervention. For instance, Moreno and Cardemil (2018) found that older Latino/a immigrants preferred more informal religious counseling from religious authority figures rather than formal mental health services when coping with hardship. Seeking informal religious counsel from church authorities and participating in confession or *confesión* may be particularly helpful for undocumented Latino/a immigrants who can benefit from seeking counseling that does not require economic eligibility, insurance coverage, language brokering, or disclosure of documentation status (Moreno & Cardemil, 2018; Villatoro, Dixon, & Mays, 2016). Finally, future research examining religious and spiritual beliefs and practices should aim to develop more culturally responsive measurement instruments (Koss-Chioino, 2013).

References

Abo-Zena, M. M., & Barry, C. M. (2013). Religion and immigrant-origin youth: A resource and a challenge. *Research in Human Development, 10*(4), 353–371.

Abraído-Lanza, A. F., Vásquez, E., & Echeverría, S. E. (2004). En las manos de Dios [in God's hands]: Religious and other forms of coping among Latinos with arthritis. *Journal of Consulting and Clinical Psychology, 72*(1), 91.

Ai, A. L., & Park, C. L. (2005). Possibilities of the positive following violence and trauma. *Journal of Interpersonal Violence*, *20*(2), 242–250.

Aisenberg, E. (2001). The effects of exposure to community violence upon Latina mothers and preschool children. *Hispanic Journal of Behavioral Sciences*, *23*(4), 378–398.

Aisenberg, E., & Herrenkohl, T. (2008). Community violence in context: Risk and resilience in children and families. *Journal of Interpersonal Violence*, *23*(3), 296–315.

Alcántara, C., Chen, C., & Alegria, M. (2014). Do post-migration perceptions of social mobility matter for Latino immigrant health? *Social Science & Medicine*, *101*, 94–106.

Alegria, M., Canino, G., Shrout, P. E., Woo, M., Duan, N., Vila, D., … Meng, X. (2008). Prevalence of mental illness in immigrant and non-immigrant U.S. Latino groups. *American Journal of Psychiatry*, *165*, 359–369.

Androff, D. K., Ayón, C., Becerra, D., & Gurrola, M. (2011). US immigration policy and immigrant children's well-being: The impact of policy shifts. *Journal of Sociology & Social Welfare*, *38*, 77.

Aranda, M. P. (2008). Relationship between religious involvement and psychological well-being: A social justice perspective. *Health & Social Work*, *33*(1), 9–21.

Arbona, C., Olvera, N., Rodriguez, N., Hagan, J., Linares, A., & Wiesner, M. (2010). Acculturative stress among documented and undocumented Latino immigrants the United States. *Hispanic Journal of Behavioral Sciences*, *32*(3), 362–384.

Austin, J. L., & Falconier, M. K. (2013). Spirituality and common dyadic coping: Protective factors from psychological aggression in Latino immigrant couples. *Journal of Family Issues*, *34*(3), 323–346.

Ayón, C. (2016). Talking to Latino children about race, inequality, and discrimination: Raising families in an anti-immigrant political environment. *Journal of the Society for Social Work and Research*, *7*(3), 449–477.

Ayón, C., & Becerra, D. (2013). Mexican immigrant families under siege: The impact of anti-immigrant policies, discrimination, and the economic crisis. *Advances in Social Work*, *14*(1), 206–228.

Ayón, C., Marsiglia, F. F., & Bermudez-Parsai, M. (2010). Latino family mental health: Exploring the role of discrimination and familismo. *Journal of Community Psychology*, *38*(6), 742–756.

Ayón, C., Valencia-Garcia, D., & Kim, S. H. (2017). Latino immigrant families and restrictive immigration climate: Perceived experiences with discrimination, threat to family, social exclusion, children's vulnerability, and related factors. *Race and Social Problems*, *9*(4), 300–312.

Benner, A. D., & Graham, S. (2011). Latino adolescents' experiences of discrimination across the first 2 years of high school: Correlates and influences on educational outcomes. *Child Development*, *82*(2), 508–519.

Benner, A. D., Wang, Y., Shen, Y., Boyle, A. E., Polk, R., & Cheng, Y. P. (2018). Racial/ethnic discrimination and well-being during adolescence: A meta-analytic review. *American Psychologist*, *73*(7), 855.

Berry, J. W. (1997). Immigration, acculturation, and adaptation. *Applied Psychology*, *46*, 5–68.

Beyene, Y., Becker, G., & Mayen, N. (2002). Perception of aging and sense of well-being among Latino elderly. *Journal of Cross-cultural Gerontology*, *17*(2), 155–172.

Brabeck, K., & Xu, Q. (2010). The impact of detention and deportation on Latino immigrant children and families: A quantitative exploration. *Hispanic Journal of Behavioral Sciences*, *32*(3), 341–361.

Burke, D. (2019). *The Evangelical Lutheran Church in America just became the country's first 'sanctuary church body*. CNN. Retrieved from www.cnn.com.

Caballero, T. M., DeCamp, L. R., Platt, R. E., Shah, H., Johnson, S. B., Sibinga, E. M. S., & Polk, S. (2017). Addressing the mental health needs of Latino children in immigrant families. *Clinical Pediatrics*, *56*(7), 648–658. https://doi.org/10.1177/0009922816679509.

Cadge, W., & Ecklund, E. H. (2007). Immigration and religion. *Annual Review of Sociology*, *33*, 359–379.

Calvillo, J. E., & Bailey, S. R. (2015). Latino religious affiliation and ethnic identity. *Journal for the Scientific Study of Religion*, *54*(1), 57–78.

Calzada, E. J., Fernandez, Y., & Cortes, D. E. (2010). Incorporating the cultural value of respeto into a framework of Latino parenting. *Cultural Diversity and Ethnic Minority Psychology*, *16*, 77–86.

Campbell, L. A., & Kaufman, R. L. (2006). Racial differences in household wealth: Beyond black and white. *Research in Social Stratification and Mobility*, *24*(2), 131–152.

Cano, M.Á., Schwartz, S. J., Castillo, L. G., Romero, A. J., Huang, S., Lorenzo-Blanco, E. I., … Lizzi, K. M. (2015). Depressive symptoms and externalizing behaviors among Hispanic immigrant adolescents: Examining longitudinal effects of cultural stress. *Journal of Adolescence*, *42*, 31–39.

Catanzarite, L., & Aguilera, M. B. (2002). Working with co-ethnics: Earnings penalties for Latino immigrants at Latino jobsites. *Social Problems*, *49*(1), 101–127.

Céspedes, Y. M., & Huey, S. J., Jr. (2008). Depression in Latino adolescents: A cultural discrepancy perspective. *Cultural Diversity and Ethnic Minority Psychology*, *14*(2), 168.

Cobb, C. L., Meca, A., Xie, D., Schwartz, S. J., & Moise, R. K. (2017). Perceptions of legal status: Associations with psychosocial experiences among undocumented Latino/a immigrants. *Journal of Counseling Psychology*, *64*(2), 167.

Comas-Díaz, L. (2006). Latino healing: The integration of ethnic psychology into psychotherapy. *Psychotherapy: Theory, Research, Practice, Training*, *43*, 436–453.

Cooley-Quille, M., Boyd, R. C., Frantz, E., & Walsh, J. (2001). Emotional and behavioral impact of exposure to community violence in inner-city adolescents. *Journal of Clinical Child Psychology*, *30*(2), 199–206.

Cooley-Strickland, M., Quille, T. J., Griffin, R. S., Stuart, E. A., Bradshaw, C. P., & Furr-Holden, D. (2009). Community violence and youth: Affect, behavior, substance use, and academics. *Clinical Child and Family Psychology Review*, *12*(2), 127–156.

Córdova, D., Jr., & Cervantes, R. C. (2010). Intergroup and within-group perceived discrimination among US-born and foreign-born Latino youth. *Hispanic Journal of Behavioral Sciences*, *32*(2), 259–274.

Cross, F. L., Medina, A., Montoro, J., Medina, M., Miller, S., Pinetta, B., … Rivas-Drake, D. (2020). Illuminating ethnic-racial socialization among undocumented Latinx parents and its implications for adolescent psychosocial functioning. *Developmental Psychology*, [in press].

Delgado, M. Y., Updegraff, K. A., Roosa, M. W., & Umaña-Taylor, A. J. (2011). Discrimination and Mexican-origin adolescents' adjustment: The moderating roles of adolescents', mothers', and fathers' cultural orientations and values. *Journal of Youth and Adolescence*, *40*(2), 125–139.

Delva, J., Horner, P., Martinez, R., Sanders, L., Lopez, W. D., & Doering-White, J. (2013). Mental health problems of children of undocumented parents in the United States: A hidden crisis. *Journal of Community Positive Practices*, *13*(3), 25–35.

Dennis, J., Basañez, T., & Farahmand, A. (2010). Intergenerational conflicts among Latinos in early adulthood: Separating values conflicts with parents from acculturation conflicts. *Hispanic Journal of Behavioral Sciences*, *32*(1), 118–135.

Dennis, J. M., Parke, R. D., Coltrane, S., Blacher, J., & Borthwick-Duffy, S. A. (2003). Economic pressure, maternal depression, and child adjustment in Latino families: An exploratory study. *Journal of Family and Economic Issues*, *24*(2), 183–202.

Denson, T. F., Marshall, G. N., Schell, T. L., & Jaycox, L. H. (2007). Predictors of posttraumatic distress 1 year after exposure to community violence: The importance of acute symptom severity. *Journal of Consulting and Clinical Psychology*, *75*(5), 683.

Dew, R. E., Daniel, S. S., Armstrong, T. D., Goldston, D. B., Triplett, M. F., & Koenig, H. G. (2008). Religion/spirituaity and adolescent psychiatric symptoms: A review. *Child Psychiatry & Human Development*, *39*, 381–398.

Djupe, P. A., & Neiheisel, J. R. (2012). How religious communities affect political participation among Latinos. *Social Science Quarterly*, *93*(2), 333–355.

Dunn, M. G., & O'Brien, K. M. (2009). Psychological health and meaning in life: Stress, social support, and religious coping in Latina/Latino immigrants. *Hispanic Journal of Behavioral Sciences*, *31*(2), 204–227.

Ellison, C. G., Burdette, A. M., & Wilcox, W. B. (2010). The couple that prays together: Race and ethnicity, religion, and relationship quality among working-age adults. *Journal of Marriage and Family*, *72*(4), 963–975.

Finch, B. K., Kolody, B., & Vega, W. A. (2000). Perceived discrimination and depression among Mexican-origin adults in California. *Journal of Health and Social behavior*, 295–313.

Fisher, C. B., Wallace, S. A., & Fenton, R. E. (2000). Discrimination distress during adolescence. *Journal of Youth and Adolescence*, *29*(6), 679–695.

Flores, E., Tschann, J. M., Dimas, J. M., Bachen, E. A., Pasch, L. A., & de Groat, C. L. (2008). Perceived discrimination, perceived stress, and mental and physical health among Mexican-origin adults. *Hispanic Journal of Behavioral Sciences*, *30*(4), 401–424.

García Coll, C., Lamberty, G., Jenkins, R., McAdoo, H. P., Crnic, K., Wasik, B. H., & Vázquez García, H. (1996). An integrative model for the study of developmental competencies in minority children. *Child Development*, *67*(5), 1891–1914. https://doi.org/10.2307/1131600.

Garcia, G., Ellison, C. G., Sunil, T. S., & Hill, T. D. (2013). Religion and selected health behaviors among Latinos in Texas. *Journal of Religion and Health*, *52*(1), 18–31.

Giles, H., Linz, D., Bonilla, D., & Gomez, M. L. (2012). Police stops of and interactions with Latino and White (non-Latino) drivers: Extensive policing and communication accommodation. *Communication Monographs*, *79*(4), 407–427.

Gómez-Barris, M., & Irazabal, C. (2009). Transnational meanings of La Virgen de Guadalupe: Religiosity, space and culture at Plaza Mexico. *Culture and Religion*, *10*(3), 339–357.

Gonzalez-Barrera, A. (2019). *Hispanics with darker skin are more likely to experience discrimination than those with lighter skin.*

Grant, B. F., Stinson, F. S., Hasin, D. S., Dawson, D. A., Chou, S. P., & Anderson, K. (2004). Immigration and lifetime prevalence of DSM-IV psychiatric disorders among Mexican Americans and non-Hispanic whites in the United States: Results from the National Epidemiologic Survey on Alcohol and Related Conditions. *Archives of General Psychiatry*, *61*, 1226–1233.

Greene, M. L., Way, N., & Pahl, K. (2006). Trajectories of perceived adult and peer discrimination among Black, Latino, and Asian American adolescents: Patterns and psychological correlates. *Developmental Psychology*, *42*(2), 218.

Gudiño, O. G., Nadeem, E., Kataoka, S. H., & Lau, A. S. (2011). Relative impact of violence exposure and immigrant stressors on Latino youth psychopathology. *Journal of Community Psychology*, *39*(3), 316–335.

Gurrola, M. A., & Ayón, C. (2018). Immigration policies and social determinants of health: Is immigrants' health at risk? *Race and Social Problems*, *10*(3), 209–220.

Guyll, M., Madon, S., Prieto, L., & Scherr, K. C. (2010). The potential roles of self-fulfilling prophecies, stigma consciousness, and stereotype threat in linking Latino/a ethnicity and educational outcomes. *Journal of Social Issues*, *66*(1), 113–130.

Hall, M., & Greenman, E. (2013). Housing and neighborhood quality among undocumented Mexican and Central American immigrants. *Social Science Research*, *42*(6), 1712–1725.

Hatzenbuehler, M. L., Prins, S. J., Flake, M., Philbin, M., Frazer, M. S., Hagen, D., & Hirsch, J. (2017). Immigration policies and mental health morbidity among Latinos: A state-level analysis. *Social Science & Medicine*, *174*, 169–178.

Hooghe, M., & Dassonneville, R. (2018). Explaining the Trump vote: The effect of racist resentment and anti-immigrant sentiments. *PS: Political Science & Politics*, *51*(3), 528–534.

Hovey, J. D. (2000). Acculturative stress, depression, and suicidal ideation in Mexican immigrants. *Cultural Diversity and Ethnic Minority Psychology*, *6*(2), 134.

Hovey, J. D., & King, C. A. (1996). Acculturative stress, depression, and suicidal ideation among immigrant and second-generation Latino adolescents. *Journal of the American Academy of Child & Adolescent Psychiatry*, *35*(9), 1183–1192.

Huynh, V. W. (2012). Ethnic microaggressions and the depressive and somatic symptoms of Latino and Asian American adolescents. *Journal of Youth and Adolescence*, *4*(7), 831–846.

Hwang, W. C., & Wood, J. J. (2009). Acculturative family distancing: Links with self-reported symptomatology among Asian Americans and Latinos. *Child Psychiatry and Human Development*, *40*(1), 123–138.

Irazábal, C., & Dyrness, G. R. (2010). Promised land? Immigration, religiosity, and space in Southern California. *Space and Culture*, *13*(4), 356–375.

Jocson, R. M., Alers-Rojas, F., Ceballo, R., & Arkin, M. (2018). Religion and spirituality: Benefits for Latino adolescents exposed to community violence. *Youth & Society*, 1–28.

Juang, L. P., Moffitt, U., Kim, S. Y., Lee, R. M., Soto, J. A., Hurley, E., … Whitbourne, S. K. (2016). Cognitive reappraisal and expressive suppression: Links to racial-ethnic discrimination and adjustment among Latino/a and Asian-heritage college students. *Journal of Adolescence*, *53*, 21–33.

Kennedy, T. M., & Ceballo, R. (2014). Who, what, when, and where? Toward a dimensional conceptualization of community violence exposure. *Review of General Psychology*, *18*(2), 69–81.

Koss-Chioino, J. (2013). Religion and spirituality in Latino life in the United States. In K. I. Pargament, J. J. Exline, & J. W. Jones (Eds.), Vol. 1. *APA handbooks in psychology®. APA handbook of psychology, religion, and spirituality (Vol. 1): Context, theory, and research* (pp. 599–615). Washington, DC: American Psychological Association. https://doi.org/10.1037/14045-033.

Kwak, K. (2003). Adolescents and their parents: A review of intergenerational family relations for immigrant and non-immigrant families. *Human Development*, *46*(2-3), 115–136.

Lau, A. S., McCabe, K. M., Yeh, M., Garland, A. F., Wood, P. A., & Hough, R. L. (2005). The acculturation gap-distress hypothesis among high-risk Mexican American families. *Journal of Family Psychology*, *19*(3), 367.

Lee, M., & Liechty, J. M. (2015). Longitudinal associations between immigrant ethnic density, neighborhood processes, and Latino immigrant youth depression. *Journal of Immigrant Minority Health*, *17*, 983–991.

Li, M. (2016). Pre-migration trauma and post-migration stressors for Asian and Latino American immigrants: Transnational stress proliferation. *Social Indicators Research*, *129*, 47–59.

Loewenthal, K. M. (2012). Religion, spirituality, and culture: Clarifying the direction of effects. In K. I. Pargament, J. J. Exline, & J. W. Jones (Eds.), Vol. 1. *APA handbook of psychology, religion, and spirituality (Vol. 1): Context, theory, and research* (pp. 239–255). Washington, DC: American Psychological Association. https://doi.org/10.1037/14045-013.

Lopez, A. B., Huynh, V. W., & Fuligni, A. J. (2011). A longitudinal study of religious identity and participation during adolescence. *Child Development*, *82*, 1297–1309.

Lopez, W. D., Kruger, D. J., Delva, J., Llanes, M., Ledón, C., Waller, A., … Israel, B. (2017). Health implications of an immigration raid: Findings from a Latino community in the Midwestern United States. *Journal of Immigrant and Minority Health*, *19*(3), 702–708.

Lynch, M. (2003). Consequences of children's exposure to community violence. *Clinical Child and Family Psychology Review*, *6*(4), 265–274.

Martinez, B. C. (2017). General strain theory, religiosity, and delinquency among young Latino adolescents. *Deviant Behavior*, *38*(11), 1223–1239.

Massey, D. S., Durand, J., & Pren, K. A. (2016). The precarious position of Latino immigrants in the United States: A comparative analysis of ethnosurvey data. *Annals of the American Academy of Political and Social Science*, *666*(1), 91–109. https://doi.org/10.1177/0002716216648999.

Mendoza, M. M., Dmitrieva, J., Perreira, K. M., Hurwich-Reiss, E., & Watamura, S. E. (2017). The effects of economic and sociocultural stressors on the well-being of children of Latino immigrants living in poverty. *Cultural Diversity and Ethnic Minority Psychology*, *23*(1), 15.

Miller, L. A. (2007). The exploitation of acculturating immigrant populations. *International Review of Victimology*, *14*(1), 11–28.

Mora, G. C. (2013). Religion and the organizational context of immigrant civic engagement: Mexican Catholicism in the US. *Ethnic and Racial Studies*, *36*(11), 1647–1665.

Moreno, O., & Cardemil, E. (2018). The role of religious attendance on mental health among Mexican populations: A contribution toward the discussion of the immigrant health paradox. *American Journal of Orthopsychiatry*, *88*(1), 10.

Moreno, O., Nelson, T., & Cardemil, E. (2017). Religiosity and attitudes towards professional mental health services: Analyzing religious coping as a mediator among Mexican origin Latinas/os in the Southwest United States. *Mental Health, Religion and Culture*, *20*(7), 626–637. https://doi.org/10.1080/13674676.2017.1372735.

Morey, B. N. (2018). Mechanisms by which anti-immigrant stigma exacerbates Racial/Ethnic health disparities. *American Journal of Public Health*, *108*(4), 460–463.

Negi, N. J. (2013). Battling discrimination and social isolation: Psychological distress among Latino day laborers. *American Journal of Community Psychology*, *51*(1-2), 164–174.

Nonnemaker, J. M., McNeely, C. A., & Blum, R. W. (2003). Public and private domains of religiosity and adolescent health risk behaviors: Evidence from the National Longitudinal Study of Adolescent Health. *Social Science & Medicine*, *57*, 2049–2054.

Ornelas, I. J., & Perreira, K. M. (2011). The role of migration in the development of depressive symptoms among Latino immigrant parents in the USA. *Social Science & Medicine*, *73*, 1169–1177. https://doi.org/10.1016/j.socscimed.2011.07.002.

Osypuk, T. L., Bates, L. M., & Acevedo-Garcia, D. (2010). Another Mexican birthweight paradox? The role of residential enclaves and neighborhood poverty in the birthweight of Mexican-origin infants. *Social Science & Medicine*, *70*(4), 550–560.

Page, M. J. L., Lindahl, K. M., & Malik, N. M. (2013). The role of religion and stress in sexual identity and mental health among lesbian, gay, and bisexual youth. *Journal of Research on Adolescence*, *23*(4), 665–677. https://doi.org/10.1111/jora.12025.

Painter, M. A., Holmes, M. D., & Bateman, J. (2015). Skin tone, race/ethnicity, and wealth inequality among new immigrants. *Social Forces*, *94*(3), 1153–1185.

Pargament, K. I., Mahoney, A., Exline, J. J., Jones, J. W., & Shafranske, E. P. (2013). Envisioning an integrative paradigm for the psychology of religion and spirituality. In K. I. Pargament, J. J. Exline, & J. W. Jones (Eds.), Vol. 1. *APA handbooks in psychology®. APA handbook of psychology, religion, and spirituality (Vol. 1): Context, theory, and research* (pp. 3–19). Washington, DC: American Psychological Association. https://doi.org/10.1037/14045-001.

Pascoe, E. A., & Smart Richman, L. (2009). Perceived discrimination and health: A meta-analytic review. *Psychological Bulletin*, *135*(4), 531.

Passel, J., & Cohn, D. (2019). *Mexicans decline to less than half the U.S. unauthorized immigrant population for the first time*. Retrieved from https://www.pewresearch.org/fact-tank/2019/06/12/us-unauthorized-immigrant-population-2017s.

Peri, G., & Sparber, C. (2009). Task specialization, immigration, and wages. *American Economic Journal: Applied Economics*, *1*(3), 135–169.

Perreira, K. M., Chapman, M. V., & Stein, G. L. (2006). Becoming an American parent: Overcoming challenges and finding strength in a new immigrant Latino community. *Journal of Family Issues*, *27*(10), 1383–1414.

Perreira, K. M., & Ornelas, I. J. (2013). Painful passages: Traumatic experiences and post-traumatic stress among U.S. immigrant Latino adolescents and their primary caregivers. *The International Migration Review*, *47*(4), 976–1005. https://doi.org/10.1111/imre.12050.

Petts, R. J. (2014). Family, religious attendance, and trajectories of psychological well-being among youth. *Journal of Family Psychology*, *28*(6), 759–768.

Pew Research Center. (2014). *The shifting religious identity of Latinos in the United States*. Washington, DC: Author. Retrieved from http://www.pewforum.org/2015/05/12/americas-changing-religious-landscape/.

Phinney, J. S., Horenczyk, G., Liebkind, K., & Vedder, P. (2001). Ethnic identity, immigration, and well-being: An interactional perspective. *Journal of Social Issues*, *57*(3), 493–510.

Purtell, K. M., & Gershoff, E. T. (2016). Poverty and mental health. *Encyclopedia of Mental Health*, *3*, 313–317. https://doi.org/10.1016/B978-0-12-397045-9.00111-7.

Reiss, F. (2013). Socioeconomic inequalities and mental health problems in children and adolescents: A systematic review. *Social Science & Medicine*, *90*, 24–31.

Reyes-Ortiz, C. A., Rodriguez, M., & Markides, K. S. (2009). The role of spirituality healing with perceptions of the medical encounter among Latinos. *Journal of General Internal Medicine*, *24*(3), 542.

Rivas-Drake, D., Syed, M., Umaña-Taylor, A., Markstrom, C., French, S., Schwartz, S. J., & Lee, R. (2014). Feeling good, happy, and proud: A meta-analysis of positive ethnic–racial affect and adjustment. *Child Development*, *85*(1), 77–102.

Roche, K. M., Vaquera, E., White, R. M., & Rivera, M. I. (2018). Impacts of immigration actions and news and the psychological distress of US Latino parents raising adolescents. *Journal of Adolescent Health*, *62*(5), 525–531.

Rojas-Flores, L., Clements, M. L., Hwang Koo, J., & London, J. (2017). Trauma and psychological distress in Latino citizen children following parental detention and deportation. *Psychological Trauma: Theory, Research, Practice, and Policy*, *9*(3), 352.

Salas-Wright, C. P., Vaughn, M. G., Hodge, D. R., & Perron, B. E. (2012). Religiosity profiles of American youth in relation to substance use, violence, and delinquency. *Journal of Youth and Adolescence*, *41*, 1560–1575.

Sanchez, M., Dillon, F., Ruffin, B., & de la Rosa, M. (2012). The influence of religious coping on the acculturative stress of recent Latino immigrants. *Journal of Ethnic and Cultural Diversity in Social Work*, *21*(3), 171–194. https://doi.org/10.1080/15313204.2012.70044.

Schmitt, M. T., Branscombe, N. R., Postmes, T., & Garcia, A. (2014). The consequences of perceived discrimination for psychological well-being: A meta-analytic review. *Psychological Bulletin*, *140*(4), 921.

Siemons, R., Raymond-Flesh, M., Auerswald, C. L., & Brindis, C. D. (2017). Coming of age on the margins: Mental health and wellbeing among Latino immigrant young adults eligible for Deferred Action for Childhood Arrivals (DACA). *Journal of Immigrant and Minority Health*, *19*(3), 543–551.

Smokowski, P. R., Rose, R., & Bacallao, M. L. (2008). Acculturation and Latino family processes: How cultural involvement, biculturalism, and acculturation gaps influence family dynamics. *Family Relations*, *57*(3), 295–308.

Stein, G. L., Gonzalez, L. M., Cupito, A. M., Kiang, L., & Supple, A. J. (2015). The protective role of familism in the lives of Latino adolescents. *Journal of Family Issues*, *36*(10), 1255–1273. https://doi.org/10.1177/0192513X13502480.

Suárez-Morales, L., & Lopez, B. (2009). The impact of acculturative stress and daily hassles on pre-adolescent psychological adjustment: Examining anxiety symptoms. *The Journal of Primary Prevention*, *30*(3-4), 335–349.

Suárez-Orozco, C., & Carhill, A. (2008). Afterword: New directions in research with immigrant families and their children. *New Directions for Child and Adolescent Development*, *2008*(121), 87–104.

Suárez-Orozco, C., Motti-Stefanidi, F., Marks, A., & Katsiaficas, D. (2018). An integrative risk and resilience model for understanding the adaptation of immigrant-origin children and youth. *American Psychologist*, *73*(6), 781–796.

Suárez-Orozco, C., Singh, S., Abo-Zena, M. M., Du, D., & Roeser, R. W. (2011). The role of religion and religious organizations in the positive youth development of immigrant youth. In A. E. A. Warren, R. M. Lerner, & E. Phelps (Eds.), *Thriving and spirituality among youth: Research perspectives and future possibilities* (pp. 255–288). Hoboken, NJ: John Wiley & Sons.

Telzer, E. H. (2010). Expanding the acculturation gap-distress model: An integrative review of research. *Human Development*, *53*(6), 313–340.

Timpane, P., & Delp, C. (2019). *Juana's story: Seeking sanctuary in a US church*. Aljazeera. Retrieved from Aljazeera.com.

Torres, J. M., & Wallace, S. P. (2013). Migration circumstances, psychological distress, and self-rated physical health for Latino immigrants in the United States. *American Journal of Public Health*, *103*(9), 1619–1627.

Tyson, D. M., Arriola, N. B., & Corvin, J. (2016). Perceptions of depression and access to mental health care among Latino immigrants: Looking beyond one size fits all. *Qualitative Health Research*, *26*(9), 1289–1302. https://doi.org/10.1177/1049732315588499.

U.S. Census Bureau. (2018). *Selected population profile in the United States: 2017 American Community Survey 1-Year estimates*.

Umaña-Taylor, A. J., & Updegraff, K. A. (2007). Latino adolescents' mental health: Exploring the interrelations among discrimination, ethnic identity, cultural orientation, self-esteem, and depressive symptoms. *Journal of Adolescence*, *30*(4), 549–567.

Villatoro, A. P., Dixon, E., & Mays, V. M. (2016). Faith-based organizations and the Affordable Care Act: Reducing Latino mental health care disparities. *Psychological Services*, *13*(1), 92.

Williams, D. R., Neighbors, H. W., & Jackson, J. S. (2003). Racial/ethnic discrimination and health: Findings from community studies. *American Journal of Public Health*, *93*(2), 200–208.

Wray-Lake, L., Wells, R., Alvis, L., Delgado, S., Syvertsen, A. K., & Metzger, A. (2018). Being a Latinx adolescent under a Trump presidency: Analysis of Latinx youth's reactions to immigration politics. *Children and Youth Services Review*, *87*, 192–204.

Yonker, J. E., Schnabelrauch, C. A., & DeHaan, L. G. (2012). The relationship between spirituality and religiosity on psychological outcomes in adolescents and emerging adults: A meta-analytic review. *Journal of Adolescence*, *35*, 299–314.

Yoshikawa, H., & Kalil, A. (2011). The effects of parental undocumented status on the developmental contexts of young children in immigrant families. *Child Development Perspectives*, *5*(4), 291–297.

Zeiders, K. H., Umaña-Taylor, A. J., & Derlan, C. L. (2013). Trajectories of depressive symptoms and self-esteem in Latino youths: Examining the role of gender and perceived discrimination. *Developmental Psychology*, *49*(5), 951–963. https://doi-org.proxy.lib.umich.edu/10.1037/a0028866.

Further reading

Sanchez, M., Dillon, F. R., Concha, M., & De La Rosa, M. (2015). The impact of religious coping on the acculturative stress and alcohol use of recent Latino immigrants. *Journal of Religion and Health*, *54*(6), 1986–2004. https://doi.org/10.1007/s10943-014-9883-6.

Chapter 8

Mental and behavioral health in immigrant populations: Assessment and interventions for culturally competent practice

Hee Yun Lee and Jessica A. Neese
School of Social Work, University of Alabama, Tuscaloosa, AL, United States

Impact immigration has on mental and behavioral health

The process of immigration is stressful in itself and increases the risk of emotional trauma in new immigrants (Pumariega, Rothe, & Pumariega, 2005; Salas-Wright, Vaughn, Goings, Miller, & Schwartz, 2018). In addition to the journey of coming to America, having previous exposure to traumatic experiences in their homeland and loss of familial connections also impacts the mental health of immigrants (Bridges, Andrews, & Deen, 2012; Pumariega et al., 2005). Exposure to political violence is recognized as being associated with mental health conditions such as posttraumatic stress disorder (PTSD) (Fortuna, Porche, & Alegria, 2008). Other stressors, such as discrimination and prejudice, are gathering recognition as negatively impacting mental health (Fortuna et al., 2008; Pumariega et al., 2005). Another taxing psychological process that is a theme throughout the immigration and mental health studies is the impact of acculturation stress. Acculturation stress is the cultural transition from a country of origin to the host country (Cervantes, Fisher, Córdova, & Napper, 2012; Fortuna et al., 2008; Pumariega et al., 2005). The definition of acculturation varies, but the overarching variables are the length of stay in the host country and proficiency of the English language (Clough, Lee, & Chae, 2013). Also, trauma as a result of migration links to symptoms of depression, anxiety, panic attacks, and PTSD in both children and adult immigrants (Caballero et al., 2017; Pumariega et al., 2005).

According to previous literature, assimilation is the most effective way to transition to a new culture, and it requires renouncing the culture of origin and fully immersing in the culture of the host country (Pumariega et al., 2005). However, more recent research suggests otherwise: Yoon et al. (2013) have indicated that

Mental and Behavioral Health of Immigrants in the United States
https://doi.org/10.1016/B978-0-12-816117-3.00008-7

assimilation results in adverse mental health more often than resulting in positive mental health. Study findings concluded that external acculturation factors such as language and behaviors and internal acculturation factors like a positive ethnic identity are essential in having a positive mental health (Yoon et al., 2013).

Contrary to popular belief, some studies have indicated that immigrants have lower rates of mental health conditions, such as depression, anxiety disorders, and PTSD, when compared to nonimmigrants (Salas-Wright et al., 2018). Researchers have created a *healthy migrant hypothesis* that suggests that individuals who decide to migrate and complete the process are more physically and psychologically healthier than nonmigrants (Salas-Wright et al., 2018). Similar to the healthy migrant hypothesis is the "immigrant paradox" that conceptualizes the resilience and overall positive behavioral health of immigrants (Cervantes, Gattamorta, & Berger-Cardoso, 2019).

A gap in research exists among older adult immigrants regarding their mental health. It is reported that older adult immigrants have mental health issues that include depressive symptoms and disorders, somatization, and culturally influenced syndromes (Kim, Jang, Chiriboga, Ma, & Schonfeld, 2010). Limited research is available on the mental health service use of older adults as well; however, findings suggest older adult immigrants have difficulty assessing services due to limited English proficiency and acculturation stress (Kim et al., 2010; Nguyen, 2011). Their stressors result from a balancing act of adhering to their culture of origin, experiencing language barriers, having limited support from family, and increasing physical ailments (Pumariega et al., 2005). As a result of these stressors, older adults are at high risk for depressive symptoms and disorders, culturally specific syndromes, and somatic ailments (Pumariega et al., 2005).

Immigration does not only affect the mental health of adults, but adolescents and youths also experience difficulties in acculturating to a new culture and are subject to similar adverse mental health symptoms as a result. Cultural adaptation is an already established factor in the mental health of immigrants and is perceived to challenge immigrant youth because of their adjustment to a new culture while also experiencing developmental issues like forming an identity associated with ethnicity (Yeh, 2003). Evidence of Yoon et al.'s (2013) study regarding the positive impact of cultural identity on mental health is strengthened through a metaanalysis of 46 studies of racial minority youth, with some being immigrants. It concluded that ethnic and racial identity (ERI) provided youth with positive mental health outcomes (Rivas-Drake et al., 2014). Moreover, positive mental health was associated with having positive regard toward ethnic or racial populations, especially among African American and Latinx youth (Rivas-Drake et al., 2014).

To address the nuances of not only immigrants' culture of origin and race and ethnicity but also the process of immigration and acculturation, culturally adapted assessment and interventions are increasingly needed and used in the field to accurately assess and treat the immigrant population for their prevalence of mental health conditions.

Major mental and behavioral health issues in prominent immigrant populations

Latinx American immigrant population

The Latinx population is one of the fastest-growing groups in the United States, and it is estimated that they will make up almost 25% of the US population by 2050 (Bridges et al., 2012; US Department of Commerce, 2003). Despite the constant influx of Latinx immigrants and the well-documented psychological impact of migration, Latinxs are less likely to use mental health services (Bridges et al., 2012). When seeking professional help for psychological distress, this population tends to utilize services provided by a primary care doctor rather than a mental health-care provider (Bridges et al., 2012; Kaltman, Hurtado de Mendoza, Gonzales, & Serrano, 2014). Acculturation, however, improves the knowledge and access to proper mental health care and has shown improvement among Latinx immigrants (Bridges et al., 2012).

As stated by Fortuna et al. (2008), political violence (PV) exposure is common among immigrants from Latin American countries, and this exposure has a profound impact on their mental health and highly associated with PTSD (Fortuna et al., 2008). Fortuna et al. (2008) found that 78% of immigrants who reported exposure to PV experienced these events before immigration. Findings also indicated that the onset of other mental health conditions such as anxiety and depression occurred after being exposed to PV in 21% of participants (Fortuna et al., 2008). For some immigrants, the decision to leave their home country is a planned process and most of the time on their account; however, of those individuals exposed to PV, nearly 59% stated they immigrated because they had to, and 67% reported PV was a significant factor in their decision to move (Fortuna et al., 2008). Trends among Latinx American older adult immigrants include a higher reporting of mood and anxiety disorder symptoms than other immigrant populations, such as Asian older adults, yet they seldom initiate mental health services (Kim et al., 2010).

Immigrant youth have also bared witness to the traumatic events of home country violence, or the distress of the immigration process (Bridges, de Arellano, Rheingold, Danielson, & Silcott, 2010; Fortuna et al., 2008). These youth also have a heightened risk for PTSD, depression, and other negative health-risk behaviors (Bridges et al., 2010). Much like adult Latinx immigrants, youth rarely seek mental health services for their symptoms, unless their parent is well acculturated to the host country's culture and can classify psychiatric and behavioral problems as needing psychiatric interventions (Bridges et al., 2010). Latinx youth share similar fears of seeking help as do their older generation counterparts such as fears of law enforcement and not having insurance (Bridges et al., 2010).

According to Glover and colleagues, out of the 2528 Latinx youth aged 11–18, foreign-born youth reported significantly higher anxiety symptoms on the Child Behavior Checklist (Glover, Pumariega, Holzer, Wise, & Rodriguez, 1999). Similarly, Latinx adolescents aged 12–17 residing in California reported youth who were less acculturated and were foreign-born had a heightened risk of depression when compared to US-born Latinx youth (Mikolajczyk, Bredehorst, Khelaifat, Maier, & Maxwell, 2007). Interestingly, findings of Degboe, BeLue, and Hillemeier (2012), indicated Latinx nonimmigrant youth reported being depressed or having anxiety at a higher prevalence than immigrant youth, but Latinx immigrant youth reported feeling worthless and withdrawn significantly more than their US-born counterparts.

Research suggests that having higher levels of cultural identity acts as a protective factor against mental illness (Yeh, 2003; Yoon et al., 2013). Findings of Rogers-Sirin and Gupta (2012) supported this suggestion as Latinx adolescents reported higher levels of cultural identity compared to their Asian counterparts, and in turn, reported lower levels of depression and withdrawal symptoms compared to the Asian adolescent participants. The study indicated that having a strong ethnic identity resulted in fewer withdrawn/depressed and somatic symptoms among the targeted youth (Rogers-Sirin & Gupta, 2012).

Asian American immigrant population

In 10 years (year 2000–10), the Asian population in the United States increased at a 43% rate from 10.2 million to 14.7 million and are labeled as the fastest-growing ethnic/racial group (US Census Bureau, 2011). A trend commonly found in the Asian immigrant population is limited contact with the health-care system, which is a result of limited English proficiency and insurance coverage (Clough et al., 2013; Nguyen & Lee, 2012). Mental health services are only used by 3%–6% of the Asian population (Nguyen & Lee, 2012). From the same study, Chinese and Vietnamese participants had the lowest English proficiency and indicated a decreased use of mental health services, increasing with age (Nguyen & Lee, 2012). Suggestions to address this issue is to increase the knowledge of health-care professionals on the traditional modes of medicine to better accommodate immigrants' preferences and to match patients with providers who speak the same language to ensure customs and beliefs compatibility (Clough et al., 2013). For Asian older adults, family conflict and stressful life events strongly predicted mental health use, which are both significant causes of mental health distress in immigrants (Nguyen, 2011).

Among adolescent immigrants, Yeh (2003) conducted a study that consisted of all Asian immigrant youth from Korean, Japanese, and Chinese subgroups and explored the impact of cultural adjustment on their mental health. Findings indicated that Korean immigrant youth had higher levels of mental health symptoms compared to their counterparts (Yeh, 2003). Age was found to be a significant predictor of mental health symptoms suggesting that older youth have been exposed to discrimination more than their younger peers, and they are experiencing more familial conflict with their parents due to the cultural conflict of opposing ideas, assumed roles, and autonomy (Yeh, 2003). As stated by Yeh (2003) and Yoon et al. (2013), cultural identity has an impact on both acculturation and mental health. Of the first- and second-generation Asian adolescents in the study by Rogers-Sirin and Gupta (2012), low levels of cultural identity were found, resulting in the 12th-grade youth reporting higher depressive and withdrawal symptoms and 10th-grade youth reporting more somatic distress symptoms. In contrast to the findings of Yeh (2003), results of Rogers-Sirin and Gupta (2012) reported that those in late adolescents reported fewer withdrawn/depressed and somatic symptoms.

African American immigrant population

In a 13-year period (2000–13), African-born immigrants in the United States increased by 137%, a total of 1.4 million (Akinsulure-Smith, 2017). Despite vast research on the mental health of immigrants, limited information is provided regarding African American immigrant population; therefore, they are of utmost importance in receiving culturally tailored interventions (Akinsulure-Smith, 2017). In the study of Ahmed and Rasmussen (2019), immigrants from the West African region were asked to complete a checklist that measured their exposure to traumatic events, as well as mental health measures to determine their postmigration mental health. Findings indicated that depression scores were influenced by exposure to traumatic events; other variables residency status was associated with PTSD symptoms (Ahmed & Rasmussen, 2019). Thirty-eight West African immigrants participated in the study of Akinsulure-Smith (2017) to determine psychological/emotional stressors. Similar to other immigrant groups, participants indicated that language barriers and immigrant status were common stressors, but they also reported racial/cultural discrimination to be the top stressor (Akinsulure-Smith, 2017). When asked what services they used to address their mental health, only two participants stated they have sought out professional counseling services, and both had negative interactions (Akinsulure-Smith, 2017). Many participants of Akinsulure-Smith's (2017) study utilized traditional methods instead; furthermore, Chaumba (2011) reported that Nigerian and Ethiopian immigrants tend to rely on spiritual healing and prayer when faced with an illness. Variables that were important in seeking mental health services were language compatibility with medical providers and services located within African-immigrant-serving community-based organizations (Akinsulure-Smith, 2017).

Assessment for mental health

As established throughout the chapter, the immigrant population varies significantly from the general population, and practitioners should tailor scales to fit the mental health needs and experiences of immigrants. Table 1 provides a summary of common assessment tools used for the immigrant population that is broken down by mental health conditions and other migration-related factors and population. Despite an array of assessment measures used among the immigrant

TABLE 1 Assessment tools used to measure mental health conditions and other factors impacting the mental health of immigrants.

Assessment tools used to measure mental health conditions and other factors impacting the mental health of immigrants			
Measurement tool	**Mental health condition measured**	**Population**	**References**
AC-OK	Various co-occurring mental health and substance abuse disorders	Latinx immigrants	Chavez et al. (2017) and Cherry, Dillon, Hellman, and Barney (2008)
Computerized Adaptive Test for Mental Health (CAT-MH)	Depression/anxiety/mania-hypomania/suicidality	Latinx immigrants in both United States and Spain	Gibbons et al. (2018)
Mini-International Neuropsychiatric Interview (MINI)	Anxiety, PTSD, and major depression (MD)	Latinx immigrants	Bridges et al. (2012) and Sheehan et al. (1998)
Hispanic Stress Inventory	Life event stress	Latinx immigrants-adults and adolescents	Cervantes et al. (2012, 2019)
Youth Self Report	Withdrawn-depressed symptoms/anxiety symptoms/somatic symptoms	Immigrant youth	Achenbach (1991), Cervantes et al. (2012), Rogers-Sirin and Gupta (2012), and Sirin et al. (2013)
Symptom Checklist-90-R (SCL-90-R)	Various mental health symptoms and distress levels	Asian immigrant youth	Derogatis (1994) and Yeh (2003)
Geriatric Depression Scale (GDS)	Depression	Older adult Asian immigrants	Mui et al. (2003)
World Health Organization (WHO) Composite International Diagnostic Interview (CIDI)	Depression, anxiety, PTSD, political violence	Latinx and Asian older adult immigrants, Latina, Asian, South Asian women immigrants	Fortuna et al. (2008), Kim et al. (2010), Lau et al. (2013), and Masood et al. (2009)
Primary Care Evaluation of Mental Disorders (PRIME-MD)	Somatic symptoms and major depressive disorder	African immigrant women	Miranda, Siddique, Belin, and Kohn-Wood (2005)

Posttraumatic Stress Disorder Checklist-Civilian (PCL-C)	Posttraumatic stress disorder (PTSD)	Latinx immigrants	Fortuna et al. (2016) and Wilkins et al. (2011)
World Mental Health Composite International Diagnostic Interview (WMH-CIDI)	Exposure to traumatic events	Voluntary migrants	Rasmussen et al. (2012)
Life Events Checklist	Exposure to traumatic events	West African immigrants	Ahmed and Rasmussen (2019) and Blake et al. (1995)
Stressful Life Events Questionnaire (SLESQ)	Trauma	Latina immigrants	Green et al. (2006) and Kaltman et al. (2014)
Brief Trauma Questionnaire	Trauma	Latinx immigrants	Fortuna et al. (2016) and Schnurr et al. (1999)
Mexican American Prevalence and Services Survey	Acculturation stress	Asian immigrants (adapted), latinx immigrants	Gong et al. (2011) and Vega et al. (1998)
Societal, Attitudinal, Familial, and Environmental-Revised-Short Form (SAFE-Short)	Acculturation stress	Immigrant adolescents	Mena et al. (1987) and Sirin et al. (2013)
Cultural Adjustment Difficulties Checklist (CADC)	Acculturation stress	Asian immigrant youth	Sodowsky and Wai Ming Lai (1997) and Yeh (2003)

population, researchers suggest that commonly used assessments are not culturally adapted to thoroughly assess the nuances of different ethnic cultures. Certain cultures such as Asian culture, typically report somatic symptoms when experiencing psychological conditions (Hall, Ibaraki, Huang, Marti, & Stice, 2016). Efforts have been made to improve culturally adapted interventions, but improvements to assessment measures are lacking. Several studies conducted by Hinton and colleagues used culturally based symptoms and effect sizes were shown to indicate cultural competence, but other factors could have also contributed to the large effect sizes such as having the same therapist throughout who spoke the native language (Hall et al., 2016; Hinton et al., 2004, 2005; Hinton, Hofmann, Pollack, & Otto, 2009; Hinton, Hofmann, Rivera, Otto, & Pollack, 2011). Silva, Paris, and Añez (2017) created a new assessment tool to measure mental health in immigrant Latinx, named CAMINO. CAMINO is an acronym that measures the immigration process through open-ended questions provided to the participant in either English or Spanish (Silva et al., 2017). This measurement tool also uses concepts of traditional idioms used in the culture to describe psychological or somatic symptoms (Silva et al., 2017). For the Latinx community, common idioms used are *nervios* for nerves and *susto* for fright (Silva et al., 2017). Silva et al. (2017) also stress the importance of knowing where the distress stems from and culturally sensitive treatment options.

As mentioned, culturally adapted assessment measures are rising in popularity, but lagging behind adapted interventions. Commonly used assessment measures have been used on the immigrant populations, and some alterations such as translation to native language have been made and have measured mental health adequality despite not being completely culturally adapted. Chavez et al. (2017) tested the adaptability of the Spanish version of the AC-OK Screen on the Latinx immigrant population, and results indicated that the Spanish version was comparable to the English version. The Computerized Adaptive Test for Mental Health (CAT-MH) was tested on Latin American migrants in both the United States and Spain (Gibbons et al., 2018). Findings indicated that the Spanish version of CAT-MH is reliable in measuring depression, anxiety, and mania and can be used as an international scale (Gibbons et al., 2018). The Mini-International Neuropsychiatric Interview (MINI), available in Spanish, is also commonly used among Latinx immigrants to assess anxiety, PTSD, and major depression (Bridges et al., 2012; Sheehan et al., 1998). To address the issue of limited culturally adapted assessment tools for the Latinx immigrant population, Cervantes et al. (2012) have created the Latino Stress Inventory-Adolescent Version to accurately measure psychological symptoms.

Other scales used among adolescent immigrants include the Youth Self Report (YSR) which includes questions pertaining to somatic symptoms commonly found in the Asian and Latinx immigrant population in addition to measuring symptoms of withdrawn-depression and anxiety (Achenbach, 1991; Rogers-Sirin & Gupta, 2012; Sirin, Ryce, Gupta, & Rogers-Sirin, 2013). Asian youth mental health symptoms have also been measured by using the Symptom

Checklist-90-R (SCL-90-R), which has been proven to be reliable among the Asian population through its ability to be translated into many Asian languages (Derogatis, 1994; Yeh, 2003).

For older adult immigrants, the Geriatric Depression Scale (GDS) was found to be reliable in assessing older adult Asian immigrants, as well as the short version of the scale (Mui, Kang, Chen, & Domanski, 2003). The GDS has been tested multiple times across many cultures and ethnicities and is considered a reliable cross-cultural measurement (Mui et al., 2003). The World Health Organization World Mental Health Composite International Diagnostic Interview (WHO WMH-CIDI, or WHO-CIDI, or WMH-CIDI) was used to assess mental health in a wide range of Latinx and Asian immigrant older adults (Kim et al., 2010), Latinx immigrants (Fortuna et al., 2008), Asian women (Lau et al., 2013), and South Asian women (Masood, Okazaki, & Takeuchi, 2009).

Traumatic events and acculturation stress

Research has shown that exposure to trauma significantly impacts the mental health of voluntary migrants, so multiple studies included assessments, such as the WMH-CIDI, that measured participants' exposure to traumatic events for voluntary migrants (Rasmussen, Crager, Baser, Chu, & Gany, 2012) or political violence in Latinx immigrants (Fortuna et al., 2008). Some measures, such as the PCL-C (Wilkins, Lang, & Norman, 2011) and Brief Trauma Questionnaire created by Schnurr, Vielhauer, Weathers, and Findler (1999) were used across two countries, Spain and the United States (Fortuna et al., 2016). Life Events Checklist, developed by Blake et al. (1995), was used to assess West African immigrants' exposure to traumatic events (Ahmed & Rasmussen, 2019). In addition, the Stressful Life Events Questionnaire (SLESQ) (Green, Chung, Daroowalla, Kaltman, & DeBenedictis, 2006) measured traumas experienced by Latina immigrants from Central and South America and Mexico (Kaltman et al., 2014).

Acculturation stress also received recognition as a significant factor in the mental health of immigrants. In the study of Gong, Xu, Fujishiro, and Takeuchi (2011), acculturation stress of Asian immigrants was measured with an adapted version of the Mexican American Prevalence and Services Survey (Vega et al., 1998). Measured mostly among immigrant youth, adolescents of Sirin et al. (2013) were assessed by the Societal, Attitudinal, Familial, and Environmental-Revised-Short Form (SAFE-Short) developed by Mena, Padilla, and Maldonado (1987) and Yeh (2003) endorsed the Cultural Adjustment Difficulties Checklist (CADC) created by Sodowsky and Wai Ming Lai (1997) to use among Asian youth.

Interventions for mental health

A metaanalysis consisting of 78 articles regarding culturally adapted interventions concluded that although efforts have been made to provide culturally sensitive treatment, more effort is needed (Hall et al., 2016). A similar study by Smith and Trimble (2016), believes that traditional treatment methods have not included or considered factors such as culture and race and ethnicity as well as other related factors. To practice culturally adapted treatments means to alter the delivery, context, and concepts to fit a clients' "cultural worldview" according to Smith and Trimble (2016). Findings of Hall et al. (2016) suggested that culturally adapted interventions reduced psychopathology symptoms more so than traditional interventions; in addition, Smith and Trimble (2016) concluded that adapted treatments offer better outcomes for people of color than traditional methods. Furthermore, findings were similar in terms of results formulated by traditional psychopathology interventions (Hall et al., 2016). Hall and colleagues identified challenges in providing culturally adapted interventions that stemmed from commonly used assessment tools failing to use culturally sensitive terminology and somatic symptoms which other ethnic cultures tend to use when expressing psychological symptoms. Other commonly known issues are the translation of interventions to non-English language and the idea of a cultural match between clinician and client (Hall et al., 2016). The meta-analysis concluded that evidence-based interventions can be translated to other non-English languages as long as the translation process included back translation as well (Hall et al., 2016). It is also suggested that ethnic match might be helpful in the beginning stages for adherence concerns but is not necessary as the therapeutic alliance begins to form (Hall et al., 2016). Effective treatments, in Smith and Trimble's (2016) study consisted of client-focused goals, appropriate cultural contexts, and clients' preferred language.

Traditional intervention approaches

Psychopharmacological approaches

Psychopharmacological approaches are commonly prescribed to individuals experiencing depression. Medication treatment adherence among depressed Latinx Americans was high (80%) among the participants of Green et al. (2017); moreover, reports indicated participants viewed the medications as helpful, and improvements were shown in their Patient Health Questionnaire (PHQ) scores. In contrast, Latinx women in the study of Kaltman et al. (2014) reported medication as the least favorable modality. Other ethnic groups showed varied preferences for pharmacological approaches. Nadeem, Lange, and Miranda (2008) conducted a study comparing treatment preferences among US-born white, Latinx, and African Americans and immigrant Latinx and African participants. Compared to US-born white, both US-born and immigrant Latinx and African participants were not as likely to label medication as helpful, which is contrary to the findings of Green et al. (2017) (Nadeem et al., 2008). However, those who reported somatic symptoms were more likely to suggest medication as a preferred treatment option, and findings suggest that symptoms that begin as physical symptoms are typically treated with a biomedical intervention method, such as medicine (Nadeem et al., 2008). Existing literature regarding the use of pharmacological approaches by African American immigrant population was limited to studies that included other immigrant populations. Therefore, research exploring their views and adherence to medication without the inclusion of other groups is needed to further create viable culturally informed treatment options.

An issue to the adherence of medication is the stigma associated with mental health as well as the preference for traditional cultural approaches to health. Over half (53%) of first-generation Korean Americans in the study of Kim-Goh, Choi, and Yoon (2015) indicated they were least willing and most ashamed to try antidepressants as a treatment option.

Psychotherapy and counseling approaches

In a study examining the treatment preferences of Latinx Americans who were diagnosed with PTSD, nearly all participants stated they would prefer some form of talk therapy in a primary care setting because of the perceived link between psychological distress and physical health (Eisenman et al., 2008). A derivative of talk therapy, narrative therapy (use of client stories or narrative to describe perceived problem behavior) is discussed by Gibbons and Farrell (2019) as a treatment method among college-aged Latinx immigrants who have a range of mental health concerns, such as acculturation stress, depression, and anxiety. Also, second-generation Latinas with depressive symptoms perceived therapy in a positive way and reported appreciation on their needs being quickly addressed; however, gender-based violence or family's disapproval significantly impacted therapy adherence (Heilemann, Pieters, & Dornig, 2016). In a study conducted among Latinx women examining the preferred intervention methods for trauma-related mental health services, the majority of the women indicated a preference for individual therapy followed by family therapy (Kaltman et al., 2014). Individual therapy was perceived to be more beneficial for the women since it would give them an opportunity to discuss themselves and a chance to decompress from stressors and receive professional guidance in a confidential setting (Kaltman et al., 2014). As for psychotherapy, supportive psychotherapy and cognitive-behavioral therapy (CBT) were selected as the most preferred type (Kaltman et al., 2014).

According to Hall et al. (2016), CBT was one of the commonly used culturally adapted treatment methods used across multiple cultures and ethnicities. CBT has also been acknowledged to be a suitable treatment method for bilingual Latinx older adults with late-life depression (Alvarez, Rengifo, Emrani, & Gallagher-Thompson, 2014). CBT was also a preferred method among Asian Americans suggested by clinicians (Kim-Goh et al., 2015). Practitioners also stated blending in other family members throughout the therapeutic process and utilizing the hierarchical structure of the counselor-client relationship were also ways to bridge in cultural approaches to the intervention (Kim-Goh et al., 2015). Another potential culturally informed treatment modality for Asian

Americans would be mindfulness-based therapy, which incorporates concepts from Buddhism and has links to the Asian culture and their perception of mental health (Kim-Goh et al., 2015).

Like pharmacological approaches, limited research is available on mental health treatment for African immigrants. However, one study devised a CBT group that consisted of Somali immigrant women. Living Life to the Full (LLTTF) incorporated building skills for positive mental well-being with a context of life stressors (Pratt et al., 2017). Somali women were trained to facilitate the program, and participants reported positive results in their happiness levels and in turn, noticed a decrease in their anxiety levels (Pratt et al., 2017). Participants also mentioned that skills learned throughout the program would be useful for future stressful situations, and the program was beneficial in engaging these women and garnering enthusiasm for ways to cope with stress and improve overall mental health (Pratt et al., 2017).

Family group psychotherapy

Intervention approaches for immigrant youth tend to be family-based with culturally specific or transcultural focus (Kim, Schwartz, Perreira, & Juang, 2018). One important protective factor among immigrant adolescents and youth was a positive cultural identity. For instance, the Identity Project was able to improve mental health of the population by promoting identity exploration and resolution (Kim et al., 2018; Umaña-Taylor, Douglass, Updegraff, & Marsiglia, 2017).

For Latinx adolescents and their families, Entre Dos Mundos provides training on bicultural skills and addresses parent-child conflict; it has been effective in reducing child aggression and blending bicultural identity for participants (Bacallao & Smokowski, 2005; Kim et al., 2018). Another program that promotes bicultural identity is Familias Unidas; it includes concepts of communication and negotiation to address family conflict and build connections between the family unit (Kim et al., 2018; Pantin et al., 2003). Another family-based intervention for Latinx adolescents and their families is Bridges, which targets parenting, proper coping for adolescents, and family cohesion (Gonzales et al., 2014; Kim et al., 2018). Family therapy was perceived as the second most desired method of treatment among Latinx females and was seen as beneficial in improving family problems through family discussion (Kaltman et al., 2014).

For Asian youth, an option is the Parent Training (PT) program; it provides parenting skills to promote communication and involvement and was effective in reducing internalized symptoms in Asian youth (Kim et al., 2018; Lau, Fung, Ho, Liu, & Gudiño, 2011). Another is a multifamily psycho-education (MFPG), which Chow et al. (2010) conducted as a pilot study targeting Asian and Tamil immigrant families who have mental health concerns present in the family. Reduced perceived mental health burden in families was found, and the cultural approach proved to be successful as participants shared experiences and supported other families in their native language (Chow et al., 2010).

Combination of psychopharmacological and psychotherapy approaches

Although there is limited research on the combination of psychopharmacological and psychotherapy approaches in immigrant populations, the literature supports effectiveness among older immigrants. Camacho, Estrada, Lagomasino, Aranda, and Green (2018) devised a program that incorporated problem-solving treatment (PST) in a primary care setting among Latinx older adults. PST is a structured form of psychosocial therapy that includes concepts of rational problem-solving, regulating emotions, and psychoeducation on depression (Arean, Hegel, & Unützer, 1999a, 1999b; Camacho et al., 2018). Fourteen older adult immigrants were able to receive PST from a bilingual facilitator and discuss issues that brought them distress, such as family conflict, naturalization process, and medication adherence (Camacho et al., 2018). Eleven participants also took medication in addition to the PST, and overall positive feedback was reported (Camacho et al., 2018). The psychoeducation segment of the treatment method was particularly effective as this population is known to not seek mental health services (Camacho et al., 2018).

Culturally sensitive alternative treatments

It is not uncommon for immigrants to prefer alternative treatments that are more incline to their cultural beliefs. Immigrants may use spiritual folk healers, herbal medicine, acupuncture, massage therapy, or chiropractic medicine instead of Western medicine such as medication, talk therapy, or a combination of the two. Other treatment options that were suggested by immigrants include exercise for depression (Kim & Im, 2015), faith (Nadeem et al., 2008), and traditional cultural medicines (Nguyen et al., 2016). Nearly 70% of Vietnamese immigrant participants in Nguyen et al.'s (2016) study indicated that they used Traditional Vietnamese Medicine (TVM), such as herbal pills and eastern massage. Ethiopians and Nigerians participants in Chaumba's (2011) study reported spiritual healing and prayer as a common treatment approach, in which studies have found religious coping approaches reduce levels of depression symptoms.

New/emerging intervention approaches

Telemedicine

Telecommunication technology is used to close the gaps of limited health-care access of underserved populations; however, there are limited studies incorporating technology in treatment options for immigrants. George, Hamilton, and Baker (2012) conducted a study in 2012 that garnered perceptions about emerging telemedicine among urban African and Latinx Americans. Although the study did not include immigrants specifically, the sample consisted of individuals residing in an urban, low-income area, in which immigrants tend to occupy as well (Bridges et al., 2012; George et al., 2012; Pumariega et al., 2005). Distrust among the medical community and African American population is a barrier in immigrants' willingness to seek professional mental health care (Nadeem et al., 2008). African American participants reported their qualms about the stability of technology, not being able to physically see the physician, and not knowing the physician's qualifications to be of utmost concern (George et al., 2012). On the other hand, Latinx American participants were not as concerned about the lack of face-to-face physical communication and appeared to like the idea of being a consumer of medical technology advancement (George et al., 2012). Findings suggest that future telemedicine treatments should be culturally tailored, and medical personnel should take extra precautions in ensuring confidentiality (George et al., 2012).

A recent study conducted among Latinx immigrant women in Spain tested the feasibility of a text messaging component with psychosocial therapies (García, Ferrás, Rocha, & Aguilera, 2019). Previous research has used mobile phones to increase communication between therapist and client as well as provide services to populations with limited resources and improve access to services (García et al., 2019). Text messaging services have been used to provide information about treatments to other vulnerable groups, and therapists are already using technology in their everyday practice, such as video and email (García et al., 2019). Over half (65.9%) the women among the intervention group stated they felt more connected with their social environment, and 81% saved the text messages for future reference (García et al., 2019). Interventions of this type might be only helpful to those of younger age, as older women responded less (García et al., 2019). Overall, the program was met with positive feedback although some women would have liked either more personalized messages or face-to-face interaction (García et al., 2019).

Despite the lack of adherence to the intended program by older women (García et al., 2019), Jang et al. (2014) conducted a pilot study on telecounseling with older Korean immigrants who reported depression symptoms and had limited English proficiency; retention rate was very high. Among immigrants, limited English proficiency is a known barrier to mental health services; however, results from the study of Jang et al. (2014) indicated that by utilizing a telecounseling approach in their native language, participants responded well to the program and received needed treatment and education regarding their mental health condition.

Another study was conducted in Denmark that included participants of asylum, refugee, and immigrant status (Mucic, 2010). Mucic (2010) tested patient satisfaction on transcultural telepsychiatry provided in patients' native language. The telepsychiatry sessions included both assessment and treatment, and although some of the participants had other mental health conditions not mentioned thus far, the majority were assessed for PTSD and depression (Mucic, 2010). Telepsychiatry provided underserved populations with the needed language and culture components without having to travel for an "ethnic match" (Mucic, 2010).

Limited research is available to access telemedicine use among adolescents; however, a recent study conducted by Wu, Torous, and Liu (2018) measured the potential use of mental health awareness smartphone apps among Chinese immigrant parents. The pilot study found that 20% of participants expressed interest in receiving resources regarding Child Psychiatrist/Psychology counseling through smartphone applications, despite 89% being interested in child mental health applications (Wu et al., 2018). Parental education played a huge role in determining interest in these applications; parents with lower education expressed higher interest (Wu et al., 2018). An explanation could be that apps increase accessibility and affordability, suggesting that apps could be an emerging method in disseminating child mental health awareness among vulnerable populations (Wu et al., 2018).

Barriers to treatment

Barriers to treatment adherence for immigrants include location of health-care and mental health-care facilities, stigma associated with mental health (both traditional culture stigma and mainstream culture stigma), language barriers (Fortuna & Porche, 2014), legal status (Fortuna & Porche, 2014), and preference for traditional culture healing methods (Pumariega et al., 2005). Other barriers to treatment include fear of being discovered, lack of finances or health insurance, and lack of time due to working multiple jobs and long hours (Fortuna & Porche, 2014). Environmental factors such as exposure to political violence also pose a barrier to treatment as immigrants who have experienced political violence have reported very low use of mental health services (Fortuna & Porche, 2014). Gender can also act as a barrier in seeking mental health services. Immigrant men who came from countries with a history of political violence did not utilize mental health services as often as their female counterparts, even though they had similar prevalence of anxiety or depression (Fortuna & Porche, 2014).

There are also ethnic-specific barriers. For the Latinx American immigrant population, the cost of services and not having a bilingual health-care provider were the top two concerns Latinxs had regarding the logistics of seeking professional help (Bridges et al., 2012; Fortuna et al., 2008; Kaltman et al., 2014). Another barrier among the Latinx population was seeking mental health services from a primary care physician, who often lack expertise in mental health knowledge. The Latinx community tended to use the primary care physician as a "one-stop-shop" for all their medical needs, and this could also be a result of their tendency to somaticize psychological distress symptoms. Also, they may be hesitant to use mental health-care providers due to preference for traditional cultural treatment methods as well as lack of insurance or documentation status (Bridges et al., 2012; Fortuna et al., 2008). For Asian American immigrants, a barrier to seeking mental health treatment lies within the cultural aspect of suppressing emotions. They will often use less direct ways to communicate distress and exhibit somatic symptoms (Kim-Goh et al., 2015). Therefore, Western mental health treatment modalities, such as therapy, that focuses on expressing feelings may deter adherence to treatment for Asian Americans (Kim-Goh et al., 2015). A barrier to seeking mental health treatment among African American immigrants include distrust in the medical system as a result of institutional racism and a history of using African Americans for research and medical purposes without authorized consent (George et al., 2012; Nadeem et al., 2008).

Implications for social work practice, policy, and future research

To ensure best practice for mental health services to the diverse immigrant population, there are many factors to consider. First, it is important to recognize the culture of the immigrant, to tailor assessments and treatment options to the individual as well as identify known cultural barriers to maintain cultural sensitivity. Second, knowing which generational cohort the individual is, will also ensure competent practice, as first-generational immigrants tend to have different mental health concerns compared to second and even third-generation immigrants, as outlined in the healthy migrant hypothesis and the immigrant paradox (Cervantes et al., 2019; Salas-Wright et al., 2018). Thirdly, other factors such as the age of migration, reason for migration, level of acculturation, acculturation stress, and permanency status in the host country should all be examined to address mental health issues in this vulnerable population.

In response to the 2012 American Psychological Association's (APA) Presidential Task Force on Immigration, research has stressed the importance of mental health practitioners providing culturally competent services and being culturally competent in the delivery of such services [American Psychological Association (APA), 2012]. Rogers-Sirin, Melendez, Refano, and Zegarra (2015) took part in an in-depth qualitative investigation to explore how ten college students with immigrant parents from various ethnicities perceived their therapists' cultural competence. Four themes of cultural incompetence emerged: lack of clarity of what therapy entails, discrimination and microaggressions, assuming cultural knowledge, and pathologizing cultural differences (Rogers-Sirin et al., 2015). Cultural competence themes such as open to learning about clients' culture, using culture in an appropriate way, knowing when culture is not related to the presenting issue, demonstrating patience, and displaying empathy emerged as well (Rogers-Sirin et al., 2015).

Social workers and other mental health professionals also should possess these cultural competency skills and objectively assess their current approach to immigrants and clients of different race and ethnicity to determine if they are acting in a culturally sensitive manner. Cross-cultural competency skills for mental health practitioners are outlined by Arredondo et al. (1996) and focus on skill-building about concepts of understanding personal cultural beliefs and biases, awareness of client's worldview, and intervention strategies that are culturally sensitive (Rogers-Sirin et al., 2015). Providing language assistance and taking into consideration the patients' culture will ensure effective treatment delivery as well as treatment acceptability.

From a research point of view, studies consisting of prevalence data among all three populations and age groups are limited, and therefore difficult to assess how many immigrants are experiencing mental health conditions as a result of their immigrant status. In particular, studies regarding the African American immigrant population are lacking. Future research is needed to determine what mental health conditions impact each subpopulation. Also, as this chapter examined that each group responds differently to interventions because of culture, level of acculturation, and other factors, the best type of intervention for each population and age group needs to be investigated.

Conclusion

The immigrant population of the United States is expected to increase over the coming years, and the constant influx of new immigrants will mix in with previous generations of immigrants. A prominent impact that literature has proven is that immigrants are susceptible to various mental health conditions such as depression, anxiety, and posttraumatic stress disorder (PTSD) due to a wide array of psychological and emotional distress from the immigration and acculturation process. Since each population and corresponding age group are impacted differently, social workers and other mental health professionals are urged to stay up-to-date on skills that promote culturally competent practice through utilizing appropriate assessment and intervention methods that are evidenced-based and work within the clients' culture. Future research is needed to expand upon the existing literature regarding the mental and behavioral health of immigrants, especially among the Latinx, Asian, and African groups who are making up a majority of the immigrant population in the United States.

References

Achenbach, T. M. (1991). *Manual for the teacher's report form and 1991 profile*. Univ. Vermont/Department Psychiatry.

Ahmed, S., & Rasmussen, A. (2019). Changes in social status and postmigration mental health among West African immigrants. *American Journal of Orthopsychiatry*, https://doi.org/10.1037/ort0000419.

Akinsulure-Smith, A. M. (2017). Resilience in the face of adversity: African immigrants' mental health needs and the American transition. *Journal of Immigrant & Refugee Studies*, *15*(4), 428–448. https://doi.org/10.1080/15562948.2016.1238989.

Alvarez, P., Rengifo, J., Emrani, T., & Gallagher-Thompson, D. (2014). Latino older adults and mental health: A review and commentary. *Clinical Gerontologist*, *37*(1), 33–48. https://doi.org/10.1080/07317115.2013.847514.

American Psychological Association (APA). (2012). *Crossroads: The psychology of immigrantion in the new century*. Washington, DC: APA.

Arean, P., Hegel, M., & Unützer, J. (1999a). *Problem-solving therapy for older primary care patients: Maintenance group manual for Project IMPACT*. Los Angeles: University of California, Los Angeles.

Arean, P., Hegel, M., & Unützer, J. (1999b). *Problem-solving treatment in primary care: Addendum to PST-PC treatment manual for Project IMPACT*. Los Angeles: University of California, Los Angeles.

Arredondo, P., Toporek, R., Brown, S. P., Jones, J., Locke, D. C., Sanchez, J., & Stadler, H. (1996). Operationalization of the multicultural counseling competencies. *Journal of Multicultural Counseling and Development*, *24*(1), 42–78.

Bacallao, M. L., & Smokowski, P. R. (2005). "Entre dos mundos" (between two worlds): Bicultural skills training with Latino immigrant families. *Journal of Primary Prevention*, *26*(6), 485–509.

Blake, D. D., Weathers, F. W., Nagy, L. M., Kaloupek, D. G., Gusman, F. D., Charney, D. S., & Keane, T. M. (1995). The development of a clinician-administered PTSD scale. *Journal of Traumatic Stress*, *8*(1), 75–90.

Bridges, A. J., Andrews, A. R., & Deen, T. L. (2012). Mental health needs and service utilization by Hispanic immigrants residing in mid-southern United States. *Journal of Transcultural Nursing*, *23*(4), 359–368. https://doi.org/10.1177/1043659612451259.

Bridges, A. J., de Arellano, M. A., Rheingold, A. A., Danielson, C. K., & Silcott, L. (2010). Trauma exposure, mental health, and service utilization rates among immigrant and United States-born Hispanic youth: Results from the Hispanic family study. *Psychological Trauma Theory Research Practice and Policy*, *2*(1), 40–48. https://doi.org/10.1037/a0019021.

Caballero, T. M., Ross DeCamp, L., Platt, R. E., Shah, H., Johnson, S. B., Sibinga, E. M. S., & Polk, S. (2017). Addressing the mental health needs of Latino children in immigrant families. *Clinical Pediatrics*, *56*(7), 648–658. https://doi.org/10.1177/0009922816679509.

Camacho, D., Estrada, E., Lagomasino, I. T., Aranda, M. P., & Green, J. (2018). Descriptions of depression and depression treatment in older Hispanic immigrants in a geriatric collaborative care program. *Aging & Mental Health*, *22*(8), 1056–1062. https://doi.org/10.1080/13607863.2017.1332159.

Cervantes, R. C., Fisher, D. G., Córdova, D., Jr., & Napper, L. E. (2012). The Hispanic Stress Inventory—Adolescent version: A culturally informed psychosocial assessment. *Psychological Assessment*, *24*(1), 187–196. https://doi.org/10.1037/a0025280.

Cervantes, R. C., Gattamorta, K. A., & Berger-Cardoso, J. (2019). Examining difference in immigration stress, acculturation stress and mental health outcomes in six Hispanic/Latino nativity and regional groups. *Journal of Immigrant and Minority Health*, *21*(1), 14–20. https://doi.org/10.1007/s10903-018-0714-9.

Chaumba, J. (2011). Health status, use of health care resources, and treatment strategies of Ethiopian and Nigerian immigrants in the United States. *Social Work in Health Care*, *50*(6), 466–481. https://doi.org/10.1080/00981389.2011.581999.

Chavez, L. M., Shrout, P. E., Wang, Y., Collazos, F., Carmona, R., & Alegría, M. (2017). Evaluation of the AC-OK mental health and substance abuse screening measure in an international sample of Latino immigrants. *Drug & Alcohol Dependence*, *180*, 121–128. https://doi.org/10.1016/j.drugalcdep.2017.07.042.

Cherry, A. L., Dillon, M. E., Hellman, C. M., & Barney, L. (2008). The AC-COD screen: Rapid detection of people with the co-occurring disorders of substance abuse, mental illness, domestic violence, and trauma. *Journal of Dual Diagnosis*, *4*(1), 35–53.

Chow, W., Law, S., Andermann, L., Yang, J., Leszcz, M., Wong, J., & Sadavoy, J. (2010). Multi-family psycho-education group for assertive community treatment clients and families of culturally diverse background: A pilot study. *Community Mental Health Journal*, *46*(4), 364–371. https://doi.org/10.1007/s10597-010-9305-5.

Clough, J., Lee, S., & Chae, D. H. (2013). Barriers to health care among Asian immigrants in the United States: A traditional review. *Journal of Health Care for the Poor and Underserved*, *24*(1), 384–403. https://doi.org/10.1353/hpu.2013.0019.

Degboe, A., BeLue, R., & Hillemeier, M. (2012). Parental immigrant status and adolescent mental health in the United states: Do racial/ethnic differences exist? *Child and Adolescent Mental Health*, *17*(4), 209–215. https://doi.org/10.1111/j.1475-3588.2011.00636.x.

Derogatis, L. (1994). *Scl-90-r: Administration, scoring and procedures manual*. Minneapolis: National Computer Systems.

Eisenman, D. P., Meredith, L. S., Rhodes, H., Green, B. L., Kaltman, S., Cassells, A., & Tobin, J. N. (2008). PTSD in Latino patients: Illness beliefs, treatment preferences, and implications for care. *Journal of General Internal Medicine*, *23*(9), 1386–1392. https://doi.org/10.1007/s11606-008-0677-y.

Fortuna, L. R., Álvarez, K., Ramos Ortiz, Z., Wang, Y., Mozo Alegría, X., Cook, B. L., & Alegría, M. (2016). Mental health, migration stressors and suicidal ideation among Latino immigrants in Spain and the United States. *European Psychiatry*, *36*, 15–22. https://doi.org/10.1016/j.eurpsy.2016.03.001.

Fortuna, L. R., & Porche, M. V. (2014). Clinical issues and challenges in treating undocumented immigrants. *Psychiatric Times*, *31*(1), 1–5. Retrieved from: https://search.ebscohost.com/login.aspx?direct=true&db=hch&AN=94412903&site=ehost-live.

Fortuna, L., Porche, M., & Alegria, M. (2008). Political violence, psychosocial trauma, and the context of mental health services use among immigrant Latinos in the United States. *Ethnicity & Health*, *13*(5), 435–463. https://doi.org/10.1080/13557850701837286.

García, Y., Ferrás, C., Rocha, Á., & Aguilera, A. (2019). Exploratory study of psychosocial therapies with text messages to mobile phones in groups of vulnerable immigrant women. *Journal of Medical Systems*, *43*(8). N.PAG-N.PAG. https://doi.org/10.1007/s10916-019-1393-3.

George, S., Hamilton, A., & Baker, R. S. (2012). How do low-income urban African Americans and Latinos feel about telemedicine? A diffusion of innovation analysis. *International Journal of Telemedicine & Applications*, 1–9. https://doi.org/10.1155/2012/715194.

Gibbons, R. D., Alegría, M., Cai, L., Herrera, L., Markle, S. L., Collazos, F., & Baca-García, E. (2018). Successful validation of the CAT-MH Scales in a sample of Latin American migrants in the United States and Spain. *Psychological Assessment*, *30*(10), 1267–1276. https://doi.org/10.1037/pas0000569.

Gibbons, M. M., & Farrell, I. C. (2019). Using narrative therapy to assist college-age Latino immigrants. *Journal of College Counseling*, *22*(1), 83–96. https://doi.org/10.1002/jocc.12116.

Glover, S. H., Pumariega, A. J., Holzer, C. E., Wise, B. K., & Rodriguez, M. (1999). Anxiety symptomatology in Mexican-American adolescents. *Journal of Child and Family Studies*, *8*(1), 47–57.

Gong, F., Xu, J., Fujishiro, K., & Takeuchi, D. T. (2011). A life course perspective on migration and mental health among Asian immigrants: The role of human agency. *Social Science & Medicine*, *73*(11), 1618–1626. https://doi.org/10.1016/j.socscimed.2011.09.014.

Gonzales, N. A., Wong, J. J., Toomey, R. B., Millsap, R., Dumka, L. E., & Mauricio, A. M. (2014). School engagement mediates long-term prevention effects for Mexican American adolescents. *Prevention Science*, *15*(6), 929–939.

Green, B. L., Chung, J. Y., Daroowalla, A., Kaltman, S., & DeBenedictis, C. (2006). Evaluating the cultural validity of the stressful life events screening questionnaire. *Violence Against Women*, *12*(12), 1191–1213.

Green, B. L., Watson, M. R., Kaltman, S. I., Serrano, A., Talisman, N., Kirkpatrick, L., & Campoli, M. (2017). Knowledge and preferences regarding antidepressant medication among depressed Latino patients in primary care. *Journal of Nervous and Mental Disease*, *205*(12), 952–959. https://doi.org/10.1097/NMD.0000000000000754.

Hall, G. C. N., Ibaraki, A. Y., Huang, E. R., Marti, C. N., & Stice, E. (2016). A meta-analysis of cultural adaptations of psychological interventions. *Behavior Therapy*, *47*(6), 993–1014. https://doi.org/10.1016/j.beth.2016.09.005.

Heilemann, M. V., Pieters, H. C., & Dornig, K. (2016). Reflections of low-income, second-generation Latinas about experiences in depression therapy. *Qualitative Health Research, 26*(10), 1351–1365. https://doi.org/10.1177/1049732315624411.

Hinton, D. E., Chhean, D., Pich, V., Safren, S. A., Hofmann, S. G., & Pollack, M. H. (2005). A randomized controlled trial of cognitive-behavior therapy for Cambodian refugees with treatment-resistant PTSD and panic attacks: A cross-over design. *Journal of Traumatic Stress, 18*, 617–629. https://doi.org/10.1002/jts.20070.

Hinton, D. E., Hofmann, S. G., Pollack, M. H., & Otto, M. W. (2009). Mechanisms of efficacy of CBT for Cambodian refugees with PTSD: Improvement in emotion regulation and orthostatic blood pressure response. *CNS Neuroscience & Therapeutics, 15*, 255–263. https://doi.org/10.1111/j. 1755-5949.2009.00100.x.

Hinton, D. E., Hofmann, S. G., Rivera, E., Otto, M. W., & Pollack, M. H. (2011). Culturally adapted CBT (CA-CBT) for Latino women with treatment-resistant PTSD: A pilot study comparing CA-CBT to applied muscle relaxation. *Behaviour Research and Therapy, 49*, 275–280. https://doi.org/10.1016/j.brat.2011.01.005.

Hinton, D. E., Pham, T., Tran, M., Safren, S. A., Otto, M. W., & Pollack, M. H. (2004). CBT for Vietnamese refugees with treatment-resistant PTSD and panic attacks: A pilot study. *Journal of Traumatic Stress, 17*, 429–433. https://doi.org/10.1023/B:JOTS.0000048956.03529.fa.

Jang, Y., Chiriboga, D. A., Molinari, V., Roh, S., Park, Y., Kwon, S., & Cha, H. (2014). Telecounseling for the linguistically isolated: a pilot study with older Korean immigrants. *Gerontologist, 54*(2), 290–296. https://doi.org/10.1093/geront/gns196.

Kaltman, S., Hurtado de Mendoza, A., Gonzales, F. A., & Serrano, A. (2014). Preferences for trauma-related mental health services among Latina immigrants from Central America, South America, and Mexico. *Psychological Trauma: Theory, Research, Practice, and Policy, 6*(1), 83–91. https://doi.org/10.1037/a0031539.

Kim, E., & Im, E.-O. (2015). Korean-Americans' knowledge about depression and attitudes about treatment options. *Issues in Mental Health Nursing, 36*(6), 455–463. https://doi.org/10.3109/01612840.2014.997846.

Kim, G., Jang, Y., Chiriboga, D. A., Ma, G. X., & Schonfeld, L. (2010). Factors associated with mental health service use in Latino and Asian immigrant elders. *Aging & Mental Health, 14*(5), 535–542. https://doi.org/10.1080/13607860903311758.

Kim, S. Y., Schwartz, S. J., Perreira, K. M., & Juang, L. P. (2018). Culture's influence on stressors, parental socialization, and developmental processes in the mental health of children of immigrants. *Annual Review of Clinical Psychology, 14*, 343–370. https://doi.org/10.1146/annurev-clinpsy-050817-084925.

Kim-Goh, M., Choi, H., & Yoon, M. S. (2015). Culturally responsive counseling for Asian Americans: Clinician perspectives. *International Journal for the Advancement of Counselling, 37*(1), 63–76. https://doi.org/10.1007/s10447-014-9226-z.

Lau, A. S., Fung, J. J., Ho, L. Y., Liu, L. L., & Gudiño, O. G. (2011). Parent training with high-risk immigrant Chinese families: A pilot group randomized trial yielding practice-based evidence. *Behavior Therapy, 42*(3), 413–426.

Lau, A. S., Tsai, W., Shih, J., Liu, L. L., Hwang, W.-C., & Takeuchi, D. T. (2013). The immigrant paradox among Asian American women: Are disparities in the burden of depression and anxiety paradoxical or explicable? *Journal of Consulting and Clinical Psychology, 81*(5), 901–911. https://doi.org/10.1037/a0032105.

Masood, N., Okazaki, S., & Takeuchi, D. T. (2009). Gender, family, and community correlates of mental health in South Asian Americans. *Cultural Diversity and Ethnic Minority Psychology, 15*(3), 265–274. https://doi.org/10.1037/a0014301.

Mena, F. J., Padilla, A. M., & Maldonado, M. (1987). Acculturative stress and specific coping strategies among immigrant and later generation college students. *Hispanic Journal of Behavioral Sciences*, *9*(2), 207–225.

Mikolajczyk, R. T., Bredehorst, M., Khelaifat, N., Maier, C., & Maxwell, A. E. (2007). Correlates of depressive symptoms among Latino and Non-Latino White adolescents: Findings from the 2003 California Health Interview Survey. *BMC Public Health*, *7*(1), 21.

Miranda, J., Siddique, J., Belin, T. R., & Kohn-Wood, L. P. (2005). Depression prevalence in disadvantaged young black women: African and Caribbean immigrants compared to US-born African Americans. *Social Psychiatry and Psychiatric Epidemiology: The International Journal for Research in Social and Genetic Epidemiology and Mental Health Services*, *40*(4), 253–258. https://doi.org/10.1007/s00127-005-0879-0.

Mucic, D. (2010). Transcultural telepsychiatry and its impact on patient satisfaction. *Journal of Telemedicine and Telecare*, *16*(5), 237–242. https://doi.org/10.1258/jtt.2009.090811.

Mui, A. C., Kang, S.-Y., Chen, L. M., & Domanski, M. D. (2003). Reliability of the geriatric depression scale for use among elderly Asian immigrants in the USA. *International Psychogeriatrics*, *15*(3), 253–271. https://doi.org/10.1017/S1041610203009517.

Nadeem, E., Lange, J. M., & Miranda, J. (2008). Mental health care preferences among low-income and minority women. *Archives of Women's Mental Health*, *11*(2), 93–102. https://doi.org/10.1007/s00737-008-0002-0.

Nguyen, D. (2011). Acculturation and perceived mental health need among older Asian immigrants. *The Journal of Behavioral Health Services & Research*, *38*(4), 526–533. https://doi.org/10.1007/s11414-011-9245-z.

Nguyen, L. T., Kaptchuk, T. J., Davis, R. B., Nguyen, G., Pham, V., Tringale, S. M., … Gardiner, P. (2016). The use of traditional vietnamese medicine among Vietnamese immigrants attending an urban community health center in the United States. *Journal of Alternative and Complementary Medicine*, *22*(2), 145–153. https://doi.org/10.1089/acm.2014.0209.

Nguyen, D., & Lee, R. (2012). Asian immigrants' mental health service use: An application of the life course perspective. *Asian American Journal of Psychology*, *3*(1), 53–63. https://doi.org/10.1037/a0026865.

Pantin, H., Coatsworth, J. D., Feaster, D. J., Newman, F. L., Briones, E., Prado, G., … Szapocznik, J. (2003). Familias Unidas: The efficacy of an intervention to promote parental investment in Hispanic immigrant families. *Prevention Science*, *4*(3), 189–201.

Pratt, R., Ahmed, N., Noor, S., Sharif, H., Raymond, N., & Williams, C. (2017). Addressing behavioral health disparities for somali immigrants through group cognitive behavioral therapy led by community health workers. *Journal of Immigrant and Minority Health*, *19*(1), 187–193. https://doi.org/10.1007/s10903-015-0338-2.

Pumariega, A. J., Rothe, E., & Pumariega, J. B. (2005). Mental health of immigrants and refugees. *Community Mental Health Journal*, *41*(5), 581–597. https://doi.org/10.1007/s10597-005-6363-1.

Rasmussen, A., Crager, M., Baser, R. E., Chu, T., & Gany, F. (2012). Onset of posttraumatic stress disorder and major depression among refugees and voluntary migrants to the United States. *Journal of Traumatic Stress*, *25*(6), 705–712. https://doi.org/10.1002/jts.21763.

Rivas-Drake, D., Seaton, E. K., Markstrom, C., Quintana, S., Syed, M., Lee, R. M., … Yip, T. (2014). Ethnic and racial identity in adolescence: Implications for psychosocial, academic, and health outcomes. *Child Development*, *85*(1), 40–57. https://doi.org/10.1111/cdev.12200.

Rogers-Sirin, L., & Gupta, T. (2012). Cultural identity and mental health: Differing trajectories among Asian and Latino youth. *Journal of Counseling Psychology*, *59*(4), 555–566. https://doi.org/10.1037/a0029329.

Rogers-Sirin, L., Melendez, F., Refano, C., & Zegarra, Y. (2015). Immigrant perceptions of therapists' cultural competence: A qualitative investigation. *Professional Psychology: Research and Practice*, *46*(4), 258–269. https://doi.org/10.1037/pro0000033.

Salas-Wright, C. P., Vaughn, M. G., Goings, T. C., Miller, D. P., & Schwartz, S. J. (2018). Immigrants and mental disorders in the United States: New evidence on the healthy migrant hypothesis. *Psychiatry Research*, *267*, 438–445. https://doi.org/10.1016/j.psychres.2018.06.039.

Schnurr, P., Vielhauer, M., Weathers, F., & Findler, M. (1999). *The brief trauma questionnaire*. White River Junction, VT: National Center for PTSD.

Sheehan, D. V., Lecrubier, Y., Sheehan, K. H., Amorim, P., Janavs, J., Weiller, E., ... Dunbar, G. C. (1998). The Mini-International Neuropsychiatric Interview (MINI): The development and validation of a structured diagnostic psychiatric interview for DSM-IV and ICD-10. *The Journal of Clinical Psychiatry*, *59*(20), 22–33.

Silva, M. A., Paris, M., & Añez, L. M. (2017). CAMINO: Integrating context in the mental health assessment of immigrant Latinos. *Professional Psychology: Research and Practice*, *48*(6), 453–460. https://doi.org/10.1037/pro0000170.

Sirin, S. R., Ryce, P., Gupta, T., & Rogers-Sirin, L. (2013). The role of acculturative stress on mental health symptoms for immigrant adolescents: A longitudinal investigation. *Developmental Psychology*, *49*(4), 736–748. https://doi.org/10.1037/a0028398.

Smith, T. B., & Trimble, J. E. (2016). Culturally adapted mental health services: An updated meta-analysis of client outcomes. In *Foundations of multicultural psychology: Research to inform effective practice* (pp. 129–144). Washington, DC: American Psychological Association.

Sodowsky, G. R., & Wai Ming Lai, E. (1997). Asian immigrant variables and structural models of cross-cultural distress. In A. Booth, A. C. Crouter, & N. S. Landale (Eds.), *Immigration and the family: Research and policy on U.S. immigrants* (pp. 211–234). Washington, DC: Lawrence Erlbaum Associates, Inc.

Umaña-Taylor, A. J., Douglass, S., Updegraff, K. A., & Marsiglia, F. F. (2017). A small-scale randomized efficacy trial of the Identity Project: Promoting adolescents' ethnic–racial identity exploration and resolution. *Child Dev*. https://doi.org/10.1111/cdev.12755. [In press].

US Census Bureau. (2011). *Overview of race and Hispanic origin: 2010*. Washington, DC: United States Department of Commerce. Retrieved from: http://www.census.gov/prod/cen2010/briefs/c2010br-02.pdf.

US Department of Commerce. (2003). *The foreign-born population: Census brief*. US Census Bureau. Retrieved from: http://www.census.gov/prod/2003pubs/c2kbr-34.pdf.

Vega, W. A., Kolody, B., Aguilar-Gaxiola, S., Alderete, E., Catalano, R., & Caraveo-Anduaga, J. (1998). Lifetime prevalence of DSM-III-R psychiatric disorders among urban and rural Mexican Americans in California. *Archives of General Psychiatry*, *55*(9), 771–778.

Wilkins, K. C., Lang, A. J., & Norman, S. B. (2011). Synthesis of the psychometric properties of the PTSD checklist (PCL) military, civilian, and specific versions. *Depression and Anxiety*, *28*(7), 596–606.

Wu, E., Torous, J., & Liu, C. (2018). Chinese immigrant use of smartphone apps toward improving child mental health awareness and resource delivery: A pilot study. *Asian Journal of Psychiatry*, *33*, 1–6. https://doi.org/10.1016/j.ajp.2017.12.007.

Yeh, C. J. (2003). Age, acculturation, cultural adjustment, and mental health symptoms of Chinese, Korean, and Japanese immigrant youths. *Cultural Diversity and Ethnic Minority Psychology*, *9*(1), 34–48. https://doi.org/10.1037/1099-9809.9.1.34.

Yoon, E., Chih-Ting, C., Kim, S., Clawson, A., Cleary, S. E., Hansen, M., ... Gomes, A. M. (2013). A meta-analysis of acculturation/enculturation and mental health. *Journal of Counseling Psychology*, *60*(1), 15–30. https://doi.org/10.1037/a0030652.

Chapter 9

Intersectional complexities of South Asian Muslim Americans: Implications for identity and mental health

Tania Chowdhury and Sumie Okazaki
New York University, New York, NY, United States

South Asian Muslim American individuals and communities have long been a part of the fabric of multicultural America since the colonial era (Kaur, 2017), yet their contemporary experiences have been colored to a great extent by the rising tide of antiimmigrant sentiments after the attacks on September 11, 2001. In the United States and the "Global West," the bulk of the hostility has been directed toward Muslims in what has been described as globalized Islamophobia (Morgan & Poynting, 2012), as "9/11" became a synecdoche for terrorism connected to Muslim and Islam. In the US government's "War on Terror," Arabs, Muslims, and South Asians have been the prime targets of scrutiny, demonization, exclusion, and criminalization (Cainkar & Maira, 2005). Cainkar and Maira argue that both Arab Americans and South Asian Americans have been ambiguously racialized in the United States, at various times classified as "white" or "non-white," contributing to societal suspicion of their belongingness and cultural citizenship within American society. South Asian American men of Sikh faith have also been targeted with violence and hostility especially post-9/11, often as a result of being misidentified as Muslim (Ahluwalia & Pellettiere, 2010).

In this chapter, we have examined the complex intersection of immigrant, ethnic, religious, and gender identities that impact the psychosocial well-being of South Asian Muslim Americans. While an in-depth account is beyond the scope of this chapter, key historical, sociopolitical, and cultural forces that shape the experiences of South Asian Muslims in the United States are presented here. We used Crenshaw's (1989) intersectional theory as a framework to capture the complex realities of South Asian Muslim Americans, as immigrants,

Mental and Behavioral Health of Immigrants in the United States
https://doi.org/10.1016/B978-0-12-816117-3.00009-9

as Muslims, as Asians, and as South Asians, and to address the gaps in the psychological literature that contribute to the misrepresentations of their lived experiences.

Intersectional lens

Intersectionality is a framework that arose out of Black feminist activist scholarship that stresses the importance of attending to multiple, intersecting identities (e.g., race, gender, class, sexual identity) and the associated systems of power and oppression. Kimberlé Crenshaw (1989, 1991) is credited with first calling attention to intersectionality in legal scholarship surrounding antidiscrimination laws, which treated sexism and racism as independent rather than interlocking systems of oppression and in the process marginalized Black women's experiences with discrimination. Whereas insights from intersectionality theory have contributed to a fuller understanding of the experiences of discrimination and inequality within psychology (Cole, 2009), Rosenthal (2016) argued that emphases on intersectional identities have not been accompanied by activism to undo the systemic inequalities that create oppression. It is through this lens of social justice and equity agenda that undergirds intersectionality theory that we discuss the intersection of religious and ethnic identities and positionalities of South Asian Muslim Americans in the United States. That is, the psychological experiences of South Asian Muslim Americans must be understood in the context of interlocking systems of oppression against Muslims, against South Asian and other immigrants, along with gender, sexual identity, class, and so on. Moreover, these insights must be accompanied by a call to action for reducing inequality and addressing social justice issues for members of this community.

An iteration of Crenshaw's intersectional theory (1989) is germane to any effort to understand the complex and overlapping realities of South Asian Muslims living in the United States. This framework can provide a better understanding of South Asian Muslim Americans by examining the intersectional and interactional effects of ethnicity, religion, race, gender, sexual orientation, class, disability status, and other marginalized identities that contribute to the development of transnational, diasporic identities and impact their psychological experiences and overall mental health. By considering the social processes that contribute to mental health outcomes, our objective is to model intersectionality along historical, sociopolitical, cultural, and other contextual factors. For South Asian Muslim Americans, developing a diasporic identity may involve negotiating separate sets of cultural systems, navigating familial and religious pressures, intergenerational conflicts, transnational politics, and confronting structural inequalities such as discrimination within and outside their own communities (e.g., Islamophobia, xenophobia, racism, anti-Blackness, etc.) all the while determining how aspects of their own identities fit into the broader diasporic experience.

Who are the South Asian Muslim Americans?

Before we trace the histories and migration of Muslims from South Asia to the United States, however, we note that South Asian Americans are a part of the broader racial/ethnic category of Asian Americans—although not without debate (Dave et al., 2000)—and of the broader religious category of Muslim Americans and that their membership in pan-ethnic/religious coalitions adds another layer of complexity to their sense of belongingness. Broadly, the Asian American population increased by 72% between 2000 and 2015, making it the fastest-growing racial or ethnic group in the United States, and is projected to become the largest immigrant group in the United States by 2055 (Pew Research Center, 2017). Around the same time frame, the South Asian American population grew 40% in size (Pew Research Center, 2017).

According to the 2017 American Community Survey (ACS) and a 2019 demographics report put forth by South Asians Americans Leading Together (SAALT, 2019), more than 5.7 million South Asians in the United States trace their roots to Bangladesh, Bhutan, India, Maldives, Nepal, Pakistan, and Sri Lanka. While Asian Indians comprise the largest segment of the South Asian population in the United States, making up over 80% of the total population, and more than half identify as Hindu, South Asians originate from a region that is ethnically, linguistically, culturally, and religiously diverse, which is also reflected in the diasporic composition in the United States. South Asia has the largest population of Muslims worldwide, with Islam characterized as the second largest religion in the region after Hinduism (Pew Research Center, 2015). With an estimated 3.45 million Muslims residing in the United States, South Asians account for 35% of the US Muslim population (Pew Research Center, 2017). Muslims are the fastest-growing religious group globally and according to the Pew Research Center (2017), Muslim Americans will surpass Jewish Americans to become the second largest faith-based group in the United States by 2050.

The heterogeneity of South Asian Americans is reflected across other sociodemographics. According to SAALT's demographic profile (2019), 75% of South Asians living in the United States are foreign-born. South Asians in the United States include naturalized citizens, legal permanent residents, student and worker visa holders, and undocumented immigrants, with undocumented Asian Indians being among the top 15 origin groups for unauthorized immigrants (Pew Research Center, 2017). Among Asian Americans, Asian Indians possess the highest level of educational attainment and the highest median income (Pew Research Center, 2017). That said, income inequality is considered to be the greatest among Asian Americans with Bangladeshi and Nepali households having median incomes well below the national average (Pew Research Center, 2015, 2017). Among South Asian Americans, Bhutanese, Bangladeshis, Nepalis, and Pakistanis have the highest poverty rates (SAALT, 2019). Occupationally, South Asian Americans work in a variety of settings, such as in the arts, in government, in business, in science and technology fields, etc. and at different levels, including low-wage jobs such as taxi drivers or restaurant workers.

Muslims in South Asia: Past and present

The unique, intersectional history of the South Asian subcontinent continues to play a pivotal role in the present-day dynamics in the region and in its populace's understanding of self, others, and the world. As described by Bose and Jalal (2017) in their book *Modern South Asia: History, Culture, Political Economy*, the foundation of modern-day South Asia has been "the site of fierce historical contestation" (p. 12), witnessing successive periods in transfers of power. Transformations resultant of invasions and colonial rule secured some of the cultural and religious practices existing in this heterogeneous region today. While followers of all religions can be found on the subcontinent, introduction of Islam to South Asia can be traced back to early seventh century CE when an area in Northwestern India known as Sindh, already inhabited by Hindus, Buddhists, and Jains, was invaded and the first Arab dynasty was established (Bose & Jalal, 2017). Contrary to narratives concerning Muslim invaders, early Arab rulers were not interested in conversion, but rather in extending control by allying with locals, preserving existing social structures, and imposing *zimmi* regulations, which protected locals paying a special tax in return for guaranteed safety and exemption from military service (Bose & Jalal, 2017; Metcalf, 2009). Large-scale Muslim expansion was brought on at the turn of the 11th century by Turkish and Afghan invaders who launched raids across the subcontinent and established the Delhi Sultanate, which lasted from the early 13th century to early 16th century (Metcalf, 2009). Emerging from reciprocal interactions between Islam and Hinduism following Arab, Turkish, Persian, and Afghan invasions, Indo-Islamic culture and traditions became deeply entrenched in the subcontinent and was reflected across forms of art, literature, music, architecture, and religious and philosophical customs, and continued into the late 1800s under Mughal rule (Bose & Jalal, 2017; Metcalf, 2009; Momin, 1977). Often met with resistance and spurring ethnoreligious tensions, cultural and religious exchanges that took place under Muslim rulers solidified links between language, region, and identity. Under the Delhi Sultanate rule, Persian became the official language and the use of Urdu, a language with roots in Sanskrit, Persian, and Arabic, developed in the 16–17th century as a way to secure an Islamic identity for Indian Muslims (Bose & Jalal, 2017).

After nearly a thousand years of Muslim rule, the British colonial period in India or *British Raj* was instituted following the expansion in political and administrative power of the British East India Company as a by-product of its victory in the Battle of Plassey during the Indian Rebellion of 1857 (Bose & Jalal, 2017; Metcalf, 2009). Expanded to cover much of India over the next century, the company was dissolved in 1858 and its possessions, powers, and functions were transferred to the British Crown (Metcalf, 2009). Under a British "rule of law," lines based on race, class, and religion were drawn forming racial and religious hierarchies. These colonial definitions of majority and minority were not abandoned in postcolonial South Asia. Privileging religious distinction, countries where Muslims were in the minority, like in India and Sri Lanka, fortified the belief that Muslim identity was incompatible with national identity (Bose & Jalal, 2017; Metcalf, 2009). The impact of the colonial era reverberated throughout postcolonial South Asian history, undergoing several ruptures driven by religious antagonism, dividing the populace, and forming new nation-states such as Pakistan and Bangladesh (Ganguly, 1993; Metcalf, 2009).

In present times, unparalleled rates of violence by extremist groups and corresponding hate and suspicion of Muslims command dynamics in South Asia as the reemergence of intraethnic and ethnoreligious tensions overwhelm the region. In India, the rise of Hindu nationalism in concert with growing Islamophobia has inflamed historically conflictual relationships since the election of Prime Minister Narendra Modi (Gettleman, Schultz, Raj, & Kumar, 2019), contributing to communal violence between non-Muslims and Muslims. According to Minority Rights Groups International (MRG, 2017), everyday Muslims, who make up 15% of India's population, have been increasingly targeted as anti-Muslim hate crimes surged since 2016. Reports of lynching, threats, attacks on places of worship, and forced conversions prompted Amnesty International (2017) to urge the Indian government to condemn and address rising Islamophobia in the country (MRG, 2017). More recently, the provocation of the longstanding opposition over Jammu and Kashmir has generated concerns of impending regional war (Bhat, 2019; Ganguly, 1993). Outside of India, Sri Lanka has witnessed anti-Muslim riots since 2014, which include the burning down of mosques by Buddhists in 2018, and the implementation of the ban on *niqaabs* or face covers following the Eastern Sunday terror attacks in 2019 (Slater & Farisz, 2019). Since late August 2017, almost a million Rohingya people, largely Muslims, have fled Myanmar's Rakhine State into neighboring Bangladesh to escape atrocities committed by Burmese security forces, which include mass killings, sexual violence, and widespread arson, inducing one of the fastest-growing refugee crisis in recent history (Kader & Choudhury, 2019).

Through transnational flows, politics and ideologies of the homeland may be reflected in communities across the South Asian diaspora in the United States. These historical and contemporary geopolitical issues facing Muslims in South Asia invariably impact the well-being of individuals in South Asian Muslim American communities, given the large proportion of the communities who are first-generation immigrants and their interconnectedness to their kins still in South Asia through occasional visits and frequent virtual contacts (Purkayastha, 2010). The inter-ethnic tensions and conflict within South Asia, as well as the persecution of Muslim minorities, can make for a fraught sense of pan-South Asian solidarity within the United States (Kurien, 2003). In Byng's (2017) qualitative study of second-generation Muslim American young adults in Philadelphia (families of 68% were from Bangladesh, Pakistan, and India), the young adults cited their visits to their parents' homeland and prolonged stays with their kins as accentuating their transnational and religious identity. For example, the young Muslim Americans appreciated public visibility of Islam in their parents' home countries, yet they were also keenly aware that the way they experienced these visits were mediated through their lens as Americans. In fact, they tended to view their identity as culturally American and religiously Muslim. Like other diasporic communities, South Asian Muslim American families have many transnational ties, and the geopolitical issues in the Indian subcontinent have personal significance to families and individuals.

History of South Asians in the United States

Psychological experiences of South Asian Muslim Americans must also be understood in the context of the history of migration, settlement, and treatment of South Asian Americans in the United States, which in turn are intricately tied to global historical and contemporary events. Although a comprehensive review of the groups' historical experiences is beyond the scope of the this chapter, we have highlighted key historical contexts—and the discourses around them—that are critical to understanding the present experiences of South Asian Muslim Americans. Of particular importance is the recurrent themes of South Asians being regarded as indistinguishable from one another, their presence as a security threat to the United States, and their race and identity being subject to constant questioning.

According to the historian Erika Lee (2015), migration from South Asia to the Americas began around the 1600s as part of Spain's Pacific empire and the British empire's colonization of South Asia. One of the earliest historical record is that of a South Asian Muslim sailor named Sick Keesar (likely an anglicized approximation of Sheikh Kesar) who had filed a petition on behalf of himself and his lascar crew from Bengal for redress of grievances in 1785 in Philadelphia against the captain of an Irish merchant ship (Kaur, 2017). British colonial rule in South Asia had facilitated the circulation of South Asian laborers to North America via the British colonies of Hong Kong and the West Indies to work in the lumber, railroad, fishing, and agriculture industries. A small number of Indian Muslim men had also "jumped ship" and settled in New Orleans, New York City, and various other cities in the South, making a living as peddlers and intermarrying with local African American women in the period between 1880 and 1950 (Bald, 2006). A more sizable migration of South Asians (predominantly from Punjab and Bengal regions) to North America along the Pacific Coast followed the migration and settlement of Chinese, Japanese, Korean, and Filipino laborers in the 18th and 19th century. By the time South Asians built their presence in the West Coast in the early 20th century, virulent anti-Asian sentiments had taken hold, and from the start, South Asian immigrants had had to fight for their place in the United States.

While most early South Asian immigrants were Sikh (with some Hindu and Muslim immigrants), white Americans and Canadians characterized their presence in the aggregate as "Hindu invasion" and as another of the undesirable and unassimilable migrants from Asia. Because South Asians were British colonial subjects whose outright exclusion may upset their relations with the British, Canada and the US immigration policies were devised at first to exclude South Asians through indirect measures. Importantly, many South Asians in the United States and Canada in the early 20th century were Indian nationalists who were involved in the movement for independence in India as well as for equal treatment in North America, and their activism was increasingly regarded as a threat to national security. Subsequently, the US Congress passed an act in 1917 that prohibited the migration of individuals from "Asiatic Barred Zone" that included the entire Indian subcontinent. South Asians contested their rights to own land and to naturalize.

The Supreme Court ruled in *United States v. Bhagat Singh Thind* (1923) that South Asians could not naturalize because they were not "white." Thind, who came to the United States for higher education, had served in the US Army during World War I. He applied for and was granted US citizenship through his applications in the states of Washington and Oregon but was subject to denaturalization by the federal Immigration and Naturalization Services. Thind fought his denaturalization by citing the anthropological racial theory, his upper-caste Hindu ancestry as Aryan but lost his case. Thind eventually regained his US citizenship in 1935 after new legislation enabled WWI veterans to naturalize regardless of race.

The *US v. Thind* is often cited as a historically significant legal case regarding the question of race and citizenship, but Koshy (1998) reminds us that Thind's was one of the 52 cases construing the racial prerequisite for naturalization that reached the courts. Across these cases, the petitioners from countries as varied as Burma, Syria, the Philippines, Japan, China, and Mexico, as well as India, argued that they were "white" and thus eligible to naturalize. And in repeatedly denying their claims, the United States over time developed their legal definitions of whiteness. The Thind ruling definitively barred South Asians from naturalization, which severely limited their economic and social opportunities in the United States.

It was not until the 1965 Immigration Act that reopened immigration to Asians that the South Asian American population began to take roots. Meanwhile, the British colonial rule came to an end with the partition of British India into independent nation-states of India (predominantly Hindu and Sikh) and Pakistan (predominantly Muslim) in 1947. The formerly Bengal region became East Pakistan during the partition, later gaining independence as Bangladesh in 1971. The initial wave of post-1965 South Asian immigrants to the United States was dominated by highly educated professionals, unlike the earlier wave of Punjabi Sikh male laborers, although the more recent waves of immigrants from South Asia represent more women and of more diverse socioeconomic backgrounds due to the emphasis on family-sponsored immigration. South Asian American communities grew exponentially in the ensuing decades. According to the US census data, there were a little over 370,000 South Asians in 1980; by 2010, there were nearly 3.4 million South Asians. Of significance to the contemporary experiences of South Asian Muslim Americans, the terror attacks on the World Trade Center and the Pentagon on September 11, 2001 ushered a new era of backlash against Muslim Americans and South Asian Americans, as they were subjected to racial and religious profiling, violence and other hate crimes, and heightened government monitoring of immigrant communities.

Islamophobia and racialization of Muslims in the United States

In the West, for a long time, there has been a dominant presupposition that Islam is Arabo-Persian and thus Islamophobia only affects Arabs. In the United States, however, Islamophobia and hate violence toward Muslims predates 9/11 and can be traced back to the transatlantic slave trade (Escalante, 2019). After 9/11, rising Islamophobia, state actions, and media reactions have led to a figure of "the Muslim" as not only a religious category but also a racial category that has been central to global racial formations (Rana, 2011; Selod & Embrick, 2013). In Britain, Abbas (2004) summarized that "the British discourse on racialized minorities has been transformed from 'color' in the 1950s and 1960s to 'race' in the 1960s, 1970s, and 1980s, to 'ethnicity' in the 1990s, and to 'religion' in the present climate" (p. 27). The emergence of religion as a "social signifier" is reflective of the shifts in the nation's understanding of race, which once began as "seeing minorities as homogenous entities to discerning differences within and between 'Blacks' and Asians; then, within South Asians, to differences among Indians, Pakistanis, and Bangladeshis; and finally among Muslims, Hindus, and Sikhs" (Abbas, 2004, p. 27). The racialization of Muslims has conflated perceived Muslimness with perceived foreignness and has produced a figure of the Muslim which now includes signifiers such as brown skin, accents, ethnic articles of clothing, etc. (Rana, 2011).

In her book *We Too Sing America: South Asian, Arab, Muslim, and Sikh Immigrants Shape Our Multiracial Future*, Deepa Iyer (2015) presents research and individual accounts of violence on South Asian, Arab, Muslim, and Sikh communities in post-9/11 America, essentially illustrating how the racialization of Muslims since then has broadly placed South Asians, regardless of religious identity, at a heightened risk for profiling and victimization. Acknowledging that targeting of these communities has a much longer history, Iyer begins by recounting the tragic event that took place on August 5, 2012, when a white supremacist opened gunfire in a Gurdwara or Sikh temple in Oak Creek, Wisconsin, killing six members of the Sikh faith and later himself. Iyer, who was actively engaged in response efforts in the immediate aftermath of the massacre, along with other individuals working with South Asian immigrant communities recognized this as another hate crime in "the continuum of backlash" targeting this demographic since 9/11 (p. 5). As the author notes, non-Muslim South Asian community members initially distanced themselves from Muslims after 9/11 to shield themselves from the subsequent backlash, however, a realization that perpetrators of violence were indiscriminate in attacking South Asian, Arab, Hindu, Muslim, and Sikh individuals materialized over the next decade. This realization occurred not only in response to direct experiences with violence, but also to state-sponsored policies (e.g., USA PATRIOT Act, NSEERS) that have legitimized disproportionate profiling, surveilling, policing, detaining, unfair prosecutions, and deportations of South Asians under the guise of combatting terrorism (Iyer, 2015).

As the population of Muslims continues to climb in the United States and globally, the widespread hatred and suspicion of Muslims show no signs of wavering. Given that the racialization of Muslims in recent history has victimized South Asians at alarming rates (Rana, 2011), the complex realities of South Asian Muslim Americans beg greater consideration from the psychology community and requires that we situate this community at the precarious intersection between Muslim communities, South Asian American communities, and more broadly, Asian American communities within multiple histories of religious and ethnic minorities in the United States.

South Asian Muslim American identity and well-being

Intersections of global and local forces, both distal and proximal, impinge on the construction, negotiation, and transformation of identities and meanings in these diasporic communities, in addition to the way they adapt, accommodate, and assimilate the dominant culture (Dwyer, 2000; Huang, Teo, & Yeoh, 2000). Furthermore, familial, cultural, and religious pressures can compound psychological processes and have implications on overall psychological health. While South Asian and Muslim Americans have increasingly become populations of interest in the psychological literature, over the last several decades, South Asian Muslims have often been grouped together with either other South Asians or other Muslims, depending on the identity of interest. Incomplete narratives of each respective population and limitations of approaches that generalize experiences on the basis of membership to a particular group have led to the neglect of the intersectional realities of South Asian Muslims in the United States within psychology. Although a comprehensive review of all works relevant to South Asian Muslim American identity and well-being is beyond the scope of this chapter, we covered themes and findings from existing social science literature that addresses the intersectional complexities that shape the psychological experiences of this population.

Upon examining psychological research on South Asians in the United States over three decades (1980–2012), Inman, Devdas, Spektor, and Pendse (2014) revealed that empirical articles increased by 360% from the 1980s to 1990s and by 356% from the 1990s to 2000s. Of the 133 empirical articles published on South Asians in the United States, five articles were published in the 1980s, 23 studies were published in the 1990s, and 105 articles were published from 2000 to 2012. As shown by Inman et al., the psychological literature disproportionately focused on Asian Indians, making up 61% of the articles reviewed. Content analysis revealed 13 major content categories, with the most frequently researched topics being psychological health (15%), acculturation/acculturative stress (14%), interpersonal dynamics (14%), identity (12%), and domestic violence (10%). Out of the 133 articles examined, 11 focused on "South Asians" as an identity of interest and far fewer explored South Asian Muslims as a broader identifying category. In fact, only one article in the 2000s focused on religious identity.

Increased interest in Muslim Americans is also reflected in recent psychological scholarship. In reviewing psychological research on Muslim Americans post-9/11, Amer and Bagasra (2013) found a 900% increase in the annual number of publications on Muslim Americans over the subsequent decade. A majority of the articles reviewed by Amer and Bagasra revealed an overwhelming emphasis on Muslim North Americans in the sample irrespective of the research focus and generally referred to Muslims or Islam as a unitary specifier without distinguishing between countries of origin. Content analysis of the 599 articles reviewed revealed 14 recurring categories. While 17.7% focused on intergroup relations and 14.1% on culturally responsive mental health service provision, terrorism and violence, mental health and substance use, gender and sexuality, identity and acculturation, health care, family and marriage each represented less than 10% of the total articles analyzed. The general failure of the research literature to recognize the intersectional invisibility of South Asian Muslim Americans necessitates the study of the Muslim American population in a way that is reflective of its ethnic and religious composition and the diversity in religious adherence.

Religio-cultural norms, values, and mental health

Although South Asian communities are diverse across demographic characteristics and immigration histories, South Asian cultures are commonly patriarchal and collectivistic. Values such as family piety, central of the family, obedience, interdependence, emphasis on a hierarchical social order, the importance of marriage, and respect for elders are emphasized and safeguarded through parenting practices, strict gender roles and expectations, compliance to strict moral and social standards (Das & Kemp, 1997; Inman, Ladany, Constantine, & Morano, 2001), and overlap with some of the teachings of Islam (Cook-Masaud & Wiggins, 2011). In traditional South Asian families, men typically take on the role of the head of the household, women are the primary caretakers, and parents have a strong influence on their children and emphasize educational attainment and financial success (Rahman & Witenstein, 2014). Endemic to South

Asian culture and Islam, the concept of *izzat* or family honor helps maintain the integrity of the family and involves a complex set of rules to protect the family honor, avoid bringing shame to the family, and to maintain the family's position in society (Gilbert, Gilbert, & Sanghera, 2004).

Examining the religio-cultural dimensions of mental health, overall health, and identity may provide greater clarity into how commonly held beliefs can be both sources of pride, success, and resiliency and sources of challenges. In a poll conducted by the Institute for Social Policy and Understanding in 2018, an overwhelming majority of Muslims sampled identified their Muslim identity as a source of happiness (Mogahed, Chouhoud, & Buageila, 2018). While Islamic tradition acknowledges the concept of mental health, belonging to a culture of shame and honor may discourage South Asian Muslim Americans from disclosing mental health challenges or seeking out mental health services due to the fear of discovery associated with dealing with problems outside of the nuclear family (Haque, 2004). Mental health and disability-related stigma in South Asian communities, rooted in the anticipation of disapproval and the loss of one's position in the society once a family member is identified as having a mental health issue or disability, can foster a culture of silence and further marginalize those in desperate need of psychological services (Lauber & Rössler, 2007).

Culture and faith-based values are by no means the only indicators of psychological adjustment among this demographic in the United States. Structural factors such as prejudice, discrimination, and poverty can contribute to identity crises and exacerbate existing inequalities. To understand the multifaceted and intersectional cultural profile of South Asian Muslim Americans, mental health professionals must continue to explore how the model minority perception of Asians, the depiction of Muslims as violent and intolerant, the portrayal of South Asian Muslims as victims of an oppressive religion and culture, and other stigmatized social categories in the United States impact identity formation and their overall well-being. They must also aggressively challenge their own misconceptions about Islam, Muslims, and South Asians when working with this population. Furthermore, deconstructing and decolonizing narratives of success around this population is imperative in challenging the model minority stereotype, which not only homogenizes this population but also perpetuates a divisive version of the "American dream" that categorizes immigrant communities on the basis of productivity.

Discrimination

The impact of discrimination against South Asian Muslims in the United States has been not been adequately investigated in the psychological literature. Given the growing hostility toward Muslims since the 2016 US presidential election, an intersectional understanding of the psychological toll of discrimination is necessitated (SPLC, 2016; UCR, 2016, 2017). The Southern Poverty Law Center

(SPLC, 2016) noted that 6% of the 867 hate incidents documented just 10 days after the 2016 election involved Muslims or those perceived to be Muslims, surpassing the number of hate incidents targeting Muslim Americans reported in the aftermath of September 11, 2001. Compared to the year leading up to the presidential election, SAALT (2019) reported a 45% increase in incidents of hate violence targeting South Asian, Muslim, Sikh, Hindu, Middle Eastern, and Arab American communities in the subsequent year. With the rise of anti-Muslim bias incidents and hate crimes continuing into 2017 (CAIR, 2018), the Council on American-Islamic Relations (CAIR) noted that perceived ethnicity was identified as the most prevalent trigger of reported anti-Muslim incidents, with perceived Muslimness as the second most common trigger (2018), providing insight into how the racialization of Muslims operates to ascribe characteristics of "foreignness" as inherent to Muslim group membership.

Discrimination and victimization have been shown to be psychologically harmful to individuals, contributing to the development of depression and anxiety and negatively impacting one's self-esteem and satisfaction with life (Carter, 2007; Lee, 2003; Utsey, Payne, Jackson, & Jones, 2002). In a study conducted by Kaduvettoor-Davidson and Inman (2013) examining the influence of stress on the experience of discrimination for 210 South Asians living in the United States, perceived discrimination, stress, and well-being were significantly related to one another for both first- and second-generation South Asian Americans, lending empirical support to race-related stress theoretical models. In another study examining the role of discrimination and acculturative stress in depression among 169 South Asians, Tummala-Narra, Alegria, and Chen (2012) found that perceived discrimination was positively associated with depression for the South Asian sample.

While discrimination has been examined broadly in psychological literature, less attention has been directed toward understanding the cumulative and intersecting impact of discrimination on South Asian Muslim Americans. During a point in time where South Asian Muslims are victimized within and outside of their communities, investigating the psychological impact of discrimination at the intersections of ethnicity and religion is only a first step. To prevent the perpetuation of intersectional erasure, efforts to capture the realities of individuals with marginalized status within a marginalized group, including sexual and gender minorities, Muslim converts/reverts, aging/older adults, individuals with disabilities, and individuals belonging to minority sects of Islam (e.g., Shias, Ahmaddiyas, etc.), is of equal significance given that multiple minority stressors have been linked to greater psychological distress for individuals with multiple marginalities (Meyer, 2003).

Women

The intersections of gender, culture, and religion present a unique set of challenges for some South Asian Muslim American women both inside and outside of their ethnoreligious communities. Patriarchial elements of Islam and South Asian and American culture have reduced the ability of women and young girls to assert rights to their bodies, education, health and reproductive care, and other fundamental liberties and to make decisions about their future. It is important to note that local, historical, cultural, and geopolitical factors influence the way in which Islam is interpreted and practiced. Thus, discourse on Islam and women's rights requires consideration of these varying constructs.

The syncretic relationship between South Asian culture and Islam has advanced the subordination and control of the rights of women in South Asian communities worldwide. Despite introducing reforms that improved the status of women by granting rights to participate in political matters, rights to inherit property and wealth, rights in marriage, and rights as a parent, Islamic teachings have often been cited by religious and political leaders and by individual Muslims to justify violation of women's rights and gender-based violence (Halim, 1999). Overwhelmingly tied to their chastity and virginity before marriage, the burden of carrying the family honor often falls on women and young girls in South Asian and Muslim families (Gilbert et al., 2004; Halim, 1999; Werbner, 2005). Although the potential benefits of patriarchal family hierarchy and family honor can resemble the availability of financial and familial support, they can also be sources of control and abuse. Draconian interpretations of culture and religion have condoned assaults on women and young girls in South Asia and in South Asian diasporas, which include various forms of violence, forced arranged marriages, and honor killings (Werbner, 2005).

For South Asian Muslim women living in the United States, identity formation and psychological experiences are rooted in local, cultural, religious, historical, and political and transnational contexts and must be conceptualized as such. As part of a religio-cultural institution that prefers males, women and young girls may find themselves occupying subordinate and marginalized positions and the cultural and racial realities of the United States undoubtedly influence their positionality. Misconceptions about South Asian Muslim women may obscure the serious realities that link sociocultural variables to the disproportionately high rates of domestic violence, suicide, and suicide attempts among South Asian women living in the United States and United Kingdom (Hicks & Bhugra, 2003; Jordan & Bhandari, 2016). Generational and immigration-related differences may separate the experiences of first- and second-generation immigrant women. Comparatively, while first-generation South Asian Muslim women may encounter more acculturative stress, second-generation women may be faced with navigating conflicts in the bicultural context, such as the expectation to uphold traditional cultural, religious, and family values in private while achieving success academically and financially in the dominant society (Inman, 2006; Kallivayalil, 2004). In addition to being racialized and gendered, South Asian Muslim women and young girls living in the United States, especially those who don a visible signifier of their faith identity, may experience discrimination at the intersection of gender and religion also known as gendered Islamophobia (Perry, 2014).

LGBTQ+ individuals

The dearth of psychological literature on LGBTQ+ issues among South Asian Muslim Americans is reflective of the various forms of stigma encountered by sexual and gender minorities within this population. LGBTQ+ South Asian Muslim Americans exist in ethnoreligious communities that are entrenched with oppressive and exclusionary cisheteronormative ideologies and in a dominant cultural context in which anti-Muslim sentiment remains unabated. Some LGBTQ+ South Asian Muslims originate from countries that stigmatize, discriminate, and criminalize LGBTQ+ individuals, which complicate their transnational connections. Careful and serious consideration of the cultural, religious, and political structures that illustrate the intersectionality of LGBTQ+ South Asian Muslims is long overdue in psychological research. Potential areas to explore include and are not limited to how sexual and gender minorities navigate their marginality and identities within and outside of South Asian Muslim communities, how they reconcile with cultural and religious values and practices, how social changes in their countries of origin influence their experiences here in the United States, how acculturative processes influence identity formations and expressions, the impact of multiple marginalities on psychological adaptation and outcomes, and the unique mental health needs that emerge as a consequence.

A limited number of studies have explored the intersectionality of religion, gender, and sexuality among South Asian Muslim Americans and the impact of multiple marginalizations on identity and psychological outcomes. In a study by Yip and Khalid (2010) on LGBTQI Muslims in Britain, New York, and Toronto, many of the 17 participants interviewed embraced Islam as a referential framework despite rejecting the dominant Islamic discourse on sexuality. Furthermore, participants established spiritual paths that prioritized Islamic teachings of equality, diversity, justice, and love. In a qualitative study by Minwalla, Rosser, Feldman, and Varga (2005) documenting the experiences of gay Muslim men in North America, participants similarly reconciled with being Muslim and gay by "emphasizing aspects of Islam that promote inclusion, peace, tolerance, and justice" (Minwalla et al., 2005, p. 124). A departure from the aforementioned studies, Al-Sayyad's (2010) empirical study on queer-identified Muslim women in the United States detailed how these women did not integrate their identities but rather renounced their religion in order to express their sexual identity. While the interaction between religion and sexuality was not explored, Sandil, Robinson, Brewster, Wong, and Geiger (2015) utilized minority stress and feminist multicultural theories to explore how external minority stress and internal stress contribute to the psychological well-being among 142 LGBQ-identified individuals from varying South Asian backgrounds. Encounters with heterosexist discrimination, racism, and internalized heterosexism were positively correlated with psychological distress while enculturation was negatively correlated. Moreover, the relationship between racist events and psychological distress was exacerbated for individuals who reported more openness about their sexual orientation, suggesting that one minority stress can affect the impact of a separate minority stressor. While LGBTQ+ individuals are at a heightened risk for negative mental health outcomes, cultural norms that alienate, isolate, and marginalize LGBTQ+ identified South Asians may thwart efforts to seek mental health services despite having access to them (Choudhury et al., 2009).

South Asian Muslim youth

Although the literature on South Asian Muslim youth is not extensive, two studies that were conducted before and after 9/11 illustrate the extent to which this tragedy has had an overwhelming impact on the lived experiences of this population. In a study examining the ethnic/cultural identity of South Asian Muslim young adults in the 1990s, Mohammad-Arif (2000) described several prevailing themes: immigrant parents' high expectations for the youth to achieve academically and to pursue prestigious professions; gendered expectations by families for girls and young women regarding modesty, religiosity, and marriage; struggles to maintain religious and cultural traditions and beliefs amidst acculturation to the United States; development of religious and cultural identity and community building through pan-South Asian solidarity; and the diversity of identification and practices with Islam. Mohammad-Arif observed the manner in which South Asian Muslim girls and women signaled their religious identity through *hijab* (head covering) appeared to reflect the diversity in their religious identity as well as the American context in which there were greater individual choices over their religious expression. Mohammad-Arif characterized the eclectic and diverse forms of South Asian Muslim American youths' identity as "masala identity" (in which masala refers to a particular blend of spices commonly used in South Asian cuisines).

These themes, some of which are particular to South Asian and Muslim families and some of which are shared with many other immigrant families, no doubt persist among South Asian Muslim American youth today. However, as illustrated in Maira's (2009) book, *Missing: Youth, Citizenship, and Empire after 9/11*, the aftermaths of the 9/11 tragedy have largely come to shape the contours of South Asian Muslim American youths' psychosocial experiences. In her ethnographic study of recently immigrated working class and lower middle class Muslim immigrant youth who were coming of age during America's War on Terror, Maira (2009) argued that the youths' experiences, particularly around the notions of cultural citizenship and belonging, were inextricably tied to the state's foreign and domestic policies that constantly questioned their loyalty and allegiance. Maira found that the young people's lives were transformed by national discourse about Islam that viewed Muslims as foreign, unassimilable, and potentially threatening to the American way of life. Against this hostile backdrop, Maira found the South Asian Muslim American youths expressing their resistance and dissent, critiquing state policies, and insisting on their rights and humanities.

Aging and older adults

The population of the United States is not only becoming more diverse but also older. According to the 2016 American Community Survey, the growth rate of those who are aged 65 and older has exceeded that of the total population and the population under the age of 65. Of the 13.5% of 65 and older age group who are foreign-born, a significant segment of this subpopulation is identified as Asian (US Census Bureau, 2016). With the population of Asian American older people projected to increase over the next decade, the need to attend to the mental health challenges of the aging population in the United States should correspond to these trends. As local and global factors continue to influence the immigration of aging/older South Asian Muslims into the United States, a profile of elders in this community should reflect those age-related and cross-cultural challenges that contribute to their mental health needs and barriers to receiving mental health care. While previously conducted research provides some insight into understanding this population, findings represent Asians as a homogenous group, ignoring the geographic, cultural, religious, and historical diversities.

Older South Asian Muslim immigrants are exposed to various risk factors that contribute to mental health disparities. Compared to White older people, Asian older people generally have lower median income, work low-paying jobs with no retirement benefits, and a greater number of individuals with no formal education (Leong & Lau, 2001). As with many ethnocultural minority older adults, older Asian and Muslim immigrants may experience acculturative stress, language barriers, conflict of cultural values, migratory loss and grief, poor physical health, intergenerational conflicts, conflictual family dynamics, difficult living situations, as well as undergo role changes, from being head of the households to becoming emotionally and financially dependent on their adult children or relatives, and a change in lifestyle and sense of community that lead to social isolation via decline in social support (Chen, Talwar, & Ji, 2015; Hasnain & Rana, 2010; Ross-Sheriff, 1994). In a study conducted by Abu-Bader, Tirmazi, and Ross-Sheriff (2011) examining the role of acculturation on depression among 70 older Muslim immigrants, of whom 44% identified as Asian, almost 50% of the sample reported the presence of depressive symptoms. Noting that the reported rates of depressive symptomatology among older immigrant groups range from 10% to as high as 72% in the research literature, the authors suggest that older Muslim immigrants experience depression at higher rates than other older immigrant populations (Abu-Bader et al., 2011). Furthermore, the results demonstrated that older Muslim immigrants were greatly separated and isolated from mainstream American culture, with isolation being the second greatest predictor of depression among this sample (Abu-Bader et al., 2011).

The responsibility of providing care for one's parents is laid out in both Islam and in South Asian culture and elders are regarded for their experiences and wisdom. While the right to expect respect and familial support in old age have been shown to have positive effects for South Asian elders, these values may be in a state of flux for some, further complicating their psychosocial realities (Diwan, Jonnalagadda, & Balaswamy, 2004). Strong religious and sociocultural ties can provide coping strategies to alleviate symptoms of depression and enhance the quality of life, however, religio-cultural perspectives on mental health and disabilities held by adult children and their aging parents can present as barriers to accessing mental health treatment in the United States (Chen et al., 2015; Hasnain & Rana, 2010).

Minority Muslim groups

Sectarian-based conflicts plaguing most of the Muslim world have advanced intolerance of minority Muslim groups, including Shias, Ahmaddiyas, and other minority factions. Thus, understanding the varying realities of South Asian Muslims in the United States cannot be adequately described by existing approaches that homogenize the religious identity and experiences of this subpopulation. While the dominant Sunni sect regards the Shia sect as a valid denomination of Islam, the contemporary geopolitical landscape has widened the Sunni-Shia divide and ongoing sectarian violence continues to endanger Shias within the region, particularly in Pakistan. The Ahmadiyya sect, a heterodox and reformist Islamic movement, is considered deviant and proclaimed as "non-Muslim" by the majority of Sunnis in Pakistan, and more recently in Bangladesh, due to their perceived rejection of one of the fundamental tenets of Islam—the finality of Prophet Muhammad—and members of the Ahmadiyya community have been systematically persecuted in countries across South Asia (Human Rights Watch, 2005). In some parts of South Asia, aspects of the Hindu caste system have been adopted by Muslims, dividing community members into Ashrafs, Ajlafs, Arzals, and other castes characterized by status hierarchy (Momin, 1977). Despite the overwhelming evidence on the short-term and long-term negative consequences of exposure to violence and other forms of trauma, living in fear of persecution, discrimination, and social exclusion on identity and mental health, which are further complicated by the presence of other marginalized identities (e.g., LGBTQ+, disability status, etc.), empirical data on psychological outcomes among members of these smaller sects of Islam are close to nonexistent. While not considered a sect in and of themselves, the realities of Muslim converts/reverts, who commonly experience "othering" and exclusion from the broader Muslim diaspora in the United States and disapproval from non-Muslim family and friends, have also remained unexplored in psychological studies.

Conclusion

South Asian Muslim Americans have been a part of American society from its earliest days, yet their psychosocial experiences have remained invisible for most of history. While South Asian Muslim Americans—like other Muslim communities in the United States and beyond—have been indelibly impacted by systemic and personal hostilities associated with the 9/11 attacks, relatively little scholarly attention to date has been paid to the unique experiences of being Muslims with roots in South Asia. We aimed to contextualize this population's unique psychosocial experiences within the historical contexts of Muslims in South Asia and in the United States; the historical contexts of South Asian (and Asian American) immigration, and the transnational kinship network and co-ethnic and co-religious community ties in the diaspora that shape this population's identity and well-being.

Using the lens of intersectionality, our review of key social science literature about South Asian Muslim Americans revealed particular challenges as well as the resilience of women, individuals who identify as LGBTQ+, youth, and older adults. Our review also suggests that there remains scope for further research, but existing evidence suggests that segments of this population have various unmet psychosocial needs and vulnerabilities. Importantly, an intersectional analysis must be accompanied by action to reduce systemic inequalities (Rosenthal, 2016). Thus we end our discussion with an urgent call for the profession to combat sources of oppression that have disproportionately affected this population, namely Islamophobia, xenophobia, and gender- and sexuality-based biases.

References

Abbas, T. (2004). After 9/11: British south Asian Muslims, islamophobia, multiculturalism, and the state. *American Journal of Islamic Social Sciences*, *21*(3), 26–38.

Abu-Bader, S. H., Tirmazi, M. T., & Ross-Sheriff, F. (2011). The impact of acculturation on depression among older Muslim immigrants in the United States. *Journal of Gerontological Social Work*, *54*(4), 425–448.

Ahluwalia, M. K., & Pellettiere, L. (2010). Sikh men post-9/11: Misidentification, discrimination, and coping. *Asian American Journal of Psychology*, *1*(4), 303–314.

Al-Sayyad, A. A. (2010). You're what?: Engaging narratives from diasporic Muslim women on identity and gay liberation. *Islam and Homosexuality*, *2*, 373–394.

Amer, M. M., & Bagasra, A. (2013). Psychological research with Muslim Americans in the age of islamophobia: Trends, challenges, and recommendations. *American Psychologist*, *68*(3), 134.

Amnesty International. (2017, June 28). *India: Hate crimes against Muslims and rising Islamophobia must be condemned*. Retrieved from https://www.amnesty.org/en/latest/news/2017/06/india-hate-crimes-against-muslims-and-rising-islamophobia-must-be-condemned/.

Bald, V. (2006). Overlapping diasporas, multiracial lives: South Asian Muslims in U.S. communities of color, 1880–1950. *Souls*, *8*(4), 3–18.

Bhat, S. A. (2019). The Kashmir conflict and human rights. *Race & Class*, *61*(1), 77–86. https://doi.org/10.1177/0306396819850988.

Bose, S., & Jalal, A. (2017). *Modern South Asia: History, culture, political economy*. Routledge.

Byng, M. (2017). Transnationalism among second-generation Muslim Americans: Being and belonging in their transnational social field. *Social Sciences*, *6*(4), 131.

Cainkar, L., & Maira, S. (2005). Targeting Arab/Muslim/South Asian Americans: Criminalization and cultural citizenship. *Amerasia Journal*, *31*(3), 1–28.

Carter, R. T. (2007). Racism and psychological and emotional injury: Recognizing and assessing race-based traumatic stress. *The Counseling Psychologist*, *35*, 13–105. https://doi.org/10.1177/0011000006292033.

Chen, X., Talwar, D., & Ji, Q. (2015). Social network and social support among elderly Asian immigrants in the United States. *Global Journal of Anthropology Research*, *2*, 15–21.

Choudhury, P. P., Badhan, N. S., Chand, J., Chhugani, S., Choksey, R., Husainy, S., … Wat, E. C. (2009). Community alienation and its impact on help-seeking behavior among LGBTIQ South Asians in Southern California. *Journal of Gay & Lesbian Social Services*, *21*(2–3), 247–266.

Cole, E. R. (2009). Intersectionality and research in psychology. *American Psychologist*, *64*(3), 170–180.

Cook-Masaud, C., & Wiggins, M. I. (2011). Counseling Muslim women: Navigating cultural and religious challenges. *Counseling and Values*, *55*(2), 247–256.

Council on American-Islamic Relations (CAIR). (2018). *2018 civil rights report*. Retrieved from http://www.islamophobia.org/reports/228-2018-civil-rights-report-bias-incident-data.htm.

Crenshaw, K. (1989). Demarginalizing the intersection of race and sex: A black feminist critique of antidiscrimination doctrine, feminist theory and antiracist politics. In *University of Chicago Legal Forum* (p. 139).

Crenshaw, K. W. (1991). Mapping the margins: Intersectionality, identity politics, and violence against women of color. *Stanford Law Review*, *43*(6), 1241–1299.

Das, A. K., & Kemp, S. F. (1997). Between two worlds: Counseling South Asian Americans. *Journal of Multicultural Counseling and Development*, *25*(1), 23–33.

Dave, S., Dhingra, P., Maira, S., Mazumdar, P., Shankar, L. D., Singh, J., & Srikanth, R. (2000). De-privileging positions: Indian Americans, South Asian Americans, and the politics of Asian American studies. *Journal of Asian American Studies*, *3*(1), 67–100.

Diwan, S., Jonnalagadda, S. S., & Balaswamy, S. (2004). Resources predicting positive and negative affect during the experience of stress: A study of older Asian Indian immigrants in the United States. *The Gerontologist*, *44*(5), 605–614.

Dwyer, C. (2000, July). Negotiating diasporic identities: Young British South Asian Muslim women. In Vol. 23 (4). *Women's Studies International Forum*. (pp. 475–486): Pergamon.

Escalante, A. (2019). The long arc of islamophobia: African slavery, Islam, and the Caribbean world. *Journal of Africana Religions*, *7*(1), 179–186.

Ganguly, S. (1993). Ethno-religious conflict in South Asia. *Survival*, *35*(2), 88–109.

Gettleman, J., Schultz, K., Raj, S., & Kumar, H. (2019, April 11). Under Modi, a Hindu nationalist surge has further divided India. In *The New York Times*. Retrieved from https://www.nytimes.com/2019/04/11/world/asia/modi-india-elections.html.

Gilbert, P., Gilbert, J., & Sanghera, J. (2004). A focus group exploration of the impact of Izzat, shame, subordination and entrapment on mental health and service use in South Asian women living in Derby. *Mental Health, Religion & Culture*, *7*(2), 109–130.

Halim, A. M. A. (1999). Reconciling the opposites: Equal but subordinate. In *Religious fundamentalisms and the human rights of women* (pp. 203–213). New York: Palgrave Macmillan.

Haque, A. (2004). Religion and mental health: The case of American Muslims. *Journal of Religion and Health*, *43*(1), 45–58.

Hasnain, R., & Rana, S. (2010). Unveiling Muslim voices: Aging parents with disabilities and their adult children and family caregivers in the United States. *Topics in Geriatric Rehabilitation*, *26*(1), 46–61.

Hicks, M. H. R., & Bhugra, D. (2003). Perceived causes of suicide attempts by UK South Asian women. *American Journal of Orthopsychiatry, 73*(4), 455–462.

Huang, S., Teo, P., & Yeoh, B. S. (2000, July). Diasporic subjects and identity negotiations: Women in and from Asia. In *Women's Studies International Forum*. Elsevier Science.

Human Rights Watch. (2005). *Breach of faith persecution of the Ahmadiyya community in Bangladesh*. (Vol. 17(6)). Retrieved from https://www.hrw.org/reports/2005/bangladesh0605/bangladesh0605.pdf.

Inman, A. G. (2006). South Asian women: Identities and conflicts. *Cultural Diversity and Ethnic Minority Psychology, 12*(2), 306.

Inman, A. G., Devdas, L., Spektor, V., & Pendse, A. (2014). Psychological research on South Asian Americans: A three-decade content analysis. *Asian American Journal of Psychology, 5*(4), 364.

Inman, A. G., Ladany, N., Constantine, M. G., & Morano, C. K. (2001). Development and preliminary validation of the cultural values conflict scale for South Asian women. *Journal of Counseling Psychology, 48*(1), 17.

Iyer, D. (2015). *We too sing America: South Asian, Arab, Muslim, and Sikh immigrants shape our multiracial future*. The New Press.

Jordan, A., & Bhandari, S. (2016). Lived experiences of South Asian women facing domestic violence in the United States. *Journal of Ethnic & Cultural Diversity in Social Work, 25*(3), 227–246.

Kader, M. F., & Choudhury, A. H. (2019). Historical background of the Rohingya refugee crisis and the implication of their statelessness. *International Journal of Social Sciences and Economic Review, 1*(1), 8–15.

Kaduvettoor-Davidson, A., & Inman, A. G. (2013). South Asian Americans: Perceived discrimination, stress, and well-being. *Asian American Journal of Psychology, 4*(3), 155.

Kallivayalil, D. (2004). Gender and cultural socialization in Indian immigrant families in the United States. *Feminism & Psychology, 14*(4), 535–559.

Kaur, R. (2017). The curious case of Sick Keesar: Tracing the roots of South Asian presence in the early republic. *Journal of Transnational American Studies, 8*(1), 1–26.

Koshy, S. (1998). Category crisis: South Asian Americans and questions of race and ethnicity. *Diaspora: A Journal of Transnational Studies, 7*(3), 285–320.

Kurien, P. A. (2003). To be or not to be south Asian: Contemporary Indian American politics. *Journal of Asian American Studies, 6*(3), 261–288.

Lauber, C., & Rössler, W. (2007). Stigma towards people with mental illness in developing countries in Asia. *International Review of Psychiatry, 19*(2), 157–178.

Lee, R. (2003). Do ethnic identity and other-group orientation protect against discrimination for Asian Americans? *Journal of Counseling Psychology, 50*, 133–141. https://doi.org/10.1037/0022-0167.50.2.133.

Lee, E. (2015). *The making of Asian America: A history*. NY: Simon and Schuster.

Leong, F. T., & Lau, A. S. (2001). Barriers to providing effective mental health services to Asian Americans. *Mental Health Services Research, 3*(4), 201–214.

Maira, S. M. (2009). *Missing: Youth, citizenship, and empire after 9/11*. Durham, NC: Duke University Press.

Metcalf, B. D. (Ed.), (2009). *Islam in South Asia in practice*: Princeton University Press.

Meyer, I. H. (2003). Prejudice, social stress, and mental health in lesbian, gay, and bisexual populations: Conceptual issues and research evidence. *Psychological Bulletin, 129*(5), 674.

Minority Rights Group International. (2017). *Narrowing space: Violence and discrimination against India's religious minorities*. Retrieved from https://minorityrights.org/wp-content/uploads/2017/06/MRG_Rep_India_Jun17-2.pdf.

Minwalla, O., Rosser, B. S., Feldman, J., & Varga, C. (2005). Identity experience among progressive gay Muslims in North America: A qualitative study within Al-Fatiha. *Culture, Health & Sexuality*, *7*(2), 113–128.

Mogahed, D., Chouhoud, Y., & Buageila, S. (2018). *American Muslim poll 2018: Pride and prejudice*. Institute for Social Policy and Understanding.

Mohammad-Arif, A. (2000). A masala identity: Young South Asian Muslims in the US. *Comparative Studies of South Asia, Africa and the Middle East*, *20*(1), 67–87.

Momin, A. (1977). The Indo-Islamic tradition. *Sociological Bulletin*, *26*(2), 242–258. Retrieved from http://www.jstor.org/stable/23618920.

Morgan, G. & Poynting, S. (Eds.), (2012). *Global islamophobia: Muslims and moral panic in the west*. Burlington, VT: Ashgate Publishing.

Perry, B. (2014). Gendered Islamophobia: Hate crime against Muslim women. *Social Identities*, *20*(1), 74–89.

Pew Research Center. (2015, May 19). *Projected changes in the global Muslim population*. Retrieved from https://www.pewforum.org/2015/04/02/muslims/.

Pew Research Center. (2017, September 8). *Key facts about Asian Americans*. Retrieved from https://www.pewresearch.org/fact-tank/2017/09/08/key-facts-about-asian-americans/.

Purkayastha, B. (2010). Interrogating intersectionality: Contemporary globalisation and racialised gendering in the lives of highly educated South Asian Americans and their children. *Journal of Intercultural Studies*, *31*(1), 29–47.

Rahman, Z., & Witenstein, M. A. (2014). A quantitative study of cultural conflict and gender differences in South Asian American college students. *Ethnic and Racial Studies*, *37*(6), 1121–1137.

Rana, J. (2011). *Terrifying Muslims: Race and labor in the south Asian diaspora*. Durham, NC: Duke University Press.

Rosenthal, L. (2016). Incorporating intersectionality into psychology: An opportunity to promote social justice and equity. *American Psychologist*, *71*(6), 474–485.

Ross-Sheriff, F. (1994). Elderly Muslim immigrants: Needs and challenges. *Muslim Communities in North America*, 407–421.

Sandil, R., Robinson, M., Brewster, M. E., Wong, S., & Geiger, E. (2015). Negotiating multiple marginalizations: Experiences of South Asian LGBQ individuals. *Cultural Diversity and Ethnic Minority Psychology*, *21*(1), 76.

Selod, S., & Embrick, D. G. (2013). Racialization and Muslims: Situating the Muslim experience in race scholarship. *Sociology Compass*, *7*(8), 644–655.

Slater, J., & Farisz, H. (2019, July 7). *After Sri Lankan attacks, Muslims face boycotts and violence*. Retrieved from https://www.washingtonpost.com/world/asia_pacific/after-easter-sunday-attacks-muslims-face-boycotts-and-violence-in-sri-lanka/2019/07/06/3e4a405a-91f6-11e9-956a-88c291ab5c38_story.html?noredirect=on.

South Asian Americans Leading Together. (2019). *A demographic snapshot of South Asians in the United States*. Retrieved from http://saalt.org/wp-content/uploads/2019/04/SAALT-Demographic-Snapshot-2019.pdf.

The Southern Poverty Law Center (SPLC). (2016). *Harassment and intimidation in the aftermath of the election*. Retrieved from https://www.splcenter.org/sites/default/files/com_hate_incidents_report_final.pdf.

Tummala-Narra, P., Alegria, M., & Chen, C. N. (2012). Perceived discrimination, acculturative stress, and depression among South Asians: Mixed findings. *Asian American Journal of Psychology*, *3*(1), 3.

Uniform Crime Reporting. (2016). *Hate crime statistics, 2015. US Department of Justice—Federal Bureau of Investigation*. Retrieved from https://ucr.fbi.gov/hate-crime/2016.

Uniform Crime Reporting. (2017). *Hate crime statistics, 2016. US Department of Justice—Federal Bureau of Investigation*. Retrieved from https://ucr.fbi.gov/hate-crime/2017.

United States Census Bureau. (2016). *American community survey, 1-year estimates*. Retrieved from https://www.census.gov/newsroom/press-kits/2017/acs-one-year.html.

Utsey, S. O., Payne, Y. A., Jackson, E. S., & Jones, A. M. (2002). Race-related stress, quality of life indicators, and life satisfaction among elderly African Americans. *Cultural Diversity and Ethnic Minority Psychology*, *8*(3), 224–233. https://doi.org/10.1037/1099-9809.8.3.224.

Werbner, P. (2005). Honor, shame and the politics of sexual embodiment among South Asian Muslims in Britain and beyond: An analysis of debates in the public sphere. *International Social Science Review*, *6*(1), 25–47.

Yip, A. K., & Khalid, A. (2010). *Looking for Allah: Spiritual quests of queer Muslims* (pp. 81–110). Sexuality and Sacred Places: Queer Spiritual Spaces.

Further reading

Mogahed, D., & Chouhoud, Y. (2017). *American Muslim poll 2017: Muslims at the crossroads. Vol. 21*. Institute for Social Policy and Understanding.

Rana, J. (2016). The racial infrastructure of the terror-industrial complex. *Social Text*, *34*(4 (129)), 111–138.

South Asian Americans Leading Together. (2018). *Communities on fire: Confronting hate violence and xenophobic political rhetoric*. Retrieved from http://saalt.org/wp-content/uploads/2018/01/Communities-on-Fire.pdf.

United States Census Bureau. (2017). *American community survey 5-year estimates*. Retrieved from https://www.census.gov/newsroom/press-kits/2017/acs-5-year.html.

Chapter 10

Mental health considerations for immigrants of Arab/MENA descent

Germine H. Awad, Hien Nguyen, Flor Castellanos, Taylor Payne and Hanan Hashem
The University of Texas at Austin, Austin, TX, United States

Americans of Arab, Middle Eastern and North African (MENA) descent Americans are a heterogeneous pan-ethnic group that are diverse in terms of ethnicity, religion, and cultural values (ADC, 2009; Awad, 2010; Read, 2008). In fact, the term Arab simply ties individuals whose lineage is linked to any of the 22 Arab League countries in the Middle East and North Africa. A majority of Arab Americans have ancestry from Lebanon, Egypt, Iraq, Morocco, and Somalia (Arab American Institute, 2018). Arab Americans also have ancestry from Algeria, Bahrain, the Comoros Islands, Djibouti, Jordan, Kuwait, Libya, Mauritania, Oman, Palestine, Qatar, Saudi Arabia, Sudan, Syria, Tunisia, the United Arab Emirates, and Yemen. The expanded MENA designation also includes Iran and Turkey. The absence of a Middle Eastern and North African category in the US Census is believed to result in an undercount of Arab/MENA individuals who live in the United States making it difficult to get an accurate count of this population. In light of these limitations, the Arab American Institute (2018) estimates that there are over 3.5 million Arab Americans.

Contrary to common misconceptions, approximately 63% of Arab Americans identify as Christian, with a majority identifying as Catholic, Orthodox, or Protestant and approximately 26% Arab Americans identify with the Muslim faith (Amer & Kayyali, 2016). Arabs and those of MENA descent are often assumed to be Muslim leading to a problem of conflation and misconception as it pertains to this group. Although there are differences in the experience of Muslim and Christian Arabs/MENAns in the United States (Awad, 2010; Padela & Heisler, 2010; Read, 2008), both groups are likely to experience discrimination due to Islamaphobia given that religious identity and ethnic identity are often conflated. Nevertheless, beyond experiences of discrimination, the majority of individuals in the MENA region report that religion plays at least some role in their lives (Harb, 2016).

Mental and Behavioral Health of Immigrants in the United States
https://doi.org/10.1016/B978-0-12-816117-3.00010-5

In addition to the importance of religion, immigrants from the Arab/MENA region share other cultural characteristics. These characteristics include morality, honor, hospitality, and family (Harb, 2016). The value of morality centers conceptions of justice, generosity, privacy and respect, fairness, and humility. Honor is typically linked to matters of reputation and is often a way to facilitate close family bonds. Hospitality and generosity are core cultural values that are believed to have emerged in nomadic times as a survival mechanism where people had to depend on the help and kindness of others to endure harsh conditions. Perhaps the most central value for Arab/MENA immigrants is the importance of the family. The family serves as the primary socialization mechanism, provider of social support, and protection (Abudabbeh, 1996; Haboush, 2007; Harb, 2016). It is not surprising that Arab children learn from a very young age that respect for elders is imperative (Dwairy, Achoui, Abouserie, & Farah, 2006).

Immigration from the Middle East and North Africa is thought to have occurred in three separate waves, each with its own legal and political challenges. Immigrants of MENA descent primarily emigrate for educational and economic opportunity, family reunification, political asylum, and refuge (Awad, Kia-Keating, & Amer, 2019). The first cohorts of MENA immigrants, termed the first wave of migration, can be characterized as predominantly Christian, Lebanese, and Syrian laborers and merchants that primarily emigrated for economic opportunity (Abraham, 1995; Naff, 1985). This migration was initiated in the late 1800s after a pivotal point in the US history. Up until 1870, one had to be White and free in order to become a citizen—until a new law was established in order to allow a pathway for Black people into citizenship (Tehranian, 2000). This law still denied non-White and non-Black immigrants the right to citizenship. The first wave of immigration ended in 1924 with the passing of the Johnson-Reed Immigration Act, which severely restricted immigration from Asia and other non-Western European world regions. Immigrants classified as non-White continued to be barred from citizenship eligibility until 1952 soon after the World War II (Bennett, 1966).

The establishment of the state of Israel in 1948 sparked the second wave of immigration due to the displacement of Muslims and other Arab communities caused by war. From 1948 to 1965, due to war and political upheaval in Egypt, Iraq, and Syria highly educated individuals from these countries emigrated to the United States for reasons of political asylum. In 1965, with the passing of the Immigration and Nationality Act (also known as the Hart-Cellar Act), a fundamental shift in the immigration patterns of various groups from different regions of the world occurred (Paik, Kula, Saito, Rahman, & Witenstein, 2014; Rumbaut, 2007). For one, the Act removed the quota restriction on immigrants from non-Western European regions to the United States. After the passing of this Act, the number of immigrants from MENA regions increased fourfold and this wave represents the third and largest wave of migration from MENA nations to the United States to date (Awad et al., 2019). This third wave of immigrants was primarily Muslim and fleeing the MENA region due the political instability (Abraham, 1995).

More recently, due to political upheaval in Somalia, Iraq, Syrian Arab Republic, and Sudan in the 2000s and a resulting international refugee crisis, a fourth wave of displaced MENA immigrants has emerged (Kia-Keating, Ahmed, & Modir, 2016). Since 2000, approximately 60% of the world's conflict-related deaths have been in the MENA region (Saidi, 2018). Globally, in 2012, over 51 million individuals were displaced and forced into migration from their home countries, with the majority of these individuals from MENA regions. Political refugees are individuals "outside their country of origin, and unable or unwilling to return there or avail themselves of its protection, due to a well-founded fear of persecution for reasons of race, religion, nationality, membership of a particular group, or political opinion" (Goodwin-Gill, 2008, p. 3). From 2008 to 2019, individuals of MENA descent have comprised the largest percentage (over 30%) of all refugees entering the United States (Refugee Processing Center, 2019). In contrast to MENA immigrants before the 2000s who voluntarily emigrated for economic and educational opportunity or for family reunification, the current emerging fourth wave of MENA refugees seek asylum in the United States from persecution, violence, and political conflict in their home countries. These individuals also face significant impediments in returning to their countries of origin (Kia-Keating et al., 2016). The conditions under which immigrants came to the United States have implications for acculturation processes.

Acculturation and acculturative stress

Acculturation, as classically defined by Redfield, Linton, and Herskovits (1936), p. 149) is the "phenomena which result when groups of individuals having different cultures come into continuous firsthand contact with subsequent changes in the original culture patterns of either or both groups." Acculturation describes the complex psychosocial pattern, comprising many aspects of human functioning, of how individuals raised and socialized in one cultural context (their home culture) dynamically attune and adapt to new contexts (Kim & Abreu, 2001). Although acculturation is considered a "neutral" process in that changes may take place in either or both the minority and dominant culture groups, in actuality, acculturation tends to induce more change in one group (the "acculturating group") than in the other (Berry, 1997). Acculturation on a narrower individual level is referred to as "psychological acculturation" (Graves, 1967). A more recent definition of psychological acculturation is Cuellar and Arnold's (1995), which specifies the process as change occurring at three levels of individual functioning: behavioral (e.g., language, music, food, and customs), affective (e.g., meanings attached to symbols), and cognitive (e.g., gender role beliefs and fundamental values).

For Arab/MENA Americans, greater acculturation to mainstream American society has been associated with greater life satisfaction (Faragallah, Schumm, & Webb, 1997), better overall health (Tailakh et al., 2016) but differences in acculturation outcomes have emerged based on several factors. Acculturation experiences may differ based on the reasons for immigration, length of stay in the United States, social support, religious identification, and identity factors, just to name a few. In terms of religious identification, Amer and Hovey (2007) found that integration was not associated with better mental health for Muslim Arabs in their sample but both Muslims and Christians reported that integration was their main acculturation strategy. Further, another study found that perceptions of discrimination differed by acculturation level and religious identification. Specifically, Christian Arabs who were highly acculturated reported the least amount of discrimination, whereas Muslim Arabs who were highly acculturated reported the highest level of discrimination (Awad, 2010).

On an individual level, sudden changes in cultural traditions, behaviors, and social skills due to the acculturation process result in acculturative stress. Acculturative stress, as defined by Berry, Kim, Minde, and Mok (1987) is thought to be a direct result of stressors related to the acculturation process that leads to poorer mental health outcomes and psychological distress often taking the form of anxiety and depression. For first-generation immigrants, acculturative stress is a direct, concurrent byproduct of the acculturation process (Trimble, 2003), a resulting "tension of contact" between the minority individual's ethnic culture and the dominant host culture (Roysircar & Maestas, 2002). Acculturative stress is both the psychological and physical stress of acclimating to a foreign culture in a new country. For voluntary migrants from MENA regions, acculturative stress after resettlement can result from phenomena such as loss of social networks, family separation, language difficulties, loss of employment, loss of social status, "culture shock," unfamiliarity, discrimination, and feelings of social alienation (Ahmed, Kia-Keating, & Tsai, 2011; Berry, 1997; Rudmin, 2009; Rudmin & Ahmadzadeh, 2001). In addition, for refugees of MENA descent, acculturative stressors may also include limited resources, difficulty meeting basic needs, continual uncertainty, cultural bereavement, separation from loved ones, and exposure to violence (Kia-Keating et al., 2016).

In general, for both voluntary immigrants and refugees of MENA descent, traumatic experiences that occurred in their home country, difficulties experienced during emigration, prejudice, and general negative sentiment in a hostile mainstream American culture after resettlement, may lead to greater acculturation difficulties in the United States for these groups than for other American immigrant groups (Awad et al., 2019). Thus, immigrants and refugees of MENA descent are at a significantly higher risk for stress-related mental health disorders compared to other immigrant groups. For example, in a meta-analysis of MENA immigrants' resettlement outcomes in the United States, inability to meet basic needs and lack of housing were significantly related to worse mental health outcomes compared to other groups (Porter & Haslam, 2005). For refugees of MENA descent, whose migration trajectory includes not only preflight stressors, but also may include traumatic events and significant adversities experienced during flight and after resettlement in the United States (Kia-Keating et al., 2016), significantly higher levels of acculturative stress is reported, leading to greater risk of trauma-related mental health illnesses such as psychosis, anxiety, and mood disorders (e.g., Bhugra & Becker, 2005).

In both voluntary migrant and refugee populations, acculturative stress predicts clinical depression and psychological distress above and beyond simply perceived stress. It is a stress unique only to those acculturating to a new culture, and statistically and theoretically differs from normal "everyday" stress (Berry, 1997; Hwang & Ting, 2008). In regard to MENA-American immigrants, acculturative stress is a valuable variable in assessing this population's mental health outcomes. For example, in a study examining the effects of acculturation, ethnic identity, and acculturative stress on the help-seeking attitudes of Assyrian-American immigrants (Roweiheb, 2013), acculturation level was found to be unrelated to help-seeking attitudes, while acculturative stress was a significant predictor. In a sample of Arab adolescents, acculturation stress predicted psychological adjustment and the perceived ability of adolescents to make friends in school, maintain friendships, perform well in school (Goforth, Oka, Leong, & Denis, 2014), and behavior problems (Goforth, Pham, & Oka, 2015).

Level of acculturation has been used in the previous research to identify immigrant or minority groups at higher risk for psychological distress, but level of acculturation in and of itself is a distal variable that does not necessarily directly correlate with increases or decreases in risk (Escobar & Vega, 2000). Acculturative stress may be a more proximal, direct, and therefore accurate variable than degree of acculturation in predicting psychological distress and mental health risk (Hwang & Ting, 2008).

Despite a political focus on immigration from MENA regions over recent years, there has been limited empirical data on the acculturation outcomes, the particular acculturative stressors, and the psychosocial well-being of these immigrants and refugees after resettlement into the United States (Kia-Keating et al., 2016). As displaced persons escaping war and political conflict in their home countries, many MENA refugees undoubtedly experience emigration contexts significantly more traumatic than voluntary migrants in other eras and circumstances. Immigrants and refugees escaping from war and violent political regimes often experience violence and loss of family members in their home countries. During the process of emigrating to asylum countries such as the United States, refugees may also experience traumatic events such as death of loved ones, injury, starvation, and physical and sexual violence. Many MENA-American refugees in the United States may have been traumatically separated from their families and have no realistic prospects of return to their homelands. Immigration for these individuals may be aptly described as a "complete loss of identity and familiarity" (Abbasi, 2015).

In many respects, pre-displacement trauma in the home country and trauma experienced during the migration trajectory imprints deep psychological scars on MENA-American refugees, and members of these communities may need significant mental health intervention for years beyond their initial migration (Marshall, Schell, Elliott, Berthold, & Chun, 2005). Compared to nonrefugee populations, refugees are at a significantly increased risk for chronic psychological disorders and trauma-related mental health disorders, such as depression, post-traumatic stress disorder (PTSD), and somatization (Porter & Haslam, 2005; Ringold, Burke, & Glass, 2005; Wrobel, Farrag, & Hymes, 2009). Numerous studies have linked exposure to violence to physical and mental health difficulties among refugees of MENA descent (Kia-Keating et al., 2016). Researchers have noted elevated levels of psychiatric illness among refugees as compared to voluntary migrants also from MENA regions. In one comparison study of an Iraqi refugee and an Arab nonrefugee sample at a mental health clinical site, Jamil et al. (2002) found that Iraqi refugees reported a greater likelihood of PTSD and health problems when compared to the nonrefugee Arab-American individuals. A similar survey found that approximately 50% of surveyed Iraqi refugees reported prevalence of emotional distress, anxiety, and depression and 31% were at high risk for post-traumatic stress disorder (Taylor et al., 2014). In general, many MENA-American immigrants report significant levels of psychological distress, which may be linked to their past immigration experiences and present acculturation difficulties. For example, one longitudinal study found that preimmigration trauma was associated with higher levels of PTSD and depression and predicted acculturation struggles a year later (LeMaster et al., 2018).

National context and discrimination

For both voluntary migrants and refugees of MENA descent, the acculturative stress of being "othered" and targeted through pervasive interpersonal and institutional discrimination in the United States and living within a hostile dominant American culture can create a sense of insecurity, hopelessness, and alienation (Awad et al., 2019). Chronic discrimination, prejudice, and oppressions against individuals of MENA descent can be labeled as a sort of pervasive "insidious trauma" (Holmes, Facemire, & DaFonseca, 2016). These traumas must be considered as a component of MENA immigrants' overall psychosocial well-being, levels of acculturative stress, and resettlement outcomes in the United States. In terms of acculturation outcomes for immigrants and refugees of MENA descent, studies provide evidence that postmigration stressors may be more influential than premigration stressors or in-flight trauma (e.g., Ellis, MacDonald, Lincoln, & Cabral, 2008). A study of MENA refugees in Denmark 8–9 years after resettlement found that "insidious trauma" and acculturative stressors experienced post-displacement were better predictors of individuals' psychological health than trauma experienced before migration (Montgomery, 2008). For refugees and immigrants of MENA descent resettling in the United States, experienced discrimination may be as crucial a factor in predicting psychological well-being and social outcomes as initial trauma exposure, especially years after resettlement (Ellis et al., 2008; Kia-Keating et al., 2016).

In addition to the circumstances for voluntary or involuntary migration faced by Arab/MENA immigrants, experiences of immigrants are often impacted by the national context in which they are embedded. Although the United States was resettled by immigrant groups, the country has a long history of restrictionist attitudes regarding who can enter this country (Espenshade & Hempstead, 1996). Negative rhetoric has been, and is a powerful tool used to perpetuate prejudicial anti-immigrant agendas. There tends to be a cyclical pattern of Americans perceiving immigrants as threats to the current social order (often a result of anti-immigrant rhetoric) that often results in limiting immigration to the United States. Arab/MENAns and other immigrant groups of color were not the only targets of negative rhetoric and discrimination. For example, the Anglo-Saxons perceived Irish and German immigrants as a threat, and the Irish and Germans later felt the same way toward Italians, Russian, and Jewish immigrants (Espenshade & Hempstead, 1996; Wei, Jacobson López, & Wu, 2019). Irish labor unions believed Chinese migrant workers were taking their jobs so the Chinese Exclusion Act 1882 was passed. In addition, after the bombing of Pearl Harbor, many individuals of Japanese heritage were perceived as a national security threat, and were removed from their homes and forced into concentration camps (Allport, 1954; Espenshade & Hempstead, 1996; Wei et al., 2019). Perceiving new immigrants as threats tends to be cyclical and typically leads to restrictive immigration policies (Espenshade & Hempstead, 1996).

Antiimmigrant and anti-Arab and Muslim sentiment were exacerbated by the events of September 11, 2001, which intensified a concern for national security and increased antiimmigrant rhetoric toward people from the MENA region (Awad & Amayreh, 2016; Erickson & Al-Timimi, 2001; Haboush, 2007). Immigrants and citizens with ancestry from the MENA region were often associated with terrorism and crime (Wright & Esses, 2019). Initiatives targeting noncitizens based on the race, religion, and ethnicity increased and led to civil rights concerns as Homeland Security officials arrested and deported Arab and Muslim immigrants (Wishnie, 2011). Similar to Japanese Americans after Pearl Harbor, after the events of September 11, 2001 (9/11), the Arab and MENA communities were treated as hostile foreigners (Awad et al., 2019). With the 2016 campaigns, election of Donald Trump, and influx of refugees from MENA countries, a resurgence of hateful rhetoric has reemerged and hate crimes against MENA and Muslim Americans increased once again (Abu-Ras, Suárez, & Abu-Bader, 2018; Federal Bureau of Investigation, 2016, 2018).

In addition to anti-immigration rhetoric, media portrayals of Arabs/MENA individuals continue to be negative, portraying Arabs/MENAns as terrorists, religious fanatics, and criminals (e.g., Shaheen, 2003). Although there has been some movement toward presenting a complex, multidimensional portrayal of Arabs and Middle Easterners in TV dramas and movies, these attempts are few and infrequent (Alsultany, 2012). Arab/MENA immigrants who come to the United States must contend with these negative and biased media images, which may increase psychological distress already present due to acculturation stress and circumstances surrounding their migration (Awad et al., 2019).

Institutional discrimination is the perpetuation of discriminatory practices at the structural, political, and organizational level. It impacts on individuals depending on their group membership (Awad & Amayreh, 2016; Sampson, 2008). This form of discrimination also serves to protect and maintain the current hierarchy of the system against perceived threats. In the United States, the PATRIOT Act, the "Muslim Ban" and discriminatory immigration practices, are some of the most prominent examples of institutional discrimination against MENA immigrants (Awad et al., 2019).

After the 9/11 attacks, the United States experienced a radical political shock. Arab and Muslim individuals became the targets of discriminatory governmental practices enacted in the name of national security (Cainkar, 2004; Zarrugh, 2016). In the months following 9/11, the government issued a hold on nonimmigrant visas for individuals from 26 (majority MENA) countries. The government also enacted the Special Registration Program, which denied visitor visas to those coming from MENA countries, and created the Absconder Apprehension Initiative which primarily targeted MENA individuals, who made up only 2% of visa absconders (Awad et al., 2019; Cainkar, 2004). Furthermore, the United States enacted the USA PATRIOT Act which stood for "United and Strengthening America by Providing Appropriate Tools Required to Intercept and Obstruct Terrorism" (Audi, 2008). The USA PATRIOT Act allowed the United States government to spy, detain, and deport individuals who were deemed possible threats. Arab/Middle Eastern and Muslim Americans were targeted disproportionally compared to other demographic groups (Audi, 2008). The "War on Terror" became an attack on the freedom and civil liberties of Arab and MENA individuals (Akram, 2002).

Given the wars in Iraq, and violence in Syria, Lebanon, Libya, Sudan, and Yemen a significant number of refugees from the MENA region have come to the United States to seek asylum from these dangerous conditions. As a response to the influx of refugees and anti-Muslim and Arab rhetoric, the Trump Administration released Executive Order 13769, commonly referred to as the "Muslim Ban," which suspended entry of Syrian refugees to the United States, suspended the US Refugee Admissions program for 4 months, and denied entry and travel to those from Syria, Sudan, Yeman, Somalia, Libya, Iran, and Iraq (Exec. Order No. 13769, 2017). Over 60,000 people had their visas revoked and over 700 people were detained (Hersher, 2017). Furthermore, the Trump administration dropped the refugee admission's cap from 85,000 to 30,000 from 2016 to 2019, and proposed zero admissions for fiscal year 2020 further fueling the institutional discrimination faced by this group.

The hostile environment and social biases perpetuated at the national level affect the daily interactions that may occur on the individual level (Awad et al., 2019; Dovidio, Hewstone, Glick, & Esses, 2010). Interpersonal discrimination occurs at the individual level, where an individual is treated unfairly due to their identity or membership to a group. It consists of negative experiences that can be overt such as verbal attacks and/or subtler, in the form of microaggressions (e.g., exclusion from activities, ignoring, and staring) (Singletary & Hebl, 2009). Although European immigrants may have an outgroup status in terms of perceived citizenship, immigrants of color may have to contend with multiple outgroup statuses due to their race, ethnicity, citizenship, and religion. Non-White immigrants are more likely than European immigrants to be "othered" and, therefore, experience interpersonal discrimination.

Ideological constructs such as Social Dominance Orientation (SDO) can help explain perceptions of Arab/MENA immigrants. SDO refers to the tendency for individuals to organize their worldview in terms of ingroups and outgroups, where their group is thought of as superior. Individuals high in (SDO) are more likely to endorse high levels of nationalism, lower levels of altruism, tolerance, and concern for others (Pratto, Sidanius, Stallworth, & Malle, 1994; Yakushko, 2009). SDO tends to be a strong predictor of prejudice generally and has been found to be a predictor of prejudice toward Arab and MENA individuals (Awad & Amayreh, 2016).

Arab and Muslim individuals are often portrayed as threat to national security and are targeted as scapegoats during tense political times. The most recent example is the Trump administrations continuous use of xenophobic rhetoric to reinforce prejudicial ideology. MENA individuals are often asked to apologize for terrorist attacks have to deal with people calling the police on them in the name of national security and consistently receive the message that they do not belong (Awad et al., 2019; Brown et al., 2013). The accumulation of these discrimination experiences contributes to the cumulative racial/ethnic trauma faced by Arab/MENA individuals (Awad et al., 2019).

Identity and racialization

Upon arriving to the United States, immigrants soon realize that race is a major mode of differentiation in this country (Smedley, 2018). Although race as a construct may exist to some degree in the Middle East and North Africa, like many regions around the world, it not the primary way that people are categorized. Immigrants of color slowly start to comprehend that they are differentiated from the White majority and that experiences in the United States tend to differ based on the racial background. In the United States, there are four established ethnic minority groups that are officially recognized by the government: African Americans/Blacks, Asian Americans, Latinx/Hispanics, and Native Americans. Arab/MENAns are currently classified as racially White and, therefore. Are not accorded the protections allotted to other ethnic minority groups.

Every 10 years, the United States collects information on race and ethnicity in a decennial census that is partially used to get an accurate count of residents, determine resource allocations, as well as identify disparities (e.g., education and health) based on the racial group membership. Because individuals of MENA descent are classified as White, there is currently not an accurate count of this population. Further, most institutions and organizations look to the census for how to measure race and ethnicity on demographic forms. Further, because the Office of Management and Budget (OMB) determines the minimal reporting standards for race and ethnicity for the government, the Census Bureau must adhere to the stimulations put forth by the OMB. Therefore, the Census cannot add a separate Middle Eastern and North African pan-ethnic/racial category until the OMB allows it.

Although the US Census categorizes those with Arab/MENA ancestry as White, most individuals that identify with this population believe that this racial classification does not an accurately represent their experiences (Awad et al., 2019; Awad, Amayreh, & Reilly, 2017; Cainkar, 2004). Experiences of discrimination (Ahmed et al., 2011; Awad & Amayreh, 2016), "othering" (Cainkar, 2004), negative media portrayals (Alsultany, 2012; Shaheen, 2003) contribute to hypervisibility for this group despite the simultaneous invisibility experienced by lack of official recognition. The longer that Arab/MENA immigrants reside in the United States the more they realize that the US racial classifications do not fit their experiences.

Conclusion

In short, although Middle Eastern and North African Americans, compared to other American ethnic groups, have had a relatively short history in the United States, it is one fraught with acculturation difficulties and acculturative stressors due to this population's unique sociopolitical fit within the larger context of American and global politics. It is important for researchers, policy makers, mental health practitioners, and community health advocates to be aware of the distinct and multilayered acculturative stressors affecting immigrants and refugees from MENA regions in order to best address the needs of the MENA-American community.

References

Abbasi, F. (2015, December). *Immigration, trauma, and the power of faith*. Retrieved January 4, 2017, from Care for Your mind website: http://careforyourmind.org/immigration-trauma-and-the-power-of-faith/.

Abraham, N. (1995). Arab Americans. In R. J. Vecoli, J. Galens, A. Sheets, & R. V. Young (Eds.), Vol. 1. *Gale encyclopedia of multicultural America* (pp. 84–98). New York: Gale Research.

Abudabbeh, N. (1996). Arab families. In M. McGoldrick, J. Giordano, & N. Garcia-Preto (Eds.), *Ethnicity and family therapy* (3rd ed., pp. 423–450). New York: Guilford.

Abu-Ras, W., Suárez, Z. E., & Abu-Bader, S. (2018). Muslim Americans' safety and well-being in the wake of trump: A public health and social justice crisis. *American Journal of Orthopsychiatry, 88*(5), 503–515. https://doi.org/10.1037/ort0000321.

Alsultany, E. (2012). *Arabs and Muslims in the media: Race and representation after 9/11*. New York: New York University Press.

American-Arab Anti-Discrimination Committee. (2009). *Facts about Arabs and the Arab world*. Retrieved August 17, 2017, from http://www.adc.org/2009/11/facts-about-arabs-and-the-arab-world/.

Ahmed, S. R., Kia-Keating, M., & Tsai, K. H. (2011). A structural model of racial discrimination, acculturative stress, and cultural resources among Arab American adolescents. *American Journal of Community Psychology*, *48*(3–4), 181–192. https://doi.org/10.1007/s10464-011-9424-3.

Akram, S. M. (2002). The aftermath of September 11, 2001: The targeting of Arabs and Muslims in America. *Arab Studies Quarterly*, *24*(2/3), 61–118.

Allport, G. W. (1954). *The nature of prejudice*. Boston: Addison-Wesley Pub. Co.

Amer, M. M., & Kayyali, R. A. (2016). Religion and religiosity: Christian and Muslim faiths, diverse practices, and psychological correlates. In M. M. Amer & G. H. Awad (Eds.), *Handbook of Arab American psychology* (pp. 414–427). New York, NY: Routledge/Taylor & Francis Group.

Amer, M. M., & Hovey, J. D. (2007). Socio-demographic differences in acculturation and mental health for a sample of 2nd generation/early immigrant Arab Americans. *Journal of Immigrant and Minority Health*, *9*(4), 335–347. https://doi.org/10.1007/s10903-007-9045-y.

Arab American Institute. (2018). *Demographics*. Retrieved from http://www.aaiusa.org/demographics.

Audi, G. Q. (2008). Challenges facing the Arab American community from a legal perspective. *American Studies Journal*, *1*. 5–5(1).

Awad, G. H. (2010). The impact of acculturation and religious identification on perceived discrimination for Arab/middle eastern Americans. *Cultural Diversity and Ethnic Minority Psychology*, *16*(1), 59–67. https://doi.org/10.1037/a0016675.

Awad, G. H., & Amayreh, W. M. (2016). Discrimination: Heightened prejudice post 9/11 and psychological outcomes. In *Handbook of Arab American psychology* (pp. 63–75). New York, NY: Routledge/Taylor & Francis Group.

Awad, G. H., Amayreh, W. M., & Reilly, E. D. (2017). Contemporary Arab American psychology. In A. W. Blume (Ed.), Vol. 1. *Social issues in living color: Challenges and solutions from the perspective of ethnic minority psychology: Overview and interpersonal issues* (pp. 29–47). Praeger/ABC-CLIO: Santa Barbara, CA. Retrieved from http://search.ebscohost.com/login.aspx?direct=true&db=psyh&AN=2016-51793-002&site=ehost-live.

Awad, G. H., Kia-Keating, M., & Amer, M. M. (2019). A model of cumulative racial–ethnic trauma among Americans of middle eastern and north African (MENA) descent. *American Psychologist*, *74*(1), 76–87. https://doi.org/10.1037/amp0000344.

Bennett, M. T. (1966). The immigration and nationality (McCarran-Walter) act of 1952, as amended to 1965. *The Annals of the American Academy of Political and Social Science*, *367*(1), 127–136.

Berry, J. W., Kim, U., Minde, T., & Mok, D. (1987). Comparative studies of acculturative stress. *The International Migration Review*, *21*(3), 491–511. https://doi.org/10.2307/2546607.

Berry, J. W. (1997). Immigration, acculturation, and adaptation. *Applied Psychology*, *46*(1), 5–34. https://doi.org/10.1111/j.1464-0597.1997.tb01087.x.

Bhugra, D., & Becker, M. A. (2005). Migration, cultural bereavement and cultural identity. *World Psychiatry*, *4*(1), 18–24.

Brown, L. M., Awad, G. H., Preas, E. J., Allen, V., Kenney, J., Roberts, S., & Lusk, L. B. (2013). Investigating prejudice toward men perceived to be Muslim: Cues of foreignness versus phenotype. *Journal of Applied Social Psychology*, *43*(Suppl. 2), E237–E245. https://doi.org/10.1111/jasp.12015.

Cainkar, L. (2004). Post 9/11 domestic policies affecting U. S. Arabs and Muslims: A brief review. *Comparative Studies of South Asia, Africa and the Middle East*, *24*(1), 247–251. https://doi.org/10.1215/1089201X-24-1-247.

Cuellar, I., & Arnold, B. (1995). Acculturation rating scale for Mexican Americans-II: A revision of the original ARSMA scale. *Hispanic Journal of Behavioral Sciences*, *17*(3), 275.

Dovidio, J. F., Hewstone, M., Glick, P., & Esses, V. M. (2010). Prejudice, stereotyping and discrimination: Theoretical and empirical overview. In *The SAGE handbook of prejudice, stereotyping and discrimination* (pp. 3–28). https://doi.org/10.4135/9781446200919.n1.

Dwairy, M., Achoui, M., Abouserie, R., & Farah, A. (2006). Adolescent-family connectedness among Arabs: A second cross-regional research study. *Journal of Cross-Cultural Psychology*, *37*, 248–261. https://doi.org/10.1177/0022022106286923.

Ellis, B. H., MacDonald, H. Z., Lincoln, A. K., & Cabral, H. J. (2008). Mental health of Somali adolescent refugees: The role of trauma, stress, and perceived discrimination. *Journal of Consulting and Clinical Psychology*, *76*(2), 184–193. https://doi.org/10.1037/0022-006X.76.2.184.

Escobar, J. I., & Vega, W. A. (2000). Mental health and immigration's AAAs: Where are we and where do we go from here? *Journal of Nervous and Mental Disease*, *188*(11), 736–740. https://doi.org/10.1097/00005053-200011000-00003.

Erickson, C. D., & Al-Timimi, N. R. (2001). Providing mental health services to Arab Americans: Recommendations and considerations. *Cultural Diversity & Ethnic Minority Psychology*, *7*(4), 308–327.

Espenshade, T. J., & Hempstead, K. (1996). Contemporary American attitudes toward U.S. immigration. *International Migration Review*, (2), 535–570.

Exec. Order No. 13769. (2017, February 1). *3 c.f.r, 82 FR 8977.*

Faragallah, M. H., Schumm, H. R., & Webb, F. J. (1997). Acculturation of Arab-American immigrants: An exploratory study. *Journal of Comparative Family Studies*, *28*, 182–203.

Federal Bureau of Investigation. (2016). *Hate crime statistics, 2015*. Retrieved August 30, 2019, from FBI website: https://ucr.fbi.gov/hate-crime/2015/topic-pages/victims_final.

Federal Bureau of Investigation. (2018). *Hate crime statistics, 2017*. Retrieved August 30, 2019, from FBI website: https://ucr.fbi.gov/hate-crime/2017.

Goforth, A. N., Oka, E. R., Leong, F. T. L., & Denis, D. J. (2014). Acculturation, acculturative stress, religiosity and psychological adjustment among Muslim Arab American adolescents. *Journal of Muslim Mental Health*, *8*(2), 3–19. https://doi.org/10.3998/jmmh.10381607.0008.202.

Goforth, A. N., Pham, A. V., & Oka, E. R. (2015). Parent–child conflict, acculturation gap, acculturative stress, and behavior problems in Arab American adolescents. *Journal of Cross-Cultural Psychology*, *46*(6), 821–836. https://doi.org/10.1177/0022022115585140.

Goodwin-Gill, G. S. (2008). *United Nations audiovisual library of international law*. Retrieved January 4, 2017, from http://legal.un.org/avl/ha/prsr/prsr.html.

Graves, T. D. (1967). Psychological acculturation in a tri-ethnic community. *Southwestern Journal of Anthropology*, *23*(4), 337–350.

Haboush, K. L. (2007). Working with Arab American families: Culturally competent practice for school psychologists. *Psychology in the Schools*, *44*(2), 183–198.

Harb, C. (2016). The Arab region: Cultures, values, and identities. In M. M. Amer & G. H. Awad (Eds.), *Handbook of Arab American psychology* (pp. 3–18). New York, NY: Routledge.

Hersher, R. (2017, February 3). *Federal judge stays trump travel order, but many visas already revoked*. Retrieved August 31, 2019, from NPR.org website: https://www.npr.org/sections/thetwo-way/2017/02/03/513306413/state-department-says-fewer-than-60-000-visas-revoked-under-travel-order.

Holmes, S. C., Facemire, V. C., & DaFonseca, A. M. (2016). Expanding criterion a for posttraumatic stress disorder: Considering the deleterious impact of oppression. *Traumatology*, *22*(4), 314–321. https://doi.org/10.1037/trm0000104.

Hwang, W.-C., & Ting, J. Y. (2008). Disaggregating the effects of acculturation and acculturative stress on the mental health of Asian Americans. *Cultural Diversity and Ethnic Minority Psychology*, *14*(2), 147–154. https://doi.org/10.1037/1099-9809.14.2.147.

Jamil, H., Hakim-Larson, J., Farrag, M., Kafaji, T., Duqum, I., & Jamil, L. H. (2002). A retrospective study of Arab American mental health clients: Trauma and the Iraqi refugees. *The American Journal of Orthopsychiatry*, *72*(3), 355–361.

Kia-Keating, M., Ahmed, S. R., & Modir, S. (2016). Refugees and forced migrants: Seeking asylum and acceptance. In *Handbook of Arab American psychology* (pp. 160–172). New York, NY: Routledge/Taylor & Francis Group.

Kim, B. S. K., & Abreu, J. M. (2001). Acculturation measurement: Theory, current instruments, and future directions. In J. G. Ponterotto, J. M. Casas, L. A. Suzuki, & C. M. Alexander (Eds.), *Handbook of multicultural counseling* (2nd ed., pp. 394–424). Thousand Oaks, CA: Sage Publications, Inc. [2008-00399-022].

LeMaster, J. W., Broadbridge, C. L., Lumley, M. A., Arnetz, J. E., Arfken, C., Fetters, M. D., … Arnetz, B. B. (2018). Acculturation and post-migration psychological symptoms among Iraqi refugees: A path analysis. *American Journal of Orthopsychiatry*, *88*(1), 38–47. https://doi.org/10.1037/ort0000240.

Marshall, G. N., Schell, T. L., Elliott, M. N., Berthold, S. M., & Chun, C.-A. (2005). Mental health of Cambodian refugees 2 decades after resettlement in the United States. *Journal of the American Medical Association*, *294*(5), 571–579. https://doi.org/10.1001/jama.294.5.571.

Montgomery, E. (2008). Long-term effects of organized violence on young middle eastern refugees' mental health. *Social Science & Medicine (1982)*, *67*(10), 1596–1603. https://doi.org/10.1016/j.socscimed.2008.07.020.

Naff, A. (1985). *Becoming American: The early Arab immigrant experience*. Carbondale, IL: Southern Illinois University Press.

Padela, A. I., & Heisler, M. (2010). The association of perceived abuse and discrimination after September 11, 2001, with psychological distress, level of happiness, and health status among Arab Americans. *American Journal of Public Health*, *100*(2), 284–291.

Paik, S., Kula, S., Saito, L. E., Rahman, Z., & Witenstein, M. (2014). Historical perspectives on diverse Asian American communities: Immigration, incorporation, and education. *Teachers College Record*, *116*(8), 1–45 [2014-32969-008].

Porter, M., & Haslam, N. (2005). Predisplacement and postdisplacement factors associated with mental health of refugees and internally displaced persons: A meta-analysis. *JAMA*, *294*(5), 602–612. https://doi.org/10.1001/jama.294.5.602.

Pratto, F., Sidanius, J., Stallworth, L. M., & Malle, B. F. (1994). Social dominance orientation: A personality variable predicting social and political attitudes. *Journal of Personality and Social Psychology*, *67*(4), 741.

Read, J. (2008). Discrimination and identity formation in a post-9/11 era, a comparison of Muslim and Christian Arab Americans. In A. Jamal & N. Naber (Eds.), *Race and Arab Americans before and after 9/11, from invisible citizens to visible subjects* (pp. 276–304). Syracuse, NY: Syracuse University Press.

Redfield, R., Linton, R., & Herskovits, M. J. (1936). Memorandum for the study of acculturation. *American Anthropologist*, *38*(1), 149–152. https://doi.org/10.1525/aa.1936.38.1.02a00330.

Refugee Processing Center. (2019). Retrieved September 1, 2019, from Refugee Processing Center website: http://www.wrapsnet.org.

Ringold, S., Burke, A., & Glass, R. M. (2005). Refugee mental health. *JAMA*, *294*(5), 646. https://doi.org/10.1001/jama.294.5.646.

Roweiheb, N. (2013). *The effects of acculturation and stress on willingness to seek mental health services among Assyrian Americans*. ProQuest Information & Learning, US (2013-99220-156).

Roysircar, G., & Maestas, M. L. (2002). Assessing acculturation and cultural variables. In K. S. Kurasaki, S. Okazaki, & S. Sue (Eds.), *Asian American mental health: Assessment theories and methods* (pp. 77–94). New York, NY: Kluwer Academic/Plenum Publishers [2002-06049-005].

Rudmin, F. (2009). Constructs, measurements and models of acculturation and acculturative stress. *International Journal of Intercultural Relations*, *33*(2), 106–123. https://doi.org/10.1016/j.ijintrel.2008.12.001.

Rudmin, F. W., & Ahmadzadeh, V. (2001). Psychometric critique of acculturation psychology: The case of Iranian migrants in Norway. *Scandinavian Journal of Psychology*, *42*(1).

Rumbaut, R. G. (2007). *Vietnamese Americans (SSRN scholarly paper no. ID 1878127)*. Retrieved from Social Science Research Network website: http://papers.ssrn.com/abstract=1878127.

Sampson, W. A. (2008). Institutional discrimination. In R. Schaefer (Ed.), *Encyclopedia of race, ethnicity, and society* (pp. 727–729). https://doi.org/10.4135/9781412963879.n289.

Saidi, N. (2018). *Middle East and North Africa: A new approach to MENA's refugee crisis—Qantara.de*. Retrieved August 28, 2019, from Qantara.de—Dialogue with the Islamic World website: https://en.qantara.de/content/middle-east-and-north-africa-a-new-approach-to-menas-refugee-crisis.

Shaheen, J. G. (2003). Reel bad Arabs: How Hollywood vilifies a people. *The Annals of the American Academy of Political and Social Science*, *588*(1), 171–193. https://doi.org/10.1177/0002716203588001011.

Singletary, S. L., & Hebl, M. R. (2009). Compensatory strategies for reducing interpersonal discrimination: The effectiveness of acknowledgments, increased positivity, and individuating information. *Journal of Applied Psychology*, *94*(3), 797–805. https://doi.org/10.1037/a0014185.

Smedley, A. (2018). *Race in North America: Origin and evolution of a worldview* (4th ed.). New York: Routledge.

Tailakh, A. K., Evangelista, L. S., Morisky, D. E., Mentes, J. C., Pike, N. A., & Phillips, L. R. (2016). Acculturation, medication adherence, lifestyle behaviors, and blood pressure control among Arab Americans. *Journal of Transcultural Nursing*, *27*(1), 57–64. https://doi.org/10.1177/1043659614526456.

Taylor, E. M., Yanni, E. A., Pezzi, C., Guterbock, M., Rothney, E., Harton, E., … Burke, H. (2014). Physical and mental health status of Iraqi refugees resettled in the United States. *Journal of Immigrant and Minority Health*, *16*(6), 1130–1137. https://doi.org/10.1007/s10903-013-9893-6.

Tehranian, J. (2000). Performing whiteness: Naturalization litigation and the construction of racial identity in America. *The Yale Law Journal*, *109*(4), 817.

Trimble, J. E. (2003). Introduction: Social change and acculturation. In *Acculturation: Advances in theory, measurement, and applied research*. Washington, DC: American Psychological Association.

Wei, K., Jacobson López, D., & Wu, S. (2019). The role of language in anti-immigrant prejudice: What can we learn from immigrants' historical experiences? *Social Sciences*, *8*(3), 93. https://doi.org/10.3390/socsci8030093.

Wishnie, M. J. (2011). Proportionality: The struggle for balance in U.S. immigration policy. *University of Pittsburgh Law Review*, *72*(3).

Wright, J. D., & Esses, V. M. (2019). It's security, stupid! Voters' perceptions of immigrants as a security risk predicted support for Donald Trump in the 2016 US presidential election. *Journal of Applied Social Psychology*, *49*(1), 36–49. https://doi.org/10.1111/jasp.12563.

Wrobel, N. H., Farrag, M. F., & Hymes, R. W. (2009). Acculturative stress and depression in an elderly Arabic sample. *Journal of Cross-Cultural Gerontology*, *24*(3), 273–290. https://doi.org/10.1007/s10823-009-9096-8.

Yakushko, O. (2009). Xenophobia: Understanding the roots and consequences of negative attitudes toward immigrants. *The Counseling Psychologist*, *37*(1), 36–66. https://doi.org/10.1177/0011000008316034.

Zarrugh, A. (2016). Racialized political shock: Arab American racial formation and the impact of political events. *Ethnic and Racial Studies*, *39*(15), 2722–2739. https://doi.org/10.1080/01419870.2016.1171368.

Further reading

Ainsley, J. (2019, August 21). *Trump admin weighs letting states, cities deny entry to refugees approved for resettlement in U.S.* Retrieved from https://www.nbcnews.com/politics/immigration/trump-admin-weighs-letting-states-cities-deny-entry-refugees-approved-n1044801.

Amer, M. M., & Awad, G. H. (2016). Research scholarship: Critique of the existing literature and visions for the future. In M. M. Amer & G. H. Awad (Eds.), *Handbook of Arab American psychology* (pp. 414–427). New York, NY: Routledge/Taylor & Francis Group.

Awad, G. H., Martinez, M. S., & Amer, M. M. (2013). Considerations for psychotherapy with immigrant women of Arab/middle eastern descent. *Women & Therapy*, *36*(3–4), 163–175. https://doi.org/10.1080/02703149.2013.797761.

Brown, C. L. (2009). Heritage language and ethnic identity: A case study of Korean-American college students. *International Journal of Multicultural Education*, *11*(1).

Gerstle, G. (2006). The political incorporation of immigrant groups: An historical perspective on the American experience. In *American Arabs and political participation* (pp. 27–38). Washington, DC: Woodrow Wilson International Center for Scholars.

Holliday, A. (2010). Complexity in cultural identity. *Language and Intercultural Communication*, *10*(2), 165–177.

Kayyali, R. (2013). US census classifications and Arab Americans: Contestations and definitions of identity markers. *Journal of Ethnic and Migration Studies*, *39*(8), 1299–1318.

Lee, T. L., & Fiske, S. T. (2006). Not an outgroup, not yet an ingroup: Immigrants in the stereotype content model. *International Journal of Intercultural Relations*, *30*(6), 751–768.

Martinez, O., Wu, E., Sandfort, T., Dodge, B., Carballo-Dieguez, A., Pinto, R., & Chavez-Baray, S. (2013). Evaluating the impact of immigration policies on health status among undocumented immigrants: A systematic review. *Journal of Immigrant and Minority Health*, *17*(3), 947–970.

Ngai, M. M. (2004). *Impossible subjects: Illegal aliens and the making of modern America*. Princeton University Press.

Nguyen, M. V. (2013). *The effects of psychoeducation on the help-seeking attitudes of Vietnamese refugees for post-traumatic stress disorder*. ProQuest Information & Learning, US (2015-99020-418).

Umaña-Taylor, A. J., & Updegraff, K. A. (2007). Latino adolescents' mental health: Exploring the interrelations among discrimination, ethnic identity, cultural orientation, self-esteem, and depressive symptoms. *Journal of Adolescence*, *30*(4), 549–567.

Section C

Psychopathology

Chapter 11

The immigrant mental health advantage in the US among ethnic minority and other groups: Findings and potential mechanisms

David M. Barnes[a,*], Sarah A. Lieff[b,*], Evan L. Eschliman[c], YiPing Li[d] and Lawrence H. Yang[b,e]

[a]*Department of Epidemiology, School of Global Public Health, New York University, New York, NY, United States,* [b]*Department of Social and Behavioral Sciences, School of Global Public Health, New York University, New York, NY, United States,* [c]*Department of Sociomedical Sciences, Mailman School of Public Health, Columbia University, New York, NY, United States,* [d]*Clinical Psychology (Psychology in Education), Teachers College, Columbia University, New York, NY, United States,* [e]*Department of Epidemiology, Mailman School of Public Health, Columbia University, New York, NY, United States*

Introduction

The United States has more immigrants than any other country in the world, accounting for one-fifth of the world's migrants in 2017 (Radford, 2019). In 2017, immigrants constituted 13.6% of the US population, nearly triple their share of the population in 1970 (4.7%) (Radford, 2019). Immigrants and their descendants are estimated to account for 88% of the US population growth through 2065 (Radford, 2019).

Researchers often view immigration as a major life stressor that puts immigrants at risk of poor health outcomes (Friis, Yngve, & Persson, 1998; Markides & Rote, 2015). The stressors immigrants face in their host country include discrimination, low socioeconomic status, and language barriers (Markides & Rote, 2015). Paradoxically, despite the well-proven association between lower socioeconomic status and poorer health, much evidence suggests that immigrants in the US have better health and lower mortality than the native-born population

*Co-first authors.

Mental and Behavioral Health of Immigrants in the United States
https://doi.org/10.1016/B978-0-12-816117-3.00011-7

(Abraido-Lanza, Dohrenwend, Ng-Mak, & Turner, 1999; Blanco et al., 2013; Markides & Rote, 2015; Salas-Wright, Vaughn, Schwartz, & Cordova, 2016; Vaughn, Salas-Wright, DeLisi, & Maynard, 2014). This phenomenon was originally termed the "Hispanic Epidemiologic Paradox" by Markides and Coreil (1986), based on findings that southwestern Latinxs primarily of Mexican origin demonstrated relatively good health despite poor socioeconomic status (Markides & Coreil, 1986; Markides & Rote, 2015). This chapter addresses how this paradox appears to extend to other immigrant groups and to mental health (Markides & Rote, 2015; Singh & Miller, 2004).

Consistent with this Immigrant Health Paradox (Markides & Rote, 2015), exposure to migration stressors does not necessarily result in elevated rates of psychopathology among immigrants in the US (Park & Kemp, 2006; Salas-Wright, Vaughn, Goings, Miller, & Schwartz, 2018; Suárez-Orozco & Carhill, 2008). Multiple studies show that immigrants in the US are less likely than US-born individuals to experience an array of mental disorders (Alarcón et al., 2016; Alegria, Alvarez, & DiMarzio, 2017; Alegria, Canino, Stinson, & Grant, 2006; Breslau, Borges, Hagar, Tancredi, & Gilman, 2009; Salas-Wright et al., 2018; Takeuchi, Alegría, Jackson, & Williams, 2007; Williams, Gonzalez, et al., 2007; Williams, Haile, et al., 2007).

Since the early 1980s, standardized diagnostic survey instruments have been developed and used worldwide to assess mental disorders at the population level. Using these instruments, psychiatric epidemiology studies conducted in large, nationally representative adult samples in the US have clarified the relationship between immigration and psychopathology. The **Epidemiological Catchment Area (ECA)** study in the early 1980s was conducted in five regions of the US. The **National Comorbidity Survey** (NCS) followed a decade later, and was in turn followed in the early 2000s by the Collaborative Psychiatric Epidemiology Surveys (CPES), a consortium of three studies (Alegría et al., 2008), and the **National Epidemiologic Survey on Alcohol and Related Conditions (NESARC).**

In the first section of this chapter, we report findings from the CPES consortium and NESARC studies, focusing on the prevalence of psychopathology in immigrants and their US-born counterparts within distinct race/ethnic groups (Blacks, Asians, Latinxs, and Whites). By reporting comparisons between foreign- and US-born individuals *within* racial/ethnic groups, we minimize variation in cultural differences between our comparison groups; emergent differences between the foreign- and US-born are then more likely to be attributable to the American context. The second section describes four mechanisms that have each been hypothesized to account for at least some of immigrants' mental health advantages in the US, and the dilution of those advantages in subsequent generations: selection effects and three processes of acculturation (substantive, artifactual, and stressor exposure). The third section focuses on the particular mechanisms underlying the immigrant mental health paradox among Black immigrants and their descendants in the US.

Epidemiology of mental illness among US- and foreign-born

Datasets/samples

The comparisons in psychopathology between US-born and foreign-born individuals presented in Section "Tables and summaries" for each racial/ethnic group draw from major psychiatric epidemiology studies: three concurrent psychiatric epidemiology studies sponsored by the Inter-University Consortium for Political and Social Research, and collectively called the Collaborative Psychiatric Epidemiology Surveys (Alegría et al., 2008)—National Comorbidity Survey—Replication (NCS-R), National Survey of American Life (NSAL), National Latino and Asian American Survey (NLAAS)—and the National Epidemiologic Survey on Alcohol and Related Conditions (NESARC).This section describes the data collection methods and sample characteristics of each (Table 1).

NCS-R. The NCS-R sampled the general US population of English-speaking civilians 18 and older living in noninstitutionalized settings in the 48 contiguous states and students living in campus housing. Psychiatric diagnoses were made in the NCS-R using the World Mental Health Survey Initiative Version of the World Health Organization's Composite International Diagnostic Interview (WMH-CIDI), a fully structured, lay-administered instrument based on the Diagnostic and Statistical Manual, version IV (DSM-IV) criteria (Kessler et al., 2003).

NSAL. The NSAL sampled African American, Afro-Caribbean, and non-Hispanic Whites using a four-stage probability design (Mays et al., 2018). The African American sample comprised households located in the 48 contiguous states with at least one Black adult 18 years or older (Williams, Gonzalez, et al., 2007; Williams, Haile, et al., 2007). The Caribbean Black sample was selected from the core sampling areas of the NSAL and from metropolitan segments sampled based on their concentration of Blacks of Caribbean descent (Williams, Gonzalez, et al., 2007; Williams, Haile, et al., 2007). Respondents identifying as Black who did not report Caribbean ancestry were part of the African American sample, while the sample of Caribbean Blacks comprised those who identified as Black and endorsed at least one of the following: (1) of West Indian or Caribbean descent, (2) from a Caribbean-area country, or (3) having parents or grandparents who were born in a Caribbean country (Williams, Gonzalez, et al., 2007; Williams, Haile, et al., 2007).

NLAAS. The NLAAS sampled Latinxs and Asian Americans. The CIDI (described above) was translated into Spanish, Chinese, Tagalog, and Vietnamese, and administered by bilingual lay interviewers when appropriate (Alegria et al., 2004; Alegría et al., 2008; Takeuchi, Zane, et al., 2007). The NLAAS also incorporated cultural idioms of distress (e.g., "ataque de nervios" and neurasthenia) as part of the prevalence estimates and assessed the impact of language on prevalence rates of psychiatric disorders (Alegria et al., 2004). Participants were

TABLE 1 Study characteristics.

	NCS-R (CPES)	NSAL (CPES)	NLAAS (CPES)	NESARC
Nationally representative	Yes	Yes	Yes	Yes
Response rate	70.9%	72.3%	75.5% for Latinxs, 65.5% for Asian Americans	81%
Sampling period	2001–2003	2001–2003	2002–2003	2001–2002
Data collection method	Face-to-face interviews, using laptop computer-assisted personal interview (CAPI) methods	Face-to-face interviews, using laptop computer-assisted personal interview (CAPI) methods	Face-to-face interviews, using laptop computer-assisted personal interview (CAPI) methods	Face-to-face interviews
Assessment of disorders	World Mental Health Survey Initiative Version of the World Health Organization's Composite International Diagnostic Interview (WMH-CIDI)	WMH-CIDI	WMH-CIDI, translated into Spanish, Chinese, Tagalog, and Vietnamese; adapted for cultural relevancy; and administered by bilingual lay interviewers when appropriate	Alcohol Use Disorder and Associated Disabilities Interview Schedule-DSM-IV Version (AUDADIS-IV)
Sample characteristics	9090 adults 18 years and older, including 8917 non-Hispanic Whites	3570 African Americans, 1621 Blacks of Caribbean descent, and 891 non-Hispanic Whites, 18 years and older	2095 Asian Americans and 2554 Latinx, 18 years and older	43,093 adults 18 years and older, including 24,507 non-Hispanic Whites, 8245 non-Hispanic Blacks, 8308 Latinx, and 1332 Asian Americans
Foreign born	Non-Hispanic Whites: 3.4% foreign-born	Caribbean Blacks: 65.1% foreign-born African Americans: 2.3% foreign-born	Asian Americans: 78.2% foreign-born Latinxs: 58.4% foreign-born	

classified into the following ethnic subgroups: Puerto Rican ($N=495$), Cuban ($N=577$), Mexican ($N=868$), Other Latinxs ($N=614$), Chinese ($N=600$), Vietnamese ($N=520$), Filipino ($N=508$), and Other Asians ($N=647$) (Alegría et al., 2007, 2008; Takeuchi, Zane, et al., 2007). Within "Other Asians," respondents identified as Japanese ($N=107$), Korean ($N=81$), Asian Indian ($N=141$), and Other ($N=138$) (Takeuchi, Zane, et al., 2007).

NESARC. The National Institute on Alcohol Abuse and Alcoholism (Bethesda, MD) conducted NESARC. The survey consisted of a civilian, noninstitutionalized sample of adults 18 and older living in households and group quarters, including military off-base housing, boarding houses, rooming houses, non-transient hotels and motels, shelters, facilities for housing workers, college housing, and group homes in all 50 states. The sampling frame was based on households in the Census 2000–2001 Supplementary Survey and group quarters in the Census 2000 Group Quarters Inventory. Blacks, Latinxs, and young adults (ages 18–24 years) were oversampled and data were weighted to adjust for oversampling and household- and person-level nonresponse to represent the US population not living on military bases in the 2000 census in terms of region, age, sex, race, and ethnicity. All psychiatric disorders were assessed using the Alcohol Use Disorder and Associated Disabilities Interview Schedule-DSM-IV Version (AUDADIS-IV), a structured diagnostic interview designed for lay interviewers. Diagnostic algorithms relied on the Diagnostic and Statistical Manual, version IV (DSM-IV) criteria. The primary difference between the AUDADIS-IV and CIDI diagnostic instruments is that the former generates more detail on substance use disorder onset, patterns, consequences, and treatment (Samet, Waxman, Hatzenbuehler, & Hasin, 2007). Information on the reliability and validity of the AUDADIS-IV can be found elsewhere (Grant et al., 2004), as can further information on NESARC more generally (Grant et al., 2004; Hasin, Goodwin, Stinson, & Grant, 2005; Hasin, Stinson, Ogburn, & Grant, 2007).

Tables and summaries

Our tables and discussion compare foreign- and US-born individuals within each racial/ethnic group. The foreign-born category refers to immigrants, refugees, and asylum seekers collectively. These three groups are all assumed to be permanently settled into the receiving country, though they may be quite different from one another (see Table 2) (Douglas, Cetron, & Spiegel, 2019; Schwartz, Unger, Zamboanga, & Szapocznik, 2010). We often refer collectively to the individuals in these three groups as *immigrants*, but note that this is a composite category consisting of the noted subcategories.

Blacks

Foreign-born Black individuals had a lower prevalence of any 12-month and lifetime mood (5.3%–12.67%), anxiety (7.66%–13.53%), and substance abuse

TABLE 2 Migration terminology.

Term	Definition
Migrant	Migrants consist of four categories: long-term immigrants (or emigrants), short-term immigrants (or emigrants); residents returning after (or leaving for) a period of working abroad; and nomads
Refugee	A person who, due to a well-founded fear of persecution based on race, religion, nationality, membership in a particular social group, or political opinions, is outside the country of his or her nationality and is unable or, owing to such fear, unwilling to avail him or herself of the protection of that country.
Asylum seeker	A person who seeks safety from persecution or serious harm in a country other than his or her own and awaits a decision on the application for refugee status under relevant international and national instruments

disorders (0.3%–7.3%) than US-born Blacks (16.28%–21.4%, 15.44%–30.5%, and 11.6%–33.1% for any 12-month and lifetime mood, anxiety, and substance abuse disorder, respectively). Of 20 comparisons for anxiety disorders, 16 demonstrate a protective effect of foreign-born status on mental health, while 4 do not show a protective effect. Of 22 comparisons for mood disorders, 13 demonstrate a protective effect of foreign-born status on mental health, while 9 do not show a protective effect. The protective effects of foreign-born status observed for substance use disorders was particularly robust—all 17 comparisons demonstrated a protective effect (Broman, Neighbors, Delva, Torres, & Jackson, 2008; Mays et al., 2018; Williams, Gonzalez, et al., 2007; Williams, Haile, et al., 2007).

Some comparisons do not show a protective effect of foreign-born status on mental health. First, analyses by gender subgroup show differences between men and women in the protective effect of foreign-born status. Foreign-born Caribbean women have the same odds of any 12-month and lifetime mood and anxiety disorder as US-born Caribbean women (Williams, Gonzalez, et al., 2007; Williams, Haile, et al., 2007).

Second, when African Americans are analyzed separately from Black Caribbeans, foreign-born status does not confer the same protective effect (González, Tarraf, Whitfield, & Vega, 2010). While foreign-born Caribbean Blacks experience lower rates of major depressive disorder than US-born Caribbean Blacks, the opposite is true for African Americans—foreign-born individuals experience higher rates of 12-month and lifetime major depressive disorder than US-born individuals (González et al., 2010; Williams, Gonzalez, et al., 2007; Williams, Haile, et al., 2007).

Third, rates of 12-month and lifetime bipolar I and II are higher among foreign-born Caribbean men or essentially equivalent among foreign-born and US-born Caribbean men. A protective effect is likely not observed here because Bipolar Disorder has a strong genetic component and relatively similar rates across populations (Mays et al., 2018). It is possible that ethnic identity plays less of a role for psychiatric disorders with a particularly strong genetic component (Burnett-Zeigler, Bohnert, & Ilgen, 2013).

Fourth, protective effects differ based on age at immigration; a protective effect on lifetime anxiety and mood disorders is observed for foreign-born Blacks who immigrated at an age equal to or greater than 13 but not for foreign-born Blacks who immigrated under 13 years (Breslau et al., 2009). The immigrant advantage in anxiety and mood disorders is limited to those who immigrated as an adolescent or adult (Breslau et al., 2009). This is discussed further in Section "Summary" (Table 3).

Asian Americans

Foreign-born Asian Americans (AAs) had lower odds of anxiety disorder than US-born AAs (Breslau & Chang, 2006). Statistically significant differences, however, were not found between foreign- and US-born AAs in lifetime odds of mood disorder and substance disorder.

Across gender, foreign-born AA women had lower odds of any lifetime disorder, lifetime mood disorder, lifetime substance use disorder, and 12-month anxiety disorder than US-born AA women, yet only the odds of lifetime substance use disorder was statistically significantly different between foreign- and US-born AA men (Takeuchi, Zane, et al., 2007).

Foreign-born AAs had a lower 12-month and lifetime prevalence of any psychiatric disorder (15.9%), anxiety disorder (9.1%–9.3%), mood (8.3%–11.8%), and substance use disorders (2.2%–8.0%) than US-born AAs (25.7%, 13.3%–17.8%, 13.4%–16.6%, 9.7%–26.9%, respectively) with the exception of agoraphobia without panic and bulimia nervosa (Table 4). These differences reached statistical significance for any lifetime disorder (Hong et al., 2014), any mood disorder (Hong et al., 2014), social phobia (Breslau & Chang, 2006), agoraphobia/ panic disorder (Breslau & Chang, 2006), major depression (Hong et al., 2014), and all substance use disorders (Breslau & Chang, 2006; Hong et al., 2014; Szaflarski et al., 2011; Takeuchi, Zane, et al., 2007).

Latinxs

Foreign-born status was associated with lower odds of any lifetime disorder for Latinx men and women. Additionally, foreign-born Latinxs had a lower prevalence of any disorder over their lifetimes (22.5%–27.2%) compared to US-born Latinxs (33.9%–40.0%).

There was no difference in the odds of any lifetime anxiety disorder between foreign-born and US-born Latinxs across sex. Foreign-born Latinxs had a lower prevalence than US-born Latinxs of any lifetime anxiety disorder, however (13.2%–17.3% vs. 16.2%–21.5%). Among five prevalence comparisons for anxiety disorders, two out of five showed a protective effect of foreign-born status (posttraumatic stress disorder and social phobia) while three out of five (agoraphobia without panic disorder, generalized anxiety disorder, and panic disorder) did not.

TABLE 3 12-month and Lifetime prevalence and adjusted odds ratios of mental disorders among US-born non-Hispanic Blacks vs. foreign-born non-Hispanic Blacks in the National Survey of American Life (NSAL) and the National Epidemiologic Study on Alcohol and Related Conditions (NESARC).

	Prevalence		
	Foreign-born % (SE)	US-born % (SE)	Adjusted OR (95% CI) (Ref: US-born non-Hispanic Blacks, unless noted)
Any disorder (%)			
12-month[a,f]	11.05 (2.14, Caribbean Blacks) 11.1 (3.6, Caribbean men)	25.60 (5.86, Caribbean Blacks) 38.5 (9.2, Caribbean men)	0.19 (0.06, 0.61) (Caribbean men)* 1.24 (0.67, 2.28) (Caribbean women)
Lifetime[a,f]	19.37 (2.66, Caribbean Blacks) 19.6 (4.1, Caribbean men)	43.11 (5.47, Caribbean Blacks) 52.5 (8.2, Caribbean men)	0.23 (0.09, 0.58) (Caribbean men)* 0.55 (0.30, 1.02) (Caribbean women)
Any anxiety disorder (%)			
12-month[a,f]	9.0 (4.2, Caribbean men)	23.2 (5.9, Caribbean men)	0.35 (0.09, 1.28) (Caribbean men) 1.04 (0.48, 2.28) (Caribbean women)
Lifetime[a,d,f]	13.53 (2.59, Imm < 13y) 7.66 (1.37, Imm >= 13y) 12.8 (3.9, Caribbean men)	15.44 (0.68) 30.5 (5.8, Caribbean men)	0.88 (0.58, 1.34, Imm < 13y) 0.47 (0.32, 0.67, Imm >= 13y)* 0.32 (0.12, 0.83) (Caribbean men)* 0.63 (0.34, 1.19) (Caribbean women)
PTSD			
12-month[f]	3.0 (1.8, Caribbean men)	14.4 (6.4, Caribbean men)	
Lifetime[f]	4.3 (1.9, Caribbean men)	15.9 (7.4, Caribbean men)	

Social phobia			
12-month[f]	5.0 (2.5, Caribbean men)	5.2 (3.8, Caribbean men)	
Lifetime[f]	5.7 (2.5, Caribbean men)	8.8 (3.3, Caribbean men)	
General anxiety disorder			
12-month[f]	1.6 (0.8, Caribbean men)	3.4 (3.1, Caribbean men)	
Lifetime[f]	2.1 (0.8, Caribbean men)	4.4 (3.2, Caribbean men)	
Panic disorder			
12-month[f]	1.0 (0.5, Caribbean men)	9.7 (7.7, Caribbean men)	
Lifetime[f]	1.7 (0.6, Caribbean men)	11.5 (7.4, Caribbean men)	
Panic attack			
12-month[f]	6.4 (4.0, Caribbean men)	29.6 (10.3, Caribbean men)	
Lifetime[f]	17.7 (4.8, Caribbean men)	37.2 (8.9, Caribbean men)	
Any mood disorder (%)			
12-month[a,f]	5.3 (2.3, Caribbean men)	16.5 (8.2, Caribbean men)	0.20 (0.04, 0.99) (Caribbean men)* 1.95 (0.72, 5.28) (Caribbean women)
Lifetime[a,d,f]	12.67 (3.07, Imm < 13y) 7.72 (1.31, Imm >= 13y) 9.3 (2.8, Caribbean men)	16.28 (0.62) 21.4 (8.2, Caribbean men)	0.98 (0.60, 1.60, Imm < 13y) 0.43 (0.31, 0.60, Imm >= 13y)* 0.33 (0.08, 1.43) (Caribbean men) 0.65 (0.29, 1.43) (Caribbean women)

Continued

TABLE 3 12-month and Lifetime prevalence and adjusted odds ratios of mental disorders among US-born non-Hispanic Blacks vs. foreign-born non-Hispanic Blacks in the National Survey of American Life (NSAL) and the National Epidemiologic Study on Alcohol and Related Conditions (NESARC)—cont'd

	Prevalence		
	Foreign-born % (SE)	US-born % (SE)	Adjusted OR (95% CI) (Ref: US-born non-Hispanic Blacks, unless noted)
Major depressive disorder			
12-month[e,f]	8.0 (2.9, African Americans) 4.8 (1.1, Caribbean) 4.9 (1.7, Caribbean men)	7.2 (0.4, African Americans) 13.4 (3.7, Caribbean) 16.4 (5.6, Caribbean men)	
Lifetime[c,e,f]	10.8 (3.7, African Americans) 8.9 (1.7, Caribbean) 13.4 (African Americans) 9.1 (Caribbean) 8.9 (2.8, Caribbean men)	10.4 (0.5, African Americans) 19.8 (5.0, Caribbean) 13.1 (African Americans) 24.1 (Caribbean) 21.1 (6.5, Caribbean men)	
Dysthymia			
12-month[f]	0.9 (0.8, Caribbean men)	7.6 (5.9, Caribbean men)	
Lifetime[f]	1.7 (0.9, Caribbean men)	8.0 (5.8, Caribbean men)	
Bipolar disorder I, II			
12-month[f]	0.9 (0.5, Caribbean men)	0.2 (0.2, Caribbean men)	
Lifetime[f]	1.0 (0.5, Caribbean men)	0.9 (0.5, Caribbean men)	

Any substance use disorder (%)			
12-month[a,f]	0.3 (0.2, Caribbean men)	15.0 (9.0, Caribbean men)	0.02 (0.00, 0.12) (Caribbean men)* 0.34 (0.12, 0.97) (Caribbean women)*
Lifetime[a,b,f]	1.9 (1.3, African Americans) 4.2 (1.3, Caribbean) 7.3 (2.3, Caribbean men)	11.6 (0.7, African Americans) 19.5 (5.4, Caribbean) 33.1 (7.9, Caribbean men)	0.15 (0.05, 0.50) (Caribbean men)* 0.18 (0.08, 0.37) (Caribbean women)* 0.2 (0.1, 0.5, Caribbean only)*
Alcohol abuse			
12-month[f]	–	13.9 (9.2, Caribbean men)	
Lifetime[b,f]	6.7 (2.3, Caribbean men)	32.6 (8.0, Caribbean men)	0.2 (0.1, 0.5, Caribbean only)*
Alcohol dependence			
12-month[f]	0.1 (0.1, Caribbean men)	5.1 (3.8, Caribbean men)	
Lifetime[f]	3.0 (2.6, Caribbean men)	10.5 (5.2, Caribbean men)	
Drug abuse			
12-month[f]	0.2 (0.2, Caribbean men)	8.5 (5.7, Caribbean men)	
Lifetime[b,f]	4.0 (2.5, Caribbean men)	19.7 (8.1, Caribbean men)	0.2 (0.0, 0.8, Caribbean only)*
Drug dependence			
12-month[f]	–	0.8 (0.5, Caribbean men)	
Lifetime[f]	3.2 (2.6, Caribbean men)	6.9 (3.5, Caribbean men)	

*$P<.05$.
[a]*Williams, Haile, et al. (2007) (NSAL).*
[b]*Broman et al. (2008) (NSAL).*
[c]*Williams, Gonzalez, et al. (2007), Williams, Haile, et al. (2007) (NSAL).*
[d]*Breslau et al. (2009) (NESARC).*
[e]*González et al. (2010) (NSAL).*
[f]*Mays et al. (2018) (NSAL).*

TABLE 4 12-month and Lifetime prevalence and adjusted odds ratios of mental disorders among US-born Asian Americans vs. foreign-born Asian Americans in the National Latino and Asian American Study (NLAAS) and the National Epidemiologic Study on Alcohol and Related Conditions (NESARC).

	Foreign-born	US-born	Adjusted OR (95% CI) (Ref: US-born Asian Americans)
	Prevalence % (SE)		
Any disorder			
Lifetime[a,b]	15.16 (1.55) 15.9 (CI 13.1–19.1)	24.62 (3.22) 25.7(CI 19.7–32.7)**	Men: 0.61 (0.38–1.06) Women: 0.53 (0.35–0.82)**
12 Month[a]	8.0 (0.79)	13.22 (1.96)	Men: 0.78 (0.45, 1.36) Women: 0.51 (0.26, 1.00)
Any anxiety disorder			
Lifetime[a,b,c]	9.3 (CI 7.3–11.8) 9.1 (1.3)	13.3 (8.4–20.5) 17.8 (3.5)	0.47 (0.28–0.79)* Men: 0.90 (0.46–1.73) Women: 0.47 (0.26–0.85)
12-Month[a]			Men: 0.89 (0.48–1.64) Women: 0.38 (1.17–0.84)*
Panic disorder[b] Lifetime	1.6 (CI 0.6–4.0)	4.0 (CI 2.4–6.6)	
Agoraphobia without Panic[b] Lifetime	0.4 (CI 0.2–0.9)	0.4 (CI 0.1–1.3)	
Agoraphobia/Panic[c] Lifetime	1.6 (0.5)	5.2 (1.1)*	
Social Phobia[b,c] Lifetime	4.5 (CI 3.5–5.9) 2.7 (0.6)	8.1 (CI 4.6–14.0) 5.8 (1.1)*	
Specific Phobia [c] Lifetime	5.0 (0.9)	8.6 (1.7)	

Posttraumatic Stress Disorder[b] Lifetime	1.7 (CI 0.9–3.2)	3.1 (CI 1.4–6.5)	
Generalized Anxiety[b,c] Lifetime	2.5 (CI 1.8–3.5) 2.0 (0.5)	2.6 (CI 1.4–4.8) 3.4 (1.3)	
Any mood disorder (%)[a,b,c]			
Lifetime	8.3 (CI 6.8–10.1) 11.8 (1.3)	13.4 (CI 9.8–17.9)** 16.6 (2.3)	0.61 (0.39–0.98) Men: 0.91 (0.48–1.73) Women: 0.50 (0.33–0.76)**
Any depressive disorder[a] 12-month			Men: 1.68 (0.76–3.70) Women: 0.52 (0.25–1.10)
Major depression[b,c] Lifetime	8.0 (CI 6.5–9.7) 8.2 (1.2)	13.0 (CI 9.5–17.6)** 11.7 (1.8)	
Dysthymia[b,c] Lifetime	2.0 (CI 1.2–3.6) 2.6 (0.7)	2.7 (CI 1.4–5.1) 4.3 (1.9)	
Bipolar (I or II)[c] Lifetime	2.7 (0.6)	3.5 (1.0)	
Any substance use disorder			
Lifetime[a,b,c]	2.2 (CI 1.1–4.4) 8.0 (1.0)	9.7 (CI 7.1–13.1)*** 26.9 (3.1)***	Men: 0.31 (0.12–0.77)* Women: 0.13 (0.05–0.32)*** 0.17 (0.10–0.28)
12-Month[a]			Men: 0.30 (0.05–1.69) Women: 0.33 (0.11–1.02)
Any drug use disorder			
Lifetime[b,c]	1.0 (CI 0.5–2.0) 2.3 (0.6)	5.5 (CI 3.7–8.2)*** 8.3 (1.3)**	
Any alcohol use disorder Lifetime[b,c]	2.0 (CI 0.9–4.2) 7.3 (1.0)	8.3 (CI 5.6–12.0)** 24.5 (2.9)***	

Continued

TABLE 4 12-month and Lifetime prevalence and adjusted odds ratios of mental disorders among US-born Asian Americans vs. foreign-born Asian Americans in the National Latino and Asian American Study (NLAAS) and the National Epidemiologic Study on Alcohol and Related Conditions (NESARC)—cont'd

	Foreign-born	US-born	Adjusted OR (95% CI) (Ref: US-born Asian Americans)
	Prevalence % (SE)		
Alcohol abuse or dependence 12-month[d]	1.65 (0.33)	6.75 (1.26)***	
Excessive drinking 12-month[d]	2.61 (0.43)	12.30 (1.55)***	
Intoxication 12-month[d]	1.45 (0.28)	3.70 (0.73)**	
Eating disorders			
Bulimia nervosa 12-month[e]	0.40 (0.24)	0.25 (0.25)	
Binge eating disorder 12-month[e]	1.01 (0.39)	1.02 (0.45)	
Any binge eating 12-month[e]	2.09 (0.57)	2.19 (0.61)	

*$P < .05$.
**$P < .01$.
***$P < .001$.
[a]*Takeuchi, Alegría, et al. (2007), Takeuchi, Zane, et al. (2007) (NLAAS).*
[b]*Hong, Walton, Tamaki, and Sabin (2014) (NLAAS).*
[c]*Breslau and Chang (2006) (NESARC).*
[d]*Szaflarski, Cubbins, and Ying (2011) (NESARC).*
[e]*Nicdau, Hong, and Takeuchi (2007) (NLAAS).*

Similarly, there was no difference in the odds of any lifetime mood disorder between foreign-born and US-born Latinxs across sex, but lifetime prevalence was lower among foreign-born Latinxs (12.6%–17.0%) compared to US-born Latinxs (17.3%–22.5%). For the two prevalence comparisons for mood disorders, one (dysthymia) did not show a difference in prevalence between foreign-born and US-born Latinxs and one (major depressive episode) did.

For any lifetime substance use disorder, foreign-born Latinxs had significantly lower odds compared to US-born Latinxs. Lifetime (?) prevalence among foreign-born Latinxs (5.4%–8.5%) was much lower than among US-born Latinxs (18.0%–22.9%), and this was true in all prevalence comparisons across substance use disorders (Table 5).

Whites

Foreign-born Whites had statistically significantly lower adjusted lifetime odds than US-born Whites of any disorder, any anxiety disorder, any mood disorder, any drug use disorder, and any alcohol use disorder (Alvarez et al., 2019; Grant et al., 2004). This was also true for all four specific lifetime anxiety disorders reported, for two of four specific lifetime mood disorders reported (major depression and dysthymia), and for all four specific lifetime drug and alcohol use disorders reported (Grant et al., 2004). The only exceptions were for mania and hypomania, where the adjusted lifetime odds were not statistically significantly different between foreign- and US-born Whites (Grant et al., 2004).

Foreign-born Whites had a lower lifetime *prevalence* than US-born Whites of any disorder (32.3% vs. 52.5%), any anxiety disorder (12.4% vs. 18.7%), any mood disorder (14.7% vs. 20.9%), any drug use disorder (4.8% vs. 11.6%), and any alcohol use disorder (16.2% vs. 35.0%) (Grant et al., 2004). Within strata defined by foreign-born age of arrival in the US (arriving before age 13 vs. 13 or older) and whether of Western European or Eastern European descent, for any lifetime anxiety disorder and any lifetime mood disorder the protective effects of foreign-born status disappeared or attenuated for Western Europeans of both age of arrival groups, and for Eastern Europeans arriving before age 13 (Breslau et al., 2009).

For prevalence of *specific* lifetime disorders, foreign-born status was protective for all four anxiety disorders reported, all five mood disorder findings reported, and all four substance use disorders reported (González et al., 2010; Grant et al., 2004). This pattern obtained as well for the one 12-month prevalence finding we report for major depression (González et al., 2010).

We highlight here the exceptions noted above to the general rule among Whites that foreign-born status conferred mental health advantages. The prevalence of mania and hypomania was relatively low (Grant et al., 2004), so our finding of no difference between foreign- and US-born Whites might be due to a ceiling effect. Regarding the findings of attenuated foreign-born protections for

TABLE 5 12-month and Lifetime prevalence and adjusted odds ratios of mental disorders among US-born Latinxs vs. foreign-born Latinxs in the National Latino and Asian American Study (NLAAS).

	Prevalence (95% CI)[a]		Adjusted OR (95% CI) (Ref: US-born Latinxs)[b]
	Foreign-born (N=1630)	US-born (N=924)	
Any disorder			
12-month[c]	–	19.0	Men: 0.60 (0.42,0.85)** Women: 0.74 (0.57,0.97)*
Lifetime[d]***	24.9 (22.5–27.2)	37.1 (33.9–40.0)	Men: 0.45 (0.34,0.58)** Women: 0.62 (0.50,0.79)**
Any anxiety disorder			
12-month[c]	–	10.5	Men: 0.69 (0.36,1.32) Women: 0.88 (0.60,1.29)
Lifetime[d]**	15.2 (13.2–17.3)	18.9 (16.2–21.5)	Men: 0.69 (0.42,1.12) Women: 0.81 (0.63,1.03)
Agoraphobia without panic disorder[d]	3.7 (2.7–4.8)	3.7 (2.5–5.1)	
Generalized anxiety disorder[d]	4.7 (3.6–5.8)	4.4 (3.1–5.6)	
Panic disorder[d]	3.5 (2.2–4.6)	4.5 (3.1–6.0)	
Posttraumatic stress disorder[d]*	4.0 (3.0–5.1)	5.9 (4.4–7.5)	
Social phobia[d]*	6.0 (4.6–7.2)	8.5 (6.5–10.2)	

Any mood disorder			
12-month[c]	–	9.9	Men: 0.60 (0.34,1.06) Women: 0.90 (0.63,1.31)
Lifetime[d]**	14.8 (12.6–17.0)	19.8 (17.3–22.5)	Men: 0.75 (0.46,1.25) Women: 0.81 (0.58,1.13)
Dysthymia[d]	3.1 (2.1–4.1)	3.4 (2.2–4.5)	
Major depressive episode[d]**	13.4 (11.6–15.4)	18.6 (16.1–21.1)	
Any substance use disorder			
12-month	–	–	Men: 0.34 (0.16,0.72)** Women: †
Lifetime[d]***	7.0 (5.4–8.5)	20.4 (18.0–22.9)	Men: 0.31 (0.20,0.46)** Women: 0.07 (0.03,0.17)***
Alcohol abuse[d]***	3.5 (2.3–4.8)	9.3 (7.4–11.2)	
Alcohol dependence[d]***	2.8 (1.9–3.8)	6.9 (5.2–8.6)	
Drug abuse[d]***	2.2 (1.4–3.1)	6.1 (4.5–7.8)	
Drug dependence[d]***	1.7 (0.9–2.6)	5.1 (3.6–6.8)	

*$P<.05$.
**$P<.01$.
***$P<.001$.
†No positive cases in this sample.
[a]Prevalences given are Bayesian lifetime prevalence adjusted for age, gender, and socioeconomic status (education and household income) (Alegría et al., 2008).
[b]Alegría et al. (2007) (NLAAS).
[c]Cook, Alegría, Lin, and Guo (2009) (NLAAS).
[d]Alegría et al. (2008) (NLAAS).

those of Western European descent arriving at any age in the US and of Eastern European descent arriving before age 13 (Breslau et al., 2009), culture may be an explanatory factor. To the extent American cultural norms harm mental health and shape diagnostic criteria (we discuss both factors below in Section "Mechanisms"), cultural proximity to the US (e.g., Western Europe) would reduce the apparent protective effects of foreign-born status. By contrast, greater cultural distance (e.g., the Middle East) might afford the foreign-born mental health advantages not accruing to those from Europe, particularly Western Europe. Consistent with this proposition is the finding that foreign-born Eastern Europeans arriving in the US after the age of 12 were the only one of these European subgroups with an appreciably lower prevalence of lifetime anxiety and mood disorders compared with their US-born counterparts. Because most Eastern Europeans in our study samples who arrived in the US after the age of 12 would have been socialized in a socialist/communist Eastern Europe, their development occurred in a context quite distinct from American culture (examined in greater depth in Section "Mechanisms") (Table 6).

Summary

In all four race/ethnic groups, foreign-born status generally protected across psychiatric disorder classes, for both lifetime and past 12-month prevalence. In 193 comparisons, the foreign-born never had appreciably higher odds or prevalence of disorder than their US-born counterparts, and they frequently had a meaningfully lower odds or prevalence of disorder. Of 75 comparisons of foreign- and US-born *odds* of psychiatric disorder, the foreign-born had statistically significantly lower odds in 45 instances and there were no appreciable differences between the groups in the remaining 30. Among the 118 *prevalence* findings, the foreign-born prevalence was lower in 106 instances, higher in 10, and equal in 2. Of the 10 instances in which foreign-born prevalence was higher, 8 differences were trivial and in the other 2, the prevalence of the disorder was under 1% in both groups.

In the following paragraphs, we note exceptions to the overall pattern of foreign-born status conferring protection against psychiatric disorder. We define exceptions as odds that are not statistically significantly different between the foreign- and US-born and prevalences that are higher in the foreign-born compared with their US-born counterparts. None of these prevalence differences was appreciable. For most, the foreign-born prevalence was not more than 1.12 times the US-born prevalence, and in the two cases where it was greater, prevalence in both groups was under 1%; accordingly, we use terms such as *marginally*, *modestly*, or *trivially* higher.

For *any disorder*, among Blacks, foreign- and US-born women did not have appreciably different odds of disorder. Among Asian Americans, foreign- and US-born men did not differ in their odds of any disorder. Prevalences of any disorder were always lower in the foreign-born compared with the US-born.

TABLE 6 Lifetime prevalence* and adjusted odds ratios of mental disorders among US-born non-Hispanic Whites vs. foreign-born non-Hispanic Whites in the National Comorbidity Study—Replication (NCS-R) and the National Epidemiologic Study on Alcohol and Related Conditions (NESARC).

	Foreign-born	US-born	Adjusted OR (95% CI)[†] (Ref: foreign-born non-Hispanic Whites, unless noted)
	Prevalence % (SE)		
Any lifetime disorder[d]	32.3 (2.08)	52.5 (0.21)	2.4 (2.1–2.8)
Any lifetime anxiety disorder[d,‡]	12.4 (1.03)	18.7 (0.45)	1.7 (1.4–2.0)
Western Europe, foreign-born arriving before age 13[c]	19.08	19.5	
Western Europe, foreign-born arriving age 13 or older[c]	21.02		
Eastern Europe, foreign-born arriving before age 13[c]	17.17	19.17	
Eastern Europe, foreign-born arriving age 13 or older[c]	8.14		
Lifetime Panic Disorder[d]	3.4 (0.48)	5.7 (0.19)	2.0 (1.4–2.8)
Lifetime Social Phobia[d]	3.4 (0.63)	5.7 (0.22)	1.7 (1.2–2.5)
Lifetime Specific Phobia[d]	5.9 (0.61)	10.1 (0.33)	1.8 (1.5–2.3)
Lifetime Generalized Anxiety[d]	3.2 (0.52)	4.7 (0.21)	1.5 (1.1–2.0)
Any lifetime mood disorder[d]	14.7 (1.11)	20.9 (0.39)	1.6 (1.3–1.9)
(NCS-R)[b]			0.57 (0.42–0.78)[§]
Western Europe, foreign-born arriving before age 13[c]	22.14	22.08	
Western Europe, foreign-born arriving age 13 or older[c]	19.66		
Eastern Europe, foreign-born arriving before age 13[c]	22.29	20.83	
Eastern Europe, foreign-born arriving age 13 or older[c]	7.9		

Continued

TABLE 6 Lifetime prevalence* and adjusted odds ratios of mental disorders among US-born non-Hispanic Whites vs. foreign-born non-Hispanic Whites in the National Comorbidity Study—Replication (NCS-R) and the National Epidemiologic Study on Alcohol and Related Conditions (NESARC)—cont'd

	Foreign-born	US-born	Adjusted OR (95% CI)[†] (Ref: foreign-born non-Hispanic Whites, unless noted)
	Prevalence % (SE)		
Major depression			
12-month[a]	6.8 (1.9)	10.7 (0.4)	
Lifetime[a]	17.2 (2.8)	26.1 (0.6)	
Lifetime[d]	12.0 (1.00)	18.2 (0.35)	1.7 (1.4–2.0)
Lifetime Dysthymia[d]	3.1 (0.57)	4.6 (0.16)	1.6 (1.1–2.2)
Lifetime Mania[d]	2.7 (0.64)	3.2 (0.15)	1.3 (0.7–2.1)
Lifetime Hypomania[d]	1.8 (0.38)	2.3 (0.12)	1.3 (0.8–2.0)
Any lifetime drug use disorder[d]	4.8 (0.70)	11.6 (0.33)	3.1 (2.3–4.2)
Any lifetime drug abuse[d]	3.2 (0.49)	8.9 (0.25)	3.4 (2.4–4.6)
Any lifetime drug dependence[d]	1.6 (0.50)	2.8 (0.16)	2.0 (1.1–4.0)
Any alcohol use disorder[d]	16.2 (1.64)	35.0 (0.60)	3.1 (2.5–3.8)
Any lifetime Alcohol abuse[d]	9.6 (1.24)	20.8 (0.43)	2.5 (2.0–3.2)
Any lifetime Alcohol dependence[d]	6.6 (0.85)	14.2 (0.35)	2.6 (2.0–3.3)

Unless otherwise specified.
[†]*Odds ratios adjusted for sex, age, marital status, place of residence (urban, rural, or town), region of country, education, and family income.*
[‡]*Diagnosed with any of the following: panic disorder, social phobia, specific phobia, and generalized anxiety disorder.*
[§]*Whites with no parents born in US (whether or not participant born in US) vs. (ref. group) Whites with at least one US-born parent (whether or not participant born in US); odds ratio adjusted for sex, age, census division, urbanicity, and respondent and parent education.*
[a]*González et al. (2010) (NCS-R).*
[b]*Alvarez et al. (2019) (NCS-R).*
[c]*Breslau et al. (2009) (NCS-R).*
[d]*Grant et al. (2004) (NESARC).*

For *anxiety disorders*, non-statistically significantly different odds of disorder were predominant among Blacks and Latinxs. Similar to any disorder among Blacks, there was a slight trend toward foreign- and US-born women having similar odds. Additionally, Black immigrants arriving before age 13 appear less protected from lifetime anxiety disorders than those arriving at age 13 or older. For Latinxs, all anxiety disorder odds comparisons that we reported were gender-specific and in neither 12-month nor lifetime reference periods was there a statistically significant difference between foreign- and US-born men or women. In 35 of 37 prevalence comparisons, anxiety disorder prevalence was lower in the foreign-born compared with the US-born.

For *mood disorders*, non-statistically significant differences in odds predominated in all groups except among Whites. Among Blacks, the pattern was similar to the pattern found for anxiety disorders: foreign-born women appeared less protected by foreign-born status than men were, and across genders, arriving at age 13 or older was protective against lifetime mood disorders, but arriving earlier was not. Among Asian Americans, the pattern of findings for odds ratios was similar to that for anxiety disorders: in gender-specific findings, foreign-born men appear to enjoy less protection against mood disorders than foreign-born women. Among Latinxs, the odds ratio findings replicate anxiety disorder findings: odds ratios were reported only within gender, and none of them, for 12-month or lifetime, was appreciably different between foreign- and US-born. Of the 37 prevalence comparisons we report for mood disorders, the foreign-born had a lower prevalence in 30; five of the seven exceptions occurred among Blacks. In all three prevalence comparisons among those identifying as African American, the foreign-born had a higher prevalence than did the US-born, but all differences were slight. Two mood disorder prevalence exceptions occurred among Whites: foreign-born of Western and Eastern European descent who arrived before age 13 had a trivially higher prevalence of any lifetime mood disorder than did their US-born counterparts.

For *substance use disorders*, the foreign-born in our findings always had statistically significantly lower odds of 12-month and lifetime substance use disorders than did their US-born counterparts. In 32 of 33 prevalence comparisons, the foreign-born had a lower prevalence of 12-month and lifetime substance use disorder than did their US-born peers. The one exception occurred for bulimia nervosa among Asians.

Summary. Our results suggest that immigrants to the US have better or equivalent mental health compared with their US-born counterparts. Across 193 comparisons, not one example arose of the foreign-born having appreciably worse mental health. Foreign-born status conferred the most consistent protection against substance use disorders. Exceptions to the pattern of foreign-born protection were more likely to occur for Black women than men, for Asian men than women, and were roughly equal between Latinx women and men. We found no gender-specific comparisons between foreign- and US-born Whites in the literature. We found evidence that arriving in the US before the age of 13 generally eroded the foreign-born advantage. We speculate that younger immigrants socializing in an American context that may not be conducive to mental health could explain this pattern. In the next section, we discuss several hypotheses that have been advanced to explain why the foreign-born appear to have a mental health advantage in the US.

Mechanisms

The finding that foreign-born status appears protective across psychiatric disorder classes in the four major racial/ethnic groups in the US is compelling and warrants exploration. We discuss four mechanisms in depth in the following section: (1) selection effects or the "healthy immigrant effect;" (2) acculturation to US norms, values, and beliefs; (3) acculturation stressors immigrants to the US experience; and (4) acculturation to the diagnostic procedures of US psychiatric epidemiology studies.

Selection effects

Extensive research on immigrants' health in numerous countries (including Australia, Canada, Germany, Sweden, the United Kingdom, and the United States) has demonstrated that when migrants first arrive in the host country, they have better physical health than native-born populations [US: (Cunningham, Ruben, & Narayan, 2008; Singh, Rodriguez-Lainz, & Kogan, 2013)]. This phenomenon has been labeled the "healthy immigrant effect" (HIE). In most countries, the HIE begins to dissipate a few years after arrival (Jass & Massey, 2004; Lou & Beaujot, 2005).

Selection, as a possible explanation for the above effects, occurs on two levels:

1. **Individual:** The hypothesis of positive self-selection of immigrants posits that immigrants are not a random sample of the population. Only the healthiest and most motivated individuals choose to immigrate and are able to undergo the stressful and sometimes traumatic experience of migration to a new country (Constant, García-Muñoz, Neuman, & Neuman, 2018).
2. **State:** Many destination countries impose another level of selection via migration policies favoring wealthier and more educated immigrants, who tend to be healthier than those who are poorer and less educated. Further, immigration policies in receiving countries often require medical examinations (Constant et al., 2018).

Apart from the HIE, the "salmon bias" hypothesis contends that immigrants have better health profiles relative to the native-born population because of the return migration of less healthy and less economically successful immigrants to their origin countries (Arenas, Goldman, Pebley, & Teruel, 2015). The poorer health and death of return immigrants is thus recorded in their origin country rather than the host country. Studies testing the salmon bias hypothesis have had mixed results (Palloni & Arias, 2004; Riosmena, Wong, & Palloni, 2013; Sander, 2007; Turra & Elo, 2008).

The greatest hindrance to persuasive research on the selection hypothesis has been the inadequacy of data on the health status of immigrants prior to moving to the US compared with their compatriots who did not immigrate and a lack of follow-up data on immigrants after moving. Research has also largely relied on comparisons between immigrants and receiving countries' native-born populations. Few studies have examined the health trajectories of immigrants and nonmigrants who remained in the countries of origin. Although both the HIE and salmon bias have been examined, direct evidence in support of either mechanisms is still limited and inconclusive.

Substantive acculturation

A second explanation advanced for immigrants' apparent mental health advantage over their US-born counterparts, and the US-born more generally, derives from Durkheim's proposition over a century ago that cultures promoting social integration over social isolation are protective against suicide (Coleman & Coleman, 1994; Daoud et al., 2016). This has often been expressed as a distinction between cultural traditions of collectivism vs. individualism, with collectivism's protective effects against suicide thought to extend to mental health more generally (Alvarez et al., 2019; Leong, Park, & Kalibatseva, 2013; Salas-Wright, Kagotho, & Vaughn, 2014). This argument posits that most immigrants to the US come from cultures with stronger collectivist traditions than those in the US, which is frequently considered a prototypical individualist culture (Alegria, Sribney, Woo, Torres, & Guarnaccia, 2007; Salas-Wright et al., 2014; Schwartz et al., 2010). The collectivistic practices described in the literature as protective for mental health among immigrants to the US include strong familial obligations and social attachments that provide reliable sources of positive affective relationships and instrumental and emotional support during stressful periods (Alvarez et al., 2019; Blanco et al., 2013; Leong et al., 2013; Peña, Zayas, Cabrera-Nguyen, & Vega, 2012; Pilver, Kasl, Desai, & Levy, 2011). Processes of acculturation by which individualistic US norms, values, and beliefs supplant more collectivist traditions from the countries of origin (Alvarez et al., 2019; Blanco et al., 2013; Cook et al., 2009) are thought to erode mental health across immigrant generations.

Additionally, greater religiosity among immigrants compared with those born in the US is posited to protect mental health (Pilver et al., 2011). Greater American secularism then gradually diminishes religiosity, and its protective effects, across immigrant generations (Pilver et al., 2011).

These acculturation processes theoretically exert their influence on first-generation immigrants from the time of their arrival in the US. Thus, among first-generation immigrants, more time in the US is associated with worse mental health, particularly for younger immigrants socialized in the US. Specifically, those arriving in childhood and adolescence experience their crucial socialization and identity formation in the American context, making them more susceptible to the detrimental effects of that context on mental health than their compatriots arriving at older ages. Acculturative harms to mental health are expected to deepen across later generations (Cook et al., 2009; Pilver et al., 2011), who have increasingly tenuous connections with their forebears' collectivist traditions. The cumulative result is that first-generation immigrants are less susceptible to these acculturative processes than subsequent generations by virtue of their stronger anchoring to native traditions (Cook et al., 2009).

Schwartz et al. (2010) have depicted the substantive acculturation process just described as an oversimplification because it presumes that discarding native traditions while adopting receiving-country traditions is a dependent process, whereas evidence suggests that they can be independent. That is, individuals may retain birth country traditions while simultaneously adopting traditions of their receiving country, yielding an *integration* of traditions. Thus, they propose a bidimensional model in which the discarding and uptake of traditions are independent processes. Such independence, however, does not preclude the acculturation pathway we describe above. To the extent trading native for US traditions is harmful for mental health—whereas integration of norms may be protective for mental health (Schwartz et al., 2010)—the epidemiologic data we present in this chapter suggest a nontrivial segment of the immigrant population in the US engages in this trade-off.

We contrast this substantive acculturation hypothesis with an artifactual acculturation hypothesis, which we consider below. The former posits that the true risk of psychiatric disorder increases with exposure to US culture and subsequent adoption of US norms, values, and beliefs. By contrast, an artifactual acculturation hypothesis posits that the increased risk of psychiatric disorder is only apparent, for reasons we discuss below.

Acculturation stress

A second acculturation pathway harmful for mental health specifies *stressors* immigrants to the US and their descendants experience as they adapt to and adopt American traditions. These stressors include inter-generational conflict over loyalty to homeland culture, increasing exposure and sensitivity to racial, ethnic, and anti-immigrant discrimination, and dashed hopes for an improving quality of life (Cook et al., 2009). Each stressor is expected to degrade the mental health protections afforded by immigrants' more communal cultural traditions. These factors can impact first-generation immigrants, but the impact is thought to increase in subsequent generations.

Through the process of substantive acculturation, descendant immigrant generations are more likely than predecessor generations to adopt American traditions, which can lead to inter-generational conflict. This can also occur in first-generation immigrant families, when children adopt or integrate American culture more readily than parents or grandparents. The mental health of children who experience this conflict, of any immigrant generation, may be particularly impacted, given that the conflict occurs during a vulnerable developmental stage (Blanco et al., 2013; Cook et al., 2009).

First-generation immigrants may be more likely than descendant generations to live in ethnic enclaves, the latter of which can protect mental health. Those in ethnic enclaves are buffered by the more collectivist traditions they arrive and surround themselves with, including ready access to rich networks of emotional and instrumental social support. In such enclaves, immigrants are also relatively protected from interpersonal and systemic discrimination directed at immigrants, particularly those who are non-White (Vega & Rumbaut, 1991). As descendant generations are increasingly likely to live outside these enclaves, their exposure increases to those outside their native group and to American culture and power structures, escalating their risk of exposure to racial, ethnic, and anti-immigrant interpersonal and structural discrimination (Alegría et al., 2008; Cook et al., 2009; Leong et al., 2013; Pilver et al., 2011; Takeuchi, 2016). With greater attunement to American norms and idioms comes heightened perception of and sensitivity to these discriminatory experiences, which can undermine mental health (Cook et al., 2009; Leong et al., 2013; Pilver et al., 2011). Additionally, descendant immigrant generations may have greater expectations than first-generation immigrants of socioeconomic advance and cultural acceptance in the US; when these expectations are disappointed by systemic and interpersonal discrimination, demoralization and mental disorder may follow (Leong et al., 2013).

The acculturation stress pathway to the diminution of mental health across immigrant generations in many ways is a by-product of the substantive acculturation pathway. That is, the adoption of American cultural traditions may not only *directly* make immigrants more vulnerable to mental disorder, but also *indirectly* do so by causing inter-generational conflict and exposing descendant immigrant generations to the double-edged promise of a better life in America.

Artifactual acculturation

A third acculturation mechanism posits that the mental health advantage that foreign-born immigrants to the US have is an artifact of the diagnostic procedures of the psychiatric epidemiology studies that have documented this apparent advantage. The culture an immigrant is from, or simply the experience of being an immigrant, could artifactually affect the diagnosis of mental disorders via: (i) the expression of symptoms of the disorder; (ii) the willingness to disclose personal information relevant to diagnosis; and (iii) the interpretation of the language and wording of the diagnostic questions asked (Breslau, Javaras, Blacker, Murphy, & Normand, 2008).

True of any country, the US has a unique understanding of and approach to mental health (Alegría & McGuire, 2003; Watters, 2010). Time spent in the US, then, could shift immigrants' expression of mental disorders, their willingness to disclose personal information, and their interpretation of the questions asked in diagnostic interviews. These mechanisms differ from substantive acculturation in that they assume cultural variation in the expression of psychiatric disorder, not in the actual rate of disorder. Moreover, these three artifactual mechanisms of how time spent in the US may increase the diagnosis of psychiatric disorders are not mutually exclusive. Thus, any combination of the mechanisms could lead to an undercount of disorder among immigrants to the US.

Chinese immigrants to the US, for example, are likely to experience depression as it is experienced in many parts of Chinese society: more physically than psychologically, and more as boredom than sadness (Kleinman, 2004). During diagnostic interviews, this experience or expression of depression may not be identified using the US-centric diagnostic criteria articulated in the DSM. However, with acculturation to more American norms of experiencing and talking about depression, diagnosis of Chinese immigrants and their descendants with depression becomes more likely. This artifactual acculturation can occur during individuals' lifetimes, and across generations. Regardless of the timeframe, however, artifactual acculturation provides one explanation for the decline—but only an *apparent* decline in the case of this explanation—in mental health between first and subsequent immigrant generations in the US.

Do the empirical findings favor one mechanism over another?

The race-ethnic findings we reported above do not, on their own, provide obvious or unambiguous support to one of the mechanisms we describe over the others. For example, the finding among Black and White immigrants that arriving in the US at a younger age erodes the immigrant mental health advantage (compared with arriving at older ages) is consistent with all three acculturation hypotheses as we describe them. Those arriving before age 13 would be subject to all three of the respective mechanisms. Because their early socialization occurs in the American context, they would be more likely than those arriving at older ages to adopt American norms (substantive acculturation), to adopt American attitudes and idioms around mental health (artifactual acculturation), and to live outside protective immigrant enclaves (acculturation stressors) (Breslau et al., 2009). An ideal study for teasing apart the explanatory power of the substantive acculturation, acculturation stress, and artifactual acculturation hypotheses would stratify samples by first, second, and third immigrant generation status, and examine each on measures of relinquishing country of origin norms, adopting US norms (including those around mental health), and exposure to immigrant and race/ethnicity related stressors, in addition to psychiatric outcomes. This kind of theory-driven research to simultaneously test the relative merits of two or more hypotheses is clearly warranted. To test the fourth mechanism, the healthy immigrant hypothesis, studies are needed that compare the mental health of immigrants with that of individuals in their countries of origin who do not immigrate (Breslau et al., 2009). These studies would need to assess immigrants' mental health close in time to their departure and use the same diagnostic tool in both groups. In short, the processes by which immigrants to the US appear to lose their mental health advantage over successive generations remain a rich field to explore.

Focus on black immigrants

We explore Black immigrants in detail to illuminate some of the more nuanced processes overshadowed by the overarching migration processes, and demonstrate some distinctive dynamics that influence the observed patterns within one racial/ethnic group. While a body of literature investigates the four aforementioned mechanisms among Latinx and Asian American populations individually, few studies explore the mechanisms explaining Black immigrants' mental health advantage over their US-born counterparts. The mechanisms primarily investigated among Black immigrants are substantive acculturation and acculturative stress. Even these processes, however, are largely understudied.

Among Black Americans, greater acculturation is associated with greater psychological distress. Among a sample of individuals of African descent (foreign- and US-born), respondents who endorsed an integrationist acculturative strategy had greater psychological distress than those who endorsed a traditionalist acculturative strategy (Obasi & Leong, 2009). The traditionalist strategy represents a preference toward maintaining one's ethnocultural heritage, while an integrationist strategy describes a bicultural individual who integrates cultural beliefs and practices from different ethnocultural groups (Obasi & Leong, 2009). An integrationist acculturative strategy entails facing multiple stressors, like worldview differences, racism, and discrimination, that erode mental health over time (Obasi & Leong, 2009).

Black immigrants face unique stressors in acculturating to the historical and social context in the US. The theory of tridimensional (3D) acculturation posits that triculturals, who combine three cultural worlds (Caribbean culture, mainstream European American culture, and African American culture), may experience even greater acculturative stress or "culture shock" than bi- or monoculturals do (Ferguson, Iturbide, & Gordon, 2014). In a sample of 80 middle-aged Jamaican immigrants, triculturals had higher psychological distress than both bi- and monoculturals (Ferguson et al., 2014).

For Black immigrants, the relationships between race, ethnicity, discrimination, and acculturation are important (Livingston, Neita, Riviere, & Livingston, 2007). Perceived discrimination is associated with increased psychological distress but acculturation may moderate this association for immigrants. New immigrants may be more likely to interpret discriminatory experiences as stemming from their unfamiliarity with US culture, rather than their race/ethnicity, an interpretation that is protective for mental health (Gee, Ryan, Laflamme, & Holt, 2006). First, Black immigrants may be less likely than US-born Blacks to perceive racial discrimination, even when the two groups are exposed to similar types of discriminatory treatment (Krieger, Kosheleva, Waterman, Chen, & Koenen, 2011). For example, the self-reported prevalence of personal racism and group racism was significantly higher among US-born than foreign-born Black pregnant women (Dominguez, Strong, Krieger, Gillman, & Rich-Edwards, 2009). Second, the relationship between racial discrimination and psychological distress may be moderated by nativity such that the adverse health impacts of self-reported experiences of racial discrimination may be more severe among US-born than foreign-born Black Americans (Krieger et al., 2011; Nazroo, Jackson, Karlsen, & Torres, 2007).

Maintaining a strong ethnic identity may promote positive psychological adjustment, by buffering against stressors to which immigrants and ethnic minorities are exposed (Burnett-Zeigler et al., 2013). For example, a study of foreign- and US-born Black individuals showed that stronger ethnic identity was associated with decreased odds of depression and anxiety, while high acculturation was significantly associated with an increased likelihood of depression and anxiety (Burnett-Zeigler et al., 2013). Maintaining a strong ethnic identity may also be protective in allowing Black immigrants to differentiate themselves from Black Americans. Assimilation may not be desirable for many Caribbean immigrants, for example, as they may perceive a loss of status from their dominant status in the Caribbean when they become Black Americans (Kasinitz, 1992). Some may cling to their ethnic identity, perceiving Black Americans as a stigmatized group that experiences low status in American society (Livingston et al., 2007).

The maintenance of ethnic identity through transnational ties may play a role in the relatively low rates of mental disorders among Caribbean immigrants, through increased social support and decreased perceived discrimination (Murphy & Mahalingam, 2004). Social support, ethnic identity, and perceived discrimination are all impacted by transnationalism, and have been linked to psychological outcomes (Murphy & Mahalingam, 2004). Most first-generation and some second-generation Caribbean immigrants have "sojourner" status—they keep in close contact with other West Indians in ethnic enclaves, participate in social organizations, take regular trips to the Caribbean, fund relatives, and sponsor social and political events in the Caribbean (Murphy & Mahalingam, 2004). Transnational ties socially enhance immigrants' lives by directly or indirectly promoting and maintaining social networks (Murphy & Mahalingam, 2004). The strong transnational social networks are associated with social capital, tangible resources, and emotional support, which might confer mental health protections and offset the alienating and stressful effects of immigration (Murphy & Mahalingam, 2004). Further, strong ties to home countries where Caribbean immigrants face less discrimination may be protective (Murphy & Mahalingam, 2004).

These findings warrant further exploration of the mechanisms accounting for the protective effect of foreign-born status on psychopathology among Black immigrants. To date, this research has been conducted in relatively small, homogenous samples, but should be investigated on a population scale. Further, the relationship between immigration status and perceived discrimination should be clarified—do immigrants experience less discrimination, perceive less discrimination, or interpret discrimination differently from US-born Blacks, and how do each of these differences impact mental health? Further, research is needed to examine selection effects among Black immigrants and the extent to which their apparent advantage is a function of the diagnostic procedures of the psychiatric epidemiology studies. The latter question is particularly compelling, given that Blacks (and other racial/ethnic minorities) report lower rates of mental disorders than Whites, even before immigration status is taken into account.

Conclusion

While researchers often investigate the health of immigrants from a social stress-illness perspective, psychiatric epidemiology studies in the US have suggested that immigrants in the US have better or equivalent mental health compared with their US-born counterparts. The data we present in this chapter demonstrate that, with some exceptions, being foreign-born was protective across all psychiatric disorder classes, with particularly strong effects observed for substance use disorders. There is also evidence that younger age of arrival in the US tended to erode the foreign-born advantage.

Four mechanisms have been hypothesized to account for at least some of the immigrants' mental health advantages in the US, and the dilution of those advantages in subsequent generations. First, selection effects posit that only the healthiest and most motivated individuals choose to move; that destination countries favor wealthier and more educated immigrants; and that less healthy and less economically successful immigrants return or migrate to their origin countries. Second, processes of acculturation by which individualistic US norms, values, and beliefs gradually supplant more collectivist traditions from the countries of origin erode mental health across generations. Third, the stressors immigrants to the US and their descendants experience when they adapt to American traditions increase psychopathology. Fourth, the mental health advantage may be an artifact of the diagnostic procedures of psychiatric epidemiology studies.

The processes by which immigrants to the US lose their mental health advantage over successive generations remain a rich field to explore. Future study should conduct a rigorous theory-driven testing of mechanisms. These mechanisms are particularly understudied among Black populations. Studies of acculturative processes should stratify samples by first-, second-, and third-generation status and examine relevant constructs, including relinquishing country-of-origin norms, adoption of US norms (including those around mental health), and exposure to stressors. Studies of selection effects are needed that compare the mental health of immigrants with those in their countries of origin who do not immigrate, assessing immigrants' mental health close in time to their departure and using the same diagnostic tools in both groups. In short, the findings we summarize in this chapter of a mental health advantage among immigrants to the US represent a rich opportunity to deepen our understanding of how social position and social exposures impact mental health.

References

Abraido-Lanza, A. F., Dohrenwend, B. P., Ng-Mak, D. S., & Turner, J. B. (1999). The Latino mortality paradox: A test of the "salmon bias" and healthy migrant hypotheses. *American Journal of Public Health*, *89*(10), 1543–1548.

Alarcón, R. D., Parekh, A., Wainberg, M. L., Duarte, C. S., Araya, R., & Oquendo, M. A. (2016). Hispanic immigrants in the USA: Social and mental health perspectives. *The Lancet Psychiatry*, *3*(9), 860–870. https://doi.org/10.1016/s2215-0366(16)30101-8.

Alegria, M., Alvarez, K., & DiMarzio, K. (2017). Immigration and mental health. *Current Epidemiology Reports*, *4*(2), 145–155. https://doi.org/10.1007/s40471-017-0111-2.

Alegría, M., Canino, G., Shrout, P. E., Woo, M., Duan, N., Vila, D., … Meng, X.-L. (2008). Prevalence of mental illness in immigrant and non-immigrant US Latino groups. *American Journal of Psychiatry*, *165*(3), 359–369.

Alegria, M., Canino, G., Stinson, F. S., & Grant, B. F. (2006). Nativity and DSM-IV psychiatric disorders among Puerto Ricans, Cuban Americans, and non-Latino whites in the United States: Results from the National Epidemiologic Survey on alcohol and related conditions. *The Journal of Clinical Psychiatry*.

Alegría, M., & McGuire, T. (2003). Rethinking a universal framework in the psychiatric symptom-disorder relationship. *Journal of Health and Social Behavior*, 257–274.

Alegría, M., Mulvaney-Day, N., Torres, M., Polo, A., Cao, Z., & Canino, G. (2007). Prevalence of psychiatric disorders across Latino subgroups in the United States. *American Journal of Public Health*, *97*(1), 68–75.

Alegria, M., Sribney, W., Woo, M., Torres, M., & Guarnaccia, P. (2007). Looking beyond nativity: The relation of age of immigration, length of residence, and birth cohorts to the risk of onset of psychiatric disorders for Latinos. *Research in Human Development*, *4*(1), 19–47. https://doi.org/10.1080/15427600701480980.

Alegria, M., Takeuchi, D., Canino, G., Duan, N., Shrout, P., Meng, X. L., … Woo, M. (2004). Considering context, place and culture: The National Latino and Asian American study. *International Journal of Methods in Psychiatric Research*, *13*(4), 208–220.

Alvarez, K., Fillbrunn, M., Green, J. G., Jackson, J. S., Kessler, R. C., McLaughlin, K. A., … Alegria, M. (2019). Race/ethnicity, nativity, and lifetime risk of mental disorders in US adults. *Social Psychiatry and Psychiatric Epidemiology*, *54*(5), 553–565.

Arenas, E., Goldman, N., Pebley, A. R., & Teruel, G. (2015). Return migration to Mexico: Does health matter? *Demography*, *52*(6), 1853–1868.

Blanco, C., Morcillo, C., Alegria, M., Dedios, M. C., Fernandez-Navarro, P., Regincos, R., & Wang, S. (2013). Acculturation and drug use disorders among Hispanics in the U.S. *Journal of Psychiatric Research*, *47*(2), 226–232. https://doi.org/10.1016/j.jpsychires.2012.09.019.

Breslau, J., Borges, G., Hagar, Y., Tancredi, D., & Gilman, S. (2009). Immigration to the USA and risk for mood and anxiety disorders: Variation by origin and age at immigration. *Psychological Medicine*, *39*(7), 1117–1127.

Breslau, J., & Chang, D. F. (2006). Psychiatric disorders among foreign-born and US-born Asian-Americans in a US national survey. *Social Psychiatry and Psychiatric Epidemiology*, *41*(12), 943–950.

Breslau, J., Javaras, K. N., Blacker, D., Murphy, J. M., & Normand, S.-L.T. (2008). Differential item functioning between ethnic groups in the epidemiological assessment of depression. *The Journal of Nervous and Mental Disease*, *196*(4), 297.

Broman, C. L., Neighbors, H. W., Delva, J., Torres, M., & Jackson, J. S. (2008). Prevalence of substance use disorders among African Americans and Caribbean Blacks in the National Survey of American Life. *American Journal of Public Health*, *98*(6), 1107–1114.

Burnett-Zeigler, I., Bohnert, K. M., & Ilgen, M. A. (2013). Ethnic identity, acculturation and the prevalence of lifetime psychiatric disorders among Black, Hispanic, and Asian adults in the US. *Journal of Psychiatric Research*, *47*(1), 56–63.

Coleman, J. S., & Coleman, J. S. (1994). *Foundations of social theory*. Harvard University Press.

Constant, A. F., García-Muñoz, T., Neuman, S., & Neuman, T. (2018). A "healthy immigrant effect" or a "sick immigrant effect"? Selection and policies matter. *The European Journal of Health Economics*, *19*(1), 103–121.

Cook, B., Alegría, M., Lin, J. Y., & Guo, J. (2009). Pathways and correlates connecting Latinos' mental health with exposure to the United States. *American Journal of Public Health*, *99*(12), 2247–2254.

Cunningham, S. A., Ruben, J. D., & Narayan, K. V. (2008). Health of foreign-born people in the United States: A review. *Health & Place*, *14*(4), 623–635.

Daoud, N., Haque, N., Gao, M., Nisenbaum, R., Muntaner, C., & O'Campo, P. (2016). Neighborhood settings, types of social capital and depression among immigrants in Toronto. *Social Psychiatry and Psychiatric Epidemiology*, *51*(4), 529–538. https://doi.org/10.1007/s00127-016-1173-z.

Dominguez, T. P., Strong, E. F., Krieger, N., Gillman, M. W., & Rich-Edwards, J. W. (2009). Differences in the self-reported racism experiences of US-born and foreign-born Black pregnant women. *Social Science & Medicine*, *69*(2), 258–265.

Douglas, P., Cetron, M., & Spiegel, P. (2019). Definitions matter: Migrants, immigrants, asylum seekers and refugees. *Journal of Travel Medicine*.

Ferguson, G. M., Iturbide, M. I., & Gordon, B. P. (2014). Tridimensional (3D) acculturation: Ethnic identity and psychological functioning of tricultural Jamaican immigrants. *International Perspectives in Psychology: Research, Practice, Consultation*, *3*(4), 238.

Friis, R., Yngve, A., & Persson, V. (1998). Review of social epidemiologic research on migrants' health: Findings, methodological cautions, and theoretical perspectives. *Scandinavian Journal of Social Medicine*, *26*(3), 173–180.

Gee, G. C., Ryan, A., Laflamme, D. J., & Holt, J. (2006). Self-reported discrimination and mental health status among African descendants, Mexican Americans, and other Latinos in the New Hampshire REACH 2010 Initiative: The added dimension of immigration. *American Journal of Public Health*, *96*(10), 1821–1828.

González, H. M., Tarraf, W., Whitfield, K. E., & Vega, W. A. (2010). The epidemiology of major depression and ethnicity in the United States. *Journal of Psychiatric Research*, *44*(15), 1043–1051.

Grant, B. F., Stinson, F. S., Hasin, D. S., Dawson, D. A., Chou, S. P., & Anderson, K. (2004). Immigration and lifetime prevalence of DSM-IV psychiatric disorders among Mexican Americans and non-Hispanic whites in the United States: Results from the national epidemiologic survey on alcohol and related conditions. *Archives of General Psychiatry*, *61*(12), 1226–1233.

Hasin, D. S., Goodwin, R. D., Stinson, F. S., & Grant, B. F. (2005). Epidemiology of major depressive disorder: Results from the National Epidemiologic Survey on alcoholism and related conditions. *Archives of General Psychiatry*, *62*(10), 1097–1106.

Hasin, D. S., Stinson, F. S., Ogburn, E., & Grant, B. F. (2007). Prevalence, correlates, disability, and comorbidity of DSM-IV alcohol abuse and dependence in the United States: Results from the National Epidemiologic Survey on alcohol and related conditions. *Archives of General Psychiatry*, *64*(7), 830–842.

Hong, S., Walton, E., Tamaki, E., & Sabin, J. A. (2014). Lifetime prevalence of mental disorders among Asian Americans: Nativity, gender, and sociodemographic correlates. *Asian American Journal of Psychology*, *5*(4), 353.

Jass, G., & Massey, D. S. (2004). Immigrant health: Selectivity and acculturation. In *Critical perspectives on racial and ethnic differences in health in late life*. Washington, DC: National Academies Press.

Kasinitz, P. (1992). *Caribbean New York: Black immigrants and the politics of race*. Cornell University Press.

Kessler, R. C., Berglund, P., Demler, O., Jin, R., Koretz, D., Merikangas, K. R., … Wang, P. S. (2003). The epidemiology of major depressive disorder: Results from the National Comorbidity Survey Replication (NCS-R). *JAMA*, *289*(23), 3095–3105.

Kleinman, A. (2004). Culture and depression. *New England Journal of Medicine*, *351*(10), 951–953.

Krieger, N., Kosheleva, A., Waterman, P. D., Chen, J. T., & Koenen, K. (2011). Racial discrimination, psychological distress, and self-rated health among US-born and foreign-born Black Americans. *American Journal of Public Health*, *101*(9), 1704–1713.

Leong, F., Park, Y. S., & Kalibatseva, Z. (2013). Disentangling immigrant status in mental health: Psychological protective and risk factors among Latino and Asian American immigrants. *The American Journal of Orthopsychiatry*, *83*(2 Pt 3), 361–371. https://doi.org/10.1111/ajop.12020.

Livingston, I. L., Neita, M., Riviere, L., & Livingston, S. (2007). Gender, acculturative stress and Caribbean immigrants health in the United States of America: An exploratory study. *West Indian Medical Journal*, *56*(3), 213–222.

Lou, Y., & Beaujot, R. (2005). What happens to the 'Healthy immigrant effect': The mental health of immigrants to Canada. *PSC Discussion Papers Series*, *19*(15), 1.

Markides, K. S., & Coreil, J. (1986). The health of Hispanics in the southwestern United States: An epidemiologic paradox. *Public Health Reports*, *101*(3), 253.

Markides, K. S., & Rote, S. (2015). Immigrant health paradox. In *Emerging trends in the social and behavioral sciences: An interdisciplinary, searchable, and linkable resource* (pp. 1–15) Wiley.

Mays, V. M., Jones, A. L., Cochran, S. D., Taylor, R. J., Rafferty, J., & Jackson, J. S. (2018). Chronicity and mental health service utilization for anxiety, mood, and substance use disorders among black men in the United States; ethnicity and nativity differences. *Healthcare (Basel)*, *6*(2). https://doi.org/10.3390/healthcare6020053.

Murphy, E. J., & Mahalingam, R. (2004). Transnational ties and mental health of Caribbean immigrants. *Journal of Immigrant Health*, *6*(4), 167–178.

Nazroo, J., Jackson, J., Karlsen, S., & Torres, M. (2007). The Black diaspora and health inequalities in the US and England: Does where you go and how you get there make a difference? *Sociology of Health & Illness*, *29*(6), 811–830.

Nicdau, E. G., Hong, S., & Takeuchi, D. T. (2007). Prevalence and correlates of eating disorders among Asian Americans: Results from the National Latino and Asian American Study. *Epidemiological Studies*, *40*, S22–S27.

Obasi, E. M., & Leong, F. T. (2009). Psychological distress, acculturation, and mental health-seeking attitudes among people of African descent in the United States: A preliminary investigation. *Journal of Counseling Psychology*, *56*(2), 227.

Palloni, A., & Arias, E. (2004). Paradox lost: Explaining the Hispanic adult mortality advantage. *Demography*, *41*(3), 385–415.

Park, Y., & Kemp, S. P. (2006). "Little alien colonies": Representations of immigrants and their neighborhoods in social work discourse, 1875–1924. *Social Service Review*, *80*(4), 705–734.

Peña, J. B., Zayas, L. H., Cabrera-Nguyen, P., & Vega, W. A. (2012). US cultural involvement and its association with suicidal behavior among youths in the Dominican Republic. *American Journal of Public Health*, *102*(4), 664–671.

Pilver, C. E., Kasl, S., Desai, R., & Levy, B. R. (2011). Exposure to American culture is associated with premenstrual dysphoric disorder among ethnic minority women. *Journal of Affective Disorders*, *130*(1–2), 334–341. https://doi.org/10.1016/j.jad.2010.10.013.

Radford, J. (2019). *Key findings about U.S. immigrants*. Retrieved from https://www.pewresearch.org/fact-tank/2019/06/17/key-findings-about-u-s-immigrants/.

Riosmena, F., Wong, R., & Palloni, A. (2013). Migration selection, protection, and acculturation in health: A binational perspective on older adults. *Demography*, *50*(3), 1039–1064.

Salas-Wright, C. P., Kagotho, N., & Vaughn, M. G. (2014). Mood, anxiety, and personality disorders among first and second-generation immigrants to the United States. *Psychiatry Research*, *220*(3), 1028–1036. https://doi.org/10.1016/j.psychres.2014.08.045.

Salas-Wright, C. P., Vaughn, M. G., Goings, T. C., Miller, D. P., & Schwartz, S. J. (2018). Immigrants and mental disorders in the United States: New evidence on the healthy migrant hypothesis. *Psychiatry Research*, *267*, 438–445.

Salas-Wright, C. P., Vaughn, M. G., Schwartz, S. J., & Cordova, D. (2016). An "immigrant paradox" for adolescent externalizing behavior? Evidence from a national sample. *Social Psychiatry and Psychiatric Epidemiology*, *51*(1), 27–37. https://doi.org/10.1007/s00127-015-1115-1.

Samet, S., Waxman, R., Hatzenbuehler, M., & Hasin, D. S. (2007). Assessing addiction: Concepts and instruments. *Addiction Science & Clinical Practice*, *4*(1), 19.

Sander, M. (2007). *Return migration and the 'healthy immigrant effect'*.

Schwartz, S. J., Unger, J. B., Zamboanga, B. L., & Szapocznik, J. (2010). Rethinking the concept of acculturation: Implications for theory and research. *American Psychologist*, *65*(4), 237.

Singh, G. K., & Miller, B. A. (2004). Health, life expectancy, and mortality patterns among immigrant populations in the United States. *Canadian Journal of Public Health*, *95*(3), I14–I21.

Singh, G. K., Rodriguez-Lainz, A., & Kogan, M. D. (2013). Immigrant health inequalities in the United States: Use of eight major national data systems. *The Scientific World Journal*, *2013*, 512313. https://doi.org/10.1155/2013/512313.

Suárez-Orozco, C., & Carhill, A. (2008). Afterword: New directions in research with immigrant families and their children. *New Directions for Child and Adolescent Development*, *2008*(121), 87–104.

Szaflarski, M., Cubbins, L. A., & Ying, J. (2011). Epidemiology of alcohol abuse among US immigrant populations. *Journal of Immigrant and Minority Health*, *13*(4), 647–658. https://doi.org/10.1007/s10903-010-9394-9.

Takeuchi, D. T. (2016). Vintage wine in new bottles: Infusing select ideas into the study of immigration, immigrants, and mental health. *Journal of Health and Social Behavior*, *57*(4), 423–435.

Takeuchi, D. T., Alegría, M., Jackson, J. S., & Williams, D. R. (2007). *Immigration and mental health: Diverse findings in Asian, Black, and Latino populations*. American Public Health Association.

Takeuchi, D. T., Zane, N., Hong, S., Chae, D. H., Gong, F., Gee, G. C., … Alegría, M. (2007). Immigration-related factors and mental disorders among Asian Americans. *American Journal of Public Health*, *97*(1), 84–90.

Turra, C. M., & Elo, I. T. (2008). The impact of Salmon Bias on the Hispanic mortality advantage: New evidence from social security data. *Population Research and Policy Review*, *27*(5), 515–530. https://doi.org/10.1007/s11113-008-9087-4.

Vaughn, M. G., Salas-Wright, C. P., DeLisi, M., & Maynard, B. R. (2014). The immigrant paradox: Immigrants are less antisocial than native-born Americans. *Social Psychiatry and Psychiatric Epidemiology*, *49*(7), 1129–1137. https://doi.org/10.1007/s00127-013-0799-3.

Vega, W. A., & Rumbaut, R. G. (1991). Ethnic minorities and mental health. *Annual Review of Sociology*, *17*(1), 351–383.

Watters, E. (2010). *Crazy like us: The globalization of the American psyche*. Simon and Schuster.

Williams, D. R., Gonzalez, H. M., Neighbors, H., Nesse, R., Abelson, J. M., Sweetman, J., & Jackson, J. S. (2007). Prevalence and distribution of major depressive disorder in African Americans, Caribbean blacks, and non-Hispanic whites: Results from the National Survey of American Life. *Archives of General Psychiatry*, *64*(3), 305–315.

Williams, D. R., Haile, R., Gonzalez, H. M., Neighbors, H., Baser, R., & Jackson, J. S. (2007). The mental health of Black Caribbean immigrants: Results from the National Survey of American Life. *American Journal of Public Health*, *97*(1), 52–59. https://doi.org/10.2105/AJPH.2006.088211.

Further reading

Kessler, R. C. (2000). Psychiatric epidemiology: Selected recent advances and future directions. *Bulletin of the World Health Organization*, *78*, 464–474.

Norquist, G. S., & Magruder, K. M. (2017). *Mental health epidemiology (psychiatric epidemiology)*. In *International Encyclopedia of Public Health* (pp. 54–62).

Chapter 12

Internalizing behavior problems in Latinx children: Patterns and correlates of anxiety, depressive, and somatic symptoms from pre-kindergarten through third grade

R. Gabriela Barajas-Gonzalez[a], Esther J. Calzada[b] and Keng-Yen Huang[a]
[a]*Department of Population Health, New York University School of Medicine, New York, NY, United States*, [b]*Steve Hicks School of Social Work, University of Texas at Austin, Austin, TX, United States*

Internalizing problems in childhood

Internalizing problems are characterized by symptoms of depression (e.g., excessive sadness), anxiety (e.g., excessive worry and fear), and somatization (e.g., frequent physical complaints such as stomachaches and headaches; Zahn-Waxler, Klimes-Dougan, & Slattery, 2000). Internalizing problems may develop in early childhood (Egger & Angold, 2006) and often become more prevalent from early to middle childhood to adolescence, with these problems demonstrating community prevalence rates of 7% for anxiety and 3% for depression in children ages 3–17 years (Ghandour et al., 2019). Left untreated, internalizing symptoms and disorders can have lasting effects on social and emotional well-being, including educational underachievement, social and occupational problems, reduced life satisfaction, drug use, and suicide attempts (Kessler, 2012). The reach of internalizing disorders is so vast that major depressive disorder is ranked as the leading cause of disability worldwide; anxiety disorders are ranked sixth (World Health Organization, 2017).

Knowledge about the development of internalizing disorders when they first emerge is critical for informing efforts to intervene early and effectively (e.g., Dougherty et al., 2013; Hirshfeld-Becker et al., 2010). Internalizing problems

Mental and Behavioral Health of Immigrants in the United States
https://doi.org/10.1016/B978-0-12-816117-3.00012-9

on average tend to increase gradually from infancy to early childhood (Gilliom & Shaw, 2004), but a challenge in identifying behaviors relevant to risk for psychopathology in young children is that the behaviors (e.g., crying and irritability) are developmentally normative. Emotional development involves greater social engagement (Bufferd, Dyson, Hernandez, & Wakschlag, 2016), some degree of individuation from parents and caregivers (Bufferd, Dougherty, & Olino, 2017), and the formation of self-other relations (Cicchetti, Rogosch, & Toth, 2000), and these developmental milestones are accompanied by normative angst that tends to dissipate as the child acclimates to new challenges. Research is further complicated by the challenge young children face in trying to communicate information about internally experienced affective states. Nonetheless, internalizing disorders in children do appear in typically manifesting form, with some exceptions based on duration and intensity (Beesdo, Knappe, & Pine, 2009). The work of Luby (Luby et al., 2003; Whalen, Dixon-Gordon, Belden, Barch, & Luby, 2015), for example, shows that children as young as 2- to 3-years old experience depressive symptoms of irritability, anhedonia, sleep and appetite changes, and low self-esteem.

The literature on somatic manifestations of psychological distress in children is scarce, due in part to the fact that the psychiatric diagnostic criteria of somatization were not developed for children until the early 1990s (Canino, 2004). Some scholars refute the idea that psychological distress is converted to somatic distress (Mak & Zane, 2004; Parker, Cheah, & Roy, 2001), whereas others contend that somatization is a known manifestation of distress, especially for those whom cultural factors make the expression of negative affect unacceptable (Guarnaccia, Lewis-Fernández, & Marano, 2003). These researchers point to cross-cultural variations in the perception, assessment, and behavioral and symptomatologic response to stressful events (Guarnaccia et al., 2003). Recent studies indicate that somatic symptoms predict anxiety and depressive disorders years later (Shanahan et al., 2015; Shelby et al., 2013). Somatic symptoms vary with age, so that abdominal pain and headaches are more common in early childhood, whereas pseudoneurological, menstrual, and polysymptomatic symptoms are more common in adolescence (Beidel, Christ, & Long, 1991; Eminson, Benjamin, Shortall, Woods, & Faragher, 1996).

Developmental trajectories of internalizing problems

Longitudinal data on internalizing problems during childhood comes primarily from the National Institute of Child Health and Development (NICHD) Study of Early Child Care and Youth Development multisite study in which mothers ($N = 1364$) rated their child's internalizing problems from the age of 2 to 11 using the Child Behavior Checklist (CBCL, 2–3 and CBCL, 4–18, depending on age of child). Notably, the sample was predominately White (76%) and included only 46 (3%) Latinx families. In their analysis of the data, Sterba, Prinstein, and Cox (2007) modeled internalizing symptoms across time using select items that were empirically identified as homotypical across childhood ("underactive, slow-moving, or lacks energy"; "unhappy, sad, or depressed"; "withdrawn, doesn't get along with others"; "overtired"; "nervous, high-strung, or tense"; "too fearful or anxious"; "shy or timid"; "self-conscious or easily embarrassed"). The average *T*-score for the sample was 47.77, suggesting low levels of internalizing problems for the sample as a whole. Three class models for both boys and girls were identified: *elevated stable* internalizing symptoms across childhood (13% of boys, 21% of girls), *decreasing/increasing* internalizing symptoms that declined from ages 2 to 6 and then rose until age 11 (22% of boys; 10% of girls) and *low* across childhood, declining from low to near zero (65% of boys, 69% of girls). Children in the low category had 0% chance of having a CBCL internalizing score in the clinical range at age 11, but boys in the elevated stable category had a 23% chance, and girls had a 12% chance of scoring in the clinical range when they were 11 years old. In other words, children with internalizing problems that first emerged in early childhood were the most likely to experience continuous or increasing symptoms over time (Sterba et al., 2007).

Using data from the same study, Fanti and Henrich (2010) investigated trajectories of pure and co-occurring internalizing and externalizing problems from age 2 to 12. Internalizing problems generally showed an upward trajectory, increasing at each time point with the exception of a decrease from ages 4.5 to 6 and 11 to 12. Still, based on their findings they concluded that consistent with prior research, most children exhibit low levels of internalizing problems from toddlerhood through early adolescence.

Internalizing problems in Latinx children

Despite making up 25% of the child population in the United States (Child Trends, 2018), research on the developmental trajectories of Latinx mental health is in its infancy. There is, however, solid evidence that in adolescence, Latinx are at greater risk for problems in comparison to non-Latinx White youth (Bámaca-Colbert, Umaña-Taylor, & Gayles, 2012; Kleylamp & Tienda, 2004; Polo & Lopez, 2009; Roberts, Roberts, & Chen, 1997). Latinx youth report more anxiety symptoms and are likely to meet criteria for an anxiety disorder than their non-Latinx peers (Pina & Silverman, 2004; Varela, Sanchez-Sosa, Biggs, & Luis, 2008). On the Youth Risk Behavior Surveillance Survey, more than a third of Latinx youth (47% girls; 21% boys) report feelings of depression, 16% (22% girls; 11% boys) report that they have seriously considered suicide (Kann et al., 2018), and one in ten Latinas attempts suicide (Kann et al., 2018). Zeiders, Umaña-Taylor, and Derlan (2013) found that depression decreased from age 12 to 22 among Mexican-origin males but increased over two time periods (ages 12–15; ages 20–22) among females, suggesting impaired functioning into young adulthood. Very little is known about anxiety, depression, and somatization in Latinx children, before adolescence.

Correlates of internalizing problems

The variability in rates of internalizing problems across ethnic groups may be due, in part, to disproportionate exposure to social stressors related to poverty and immigration. In a study with immigrant youth, time spent in the United States was found to be protective against anxiety and depression among first-generation Latinx adolescents, presumably due to greater fluency in English and knowledge to navigate US social systems, both of which resulted in fewer daily hassles (Potochnick & Perreira, 2010). In that sample ($n=255$; 70% Mexican), 29% of Latinx adolescents were symptomatic for anxiety and nearly 7% were symptomatic for depression. Other research shows higher rates of internalizing symptoms have been found in US-born, relative to immigrant, Mexican-American adolescents (Nair, White, Roosa, & Zeiders, 2013), and in Latinx third graders (Dawson & Williams, 2008). Acculturation stress appears to play out in immigrant and later generations, albeit in different ways.

In 2017, 25% of Latinx children lived in impoverished households, compared to 11% of non-Latinx white children, and 54% lived in immigrant homes, where rates of poverty are highest (Child Trends, 2019). Youth exposed to economic hardship are at higher risk for internalizing problems (Mendoza, Dmitrieva, Perreira, Hurwich-Reiss, & Watamura, 2017), as poverty increases risk of exposure to social stressors and the use of harsh parenting including physical discipline (Barajas-Gonzalez & Brooks-Gunn, 2014; Linver, Brooks-Gunn, & Kohen, 2002). For Latinx parents, acculturative stress and experiences of discrimination also impact parenting (Lorenzo-Blanco et al., 2017; Zeiders, Umaña-Taylor, Jahromi, Updegraff, & White, 2016). According to the family stress model, these contextual stressors compromise positive and consistent parenting due to the increased risk for mental health problems like maternal depression (Calzada, Sales, & O'Gara, 2019; White, Roosa, Weaver, & Nair, 2009).

Parenting characterized by low levels of warmth and high levels of control and overprotection has been identified as the most proximal predictor of child internalizing symptoms. Low levels of warmth are associated with higher levels of internalizing symptoms in early childhood (Bayer, Sanson, & Hemphill, 2006), middle to late childhood (Dallaire et al., 2006; Lengua, 2006), and adolescence (Gil-Rivas, Greenberger, Chen, & Montero y López-Lena, 2003; Roche et al., 2019; White, Roosa, & Zeiders, 2012; Zahn-Waxler et al., 2000). A multisite study of spanking at ages 3 and 4 showed prospective associations with internalizing problems at age 9 in a sample of 311 Latinx families (Coley, Kull, & Carrano, 2014). Spanking was also linked with internalizing problems in a national sample of Latinx 5-year olds from the Fragile Families study (Yildirim & Roopnarine, 2015). A meta-analysis of negative parenting (rejection, hostility, and control) revealed small effects on child anxiety and medium effects on childhood depression (McLeod, Weisz, & Wood, 2007; McLeod, Wood, & Weisz, 2007), and there is great potential to offset risk for internalizing problems by promoting positive parenting practices.

Latinos in context

The present study focused on internalizing behaviors in early childhood using data from a longitudinal study of 749 Dominican- (DA) and Mexican-origin (MA) families in New York City, Latinos in Contexts (LINCs). Funded by the NICHD and IES (PI, Calzada), LINCs was designed to examine an integrative developmental model that includes both universal (e.g., parenting) and culturally specific (e.g., cultural socialization practices) variables as determinants of the developmental trajectories of Latinx students from pre-Kindergarten through third grade. Details on the methods, including sample characteristics, are presented below. First, we summarize past findings from our program of research (which includes LINCs and similar but smaller studies), as relevant to the present study goals.

In a series of studies, we proposed and tested a cultural framework of Latinx parenting (Calzada, Fernandez, & Cortes, 2010) that highlights the traditional Latinx value of *respeto*, which encourages children to show respect for and deference to authority figures including parents, and the potentially incongruous Westernized value of independence, which encourages children to be assertive and autonomous. Conceptually, independence aligns with authoritative parenting practices that use scaffolding and encouragement to enforce high but reasonable demands with a child, and *respeto* aligns with authoritarian practices that place high demands on children that may not be reasonable and are enforced with limited emotional or instrumental support for the child. Variations in values and practices are believed to reflect mothers' acculturative status. We tested this model with cross-sectional data when LINCs participants were 4–5 years old and found that (1) associations between socialization messages and parenting practices were as expected, and (2) authoritarian, but not authoritative, practices were concurrently associated with a global score of internalizing problems (Calzada, Huang, Anicama, Fernandez, & Brotman, 2012).

In a follow-up test of the model (Calzada, Barajas-Gonzalez, Huang, & Brotman, 2017), we found that authoritarian practices when children were 4- to 5-years old were associated with more depression when children were 5- to 6-years old and that authoritative practices were prospectively associated with less somatization, but only in DA children. Notably, cultural socialization had direct and negative effects on children's functioning; independence predicted more anxiety in DA children, and *respeto* predicted more somatization in MA children. In a more recent study with Mexican-origin mother-child (3- to 6-year old) dyads, we found that 19% of children had significant internalizing problems and authoritarian parenting again emerged as a significant risk factor (Calzada, Sales, & O'Gara, 2019).

We also note findings with LINCs data showing the protective role of social support (emotional and instrumental) from family and the school community. Specifically, familial support was associated with positive parenting practices and with more adaptive child behavior, in both DA and MA families. In DA families, school-based support (i.e., from other parents at the child's school) was associated with less harsh parenting, which was associated with better child functioning including more adaptive behavior. We did not, however, look specifically at effects on child internalizing behaviors.

The present study

The present study builds on past LINCs findings and the broader literature to advance knowledge of internalizing behavior problems and its correlates in Latinx children. As shown in more detail below, LINCs participants appear to be at incredibly high risk for internalizing symptoms, but we have not examined rates over time. Thus, our first aim was to describe the prevalence of early childhood internalizing problems at four time points: pre-K (age 4–5), Kindergarten (K; age 5–6), first grade (G1; age 6–7), and third grade (G3; ages 8–9), focusing on symptoms of anxiety, depression, and somatization as reported by mothers and teachers. As in studies with older Latinx youth and consistent with baseline LINCs data, we expected rates of internalizing problems to be high in this community sample of young children. Importantly, we attend to two methodological limitations of the literature: First, we use longitudinal data and focus on early childhood to move beyond the historical reliance on cross-sectional studies focused on school-aged and adolescent Latinx, and second, we attend to the internal diversity of the Latinx population by considering differences based on ethnicity (i.e., country of origin) and child gender. The second aim of the present study was to examine predictors of anxiety, depression, and somatization, including family poverty status, cultural socialization and parenting practices, and social support. Based on earlier findings, we expected family poverty status and authoritarian practices to be risk factors, and authoritative practices and social support to have a protective but limited role in predicting internalizing problems.

Methods

Participants

The LINCs study took place in 24 public elementary schools in NYC, where eligible 4- and 5-year-old children were enrolled between 2010 and 2013. Children were eligible if their mothers identified as Mexican (MA) or Dominican (DA) and if they were newly enrolled in pre-K or K in one of 24 study partner schools. The final sample included 413 MA and 336 DA students (51% girls) and their mothers ($N=749$ mother-child pairs). MA and DA families differed on several demographic characteristics, as shown in Table 1. Specifically, MA mothers were more likely to be immigrants ($P<.001$), have less than a high school education ($P<.001$), and live in poverty ($P<.001$) in comparison to DA mothers.

TABLE 1 LINCs sample characteristics at baseline.

	Possible range	MA (n=413) M (SD)	DA (n=336) M (SD)	t-test/ chi-square
Child age		4.91 (0.58)	4.95 (0.56)	−1.165
Mother age		31.63 (5.63)	34.12 (7.65)	−4.917**
Child gender		47.50%	51.50%	1.204
Mother foreign-born		98.5%	84.4%	51.14***
Child foreign-born		2.5%	14.8%	37.46**
Family poverty		82.1%	56.0%	56.9***
Mother completed high school		40.2%	76.9%	100.42***
Mother's English language competence	1–5	1.8 (0.58)	2.58 (0.94)	−13.25***
Mother's Spanish language competence	1–5	3.58 (0.55)	3.7 (0.45)	−3.35**
Cultural socialization				
Independence	1–5	4.16 (0.39)	4.2 (0.42)	−1.11
Respeto	1–5	3.94 (0.46)	4.02 (0.45)	2.49*
Parenting practices				
Authoritarian parenting	1–5	1.79 (0.46)	1.71 (0.46)	2.34*
Authoritative parenting	1–5	4.01 (0.68)	4.25 (0.56)	−5.33***
Social support from family	1–7	5.9 (1.22)	6.22 (0.99)	−4.03**
Social support in school	1–7	3.71 (1.68)	3.55 (1.54)	1.3

MA, Mexican-origin; *DA*, Dominican-origin.
Note: Baseline data from time of entry in the study, either in pre-K or K.
*$P<.05$.
**$P<.01$.
***$P<.001$.

Measures

Demographic characteristics

Upon enrollment into the study, mothers reported on their sociodemographic variables, including maternal age, marital status, poverty status, maternal education (1 = high school or above), child gender (1 = male), and the number of people in the household were collected using a demographic form administered at Time 1. Poverty was calculated by comparing each respondent's reported annual household income with the US Department of Health and Human Services poverty guidelines.

Cultural socialization messages

In pre-K, K, and G1, mothers completed the Cultural Socialization of Latino Children (CSLC; Calzada et al., 2010), a measure that was developed based on Latina mothers' descriptions of the behavioral manifestations of cultural values. The *respeto* scale includes 20 items (e.g., "I tell my child to defer to adult wishes."), and the independence scale includes 17 items (e.g., "I encourage my child to tell me when he disagrees with me"), each rated on a Likert scale from "strongly disagree" to "strongly agree." Items were averaged to create a scale score, with higher scores reflecting more socialization of that value. Internal consistency was adequate for both scales, for the MA and DA samples (α were .81 and .77 for MA, and .83 and .76 for DA, for *respeto* and independence, respectively), and for those responding in English or Spanish (.85 and .87, respectively).

Parenting practices

In pre-K, K, and G1, mothers completed the Parenting Styles and Dimensions (PSD; Robinson, Mandleco, Olsen, & Hart, 1995), a 32-item measure of parenting practices with three orthogonal factors corresponding to Baumrind's (1995) authoritarian, authoritative, and permissive parenting style constructs. Parents respond to each item on a 5-point Likert scale anchored by "never" and "always." The PSD has been standardized for parents of young children and has been used with samples of various ethnic backgrounds including Latina mothers from Puerto Rico, the Dominican Republic, and Mexico (Calzada et al., 2012; Calzada & Eyberg, 2002). The permissive scale, which showed low internal consistency, was not used in the present study. Alpha coefficients were adequate for authoritative and authoritarian parenting for both ethnic groups and in both languages (.69–.87).

Social support

In pre-K, K, and G1, mothers completed the Multidimensional Scale of Perceived Social Support (MSPSS; Zimet, Dahlem, Zimet, & Farley, 1988) measures perceived social support from distinct social networks. For study purposes, we used the family scale and changed the reference from "friends" to "other parents in your school community." The family support scale had eight items of emotional (e.g., "I get the emotional help and support I need from my family") and instrumental ("I can count on relatives when things go wrong") support. The school community support scale had four items of emotional (e.g., "There are parents at this school who are a real source of comfort to me") and instrumental (e.g., "There are parents at this school who are around when I am in need") support. Items were rated on a seven-point Likert scale and averaged to obtain scale scores. Alphas for both scales, both ethnic groups, and both languages ranged from .87 to .92.

Child internalizing problems

In pre-K, K, G1, and G3 (teachers only), mothers and teachers completed the Behavior Assessment System for Children, Parent Rating Scale and Teacher Rating Scale (BASC PRS, BASC TRS; Reynolds & Kamphaus, 2004), a standardized measure of child behavior and emotional functioning for children between the ages of 2.5 and 18 years. The parent form (the PRS) is available in both English and Spanish based on translation and standardization by the measure developers with a sample of 386 Latinos (specific ethnic groups not described; Reynolds & Kamphaus, 2004). In the present study, standardized (*T*) scores from the anxiety, depression, and somatization subscales (αs ranged from .71 to.80) were used. *T*-scores 60 and above are considered in the at-risk (60–69) or clinical range (70+).

Procedure

Participant enrollment

We sampled from students entering their zoned New York City public elementary school, whether as pre-K or K students, to characterize Latinx children's experiences during the transition to formal schooling. Participant enrollment took place exclusively in the initial 3-month period of the school year. Because of the large range in the concentration of MA and DA students across schools, we did not recruit all eligible students in all schools. Instead, we randomly selected a subset of eligible students, balancing across classroom and child gender, in schools with >50% eligible students among its student population. (In contrast, all eligible students were recruited in schools with <50% eligibility in its population.) This procedure, which ensured that an equivalent number of participants were approached for enrollment in each of the 24 schools, was followed to avoid selection bias. Across schools, our recruitment rate averaged 79% (range: 59%–98%).

Assessment procedures

All research activities were conducted in the language of the mother's preference; the majority of mothers (98% of MA and 76% of DA) chose to be interviewed in Spanish. Interviews lasted approximately 2 h and mothers received a stipend for their participation. After obtaining mother consent, teachers of participating children were contacted and asked to complete child ratings. Most teachers consented (92%) and most consenting teachers returned their packets (93%), resulting in 201 teachers who provided data on 702 (of the 749) participant children. There were no differences on demographics or parent-rated child functioning between children who had teacher ratings and those who did not ($P > .05$).

Data was collected again in K (for the pre-K cohort), G1, and G3. The G3 assessment was designed to collect child outcome data and consisted only of school records and teacher ratings (no mother or child interviews) due to limited resources to recontact families for additional data collection. The present study used data from all time points.

Analytic approach

Missing data was due to our study design and attrition from the study. Among children enrolled in pre-K ($n = 326$), parent data was available for 72% at K and 64% at G1 (parent data was not collected in G3). For the pre-K sample, teacher data was available for 94% in pre-K, 67% in K, 54% in G1, and 52% in G3. Among children enrolled in K ($n = 423$), parent data was available for 75% at K and at G1 (again, parent data was not collected at G3). For the K sample, teacher data was available for 93% in K, 63% in G1, and 52% in G3. To account for cases with partial data or missing data at follow-up, multiple imputations (MI) was applied to generate 10 imputed data sets. Imputation was used to minimize the chance of biased results. Specifically, because attrition analyses showed that children with lower school readiness scores and more externalizing behavior problems were less likely to remain in the study and nonimputed model estimates were likely to be underestimated. Imputations were conducted separately for children enrolled in pre-K and K, and all 749 children were included in the analyses. Analyses were conducted using SAS software, version 9.4 of the SAS system. Proc MI and Proc MIANALYZE were used to impute, merge, and analyze data, and Proc GEE was used to study trajectories and predictors, with consideration of individual repeated nested data.

Results

Trajectories of internalizing behavior problems

Our first aim was to examine internalizing problems over time, from the start of pre-K or K through the end of G3. Rates of children in the at-risk range (T-score ≥ 60), based on GEE estimated results, are shown in Figs. 1 and 2. According to teacher ratings, 10% of children were at risk for depression in pre-K and 14% were at risk by G3; 7% of children were at risk for anxiety in pre-K and 10% were at risk by G3, and 12% of children were at risk for somatization in pre-K and 18% were at risk by G3. Scores on mother ratings were significantly higher. According to mothers, 21% of children were at risk for depression in pre-K and 13% were at risk by G3; 45% of children were at risk for anxiety in pre-K and 39% were at risk by G3, and 16% of children were at risk for somatization in pre-K and 16% were at risk in G3.

To examine whether internalizing problems changed over time, we estimated the effect of time on teacher and mother ratings. Table 1 shows the results for teacher- and mother-rated anxiety, depression, and somatization. Rates of anxiety and somatization increased from pre-K to G3 according to teacher report, but were steady according to mother report. In contrast, rates of depression

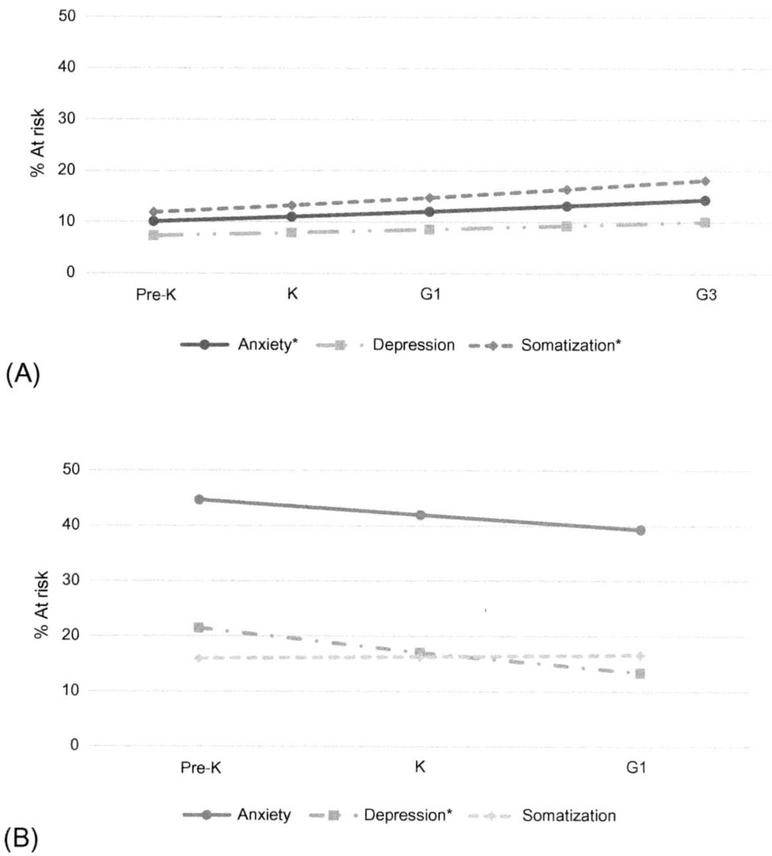

FIG. 1 (A) Teacher report of internalizing problems over time and (B) mother report of internalizing problems over time.

decreased over time according to mother report, but were steady according to teacher report.

We also examined ethnic and gender differences by including ethnicity (1 = DA, 0 = MA) and child gender (1 = male, 0 = female) in the model. For teacher-rated outcomes, we found ethnic group differences showing more depressive and somatization symptoms in DA compared to MA children. For mother-rated outcomes, we also found an ethnic group difference in somatization showing more somatization symptoms in DA children compared to MA children. To examine whether trajectories differed based on ethnicity or gender, we conducted another set of analyses by including ethnicity-by-time and gender-by-time interaction terms in the models (not shown in the table). There was one significant finding showing a decrease in somatization for DA children, and an increase in somatization for MA children (ethnicity-by-time: $E(SE) = -.40$ (.19), ($P < .05$); see Fig. 3).

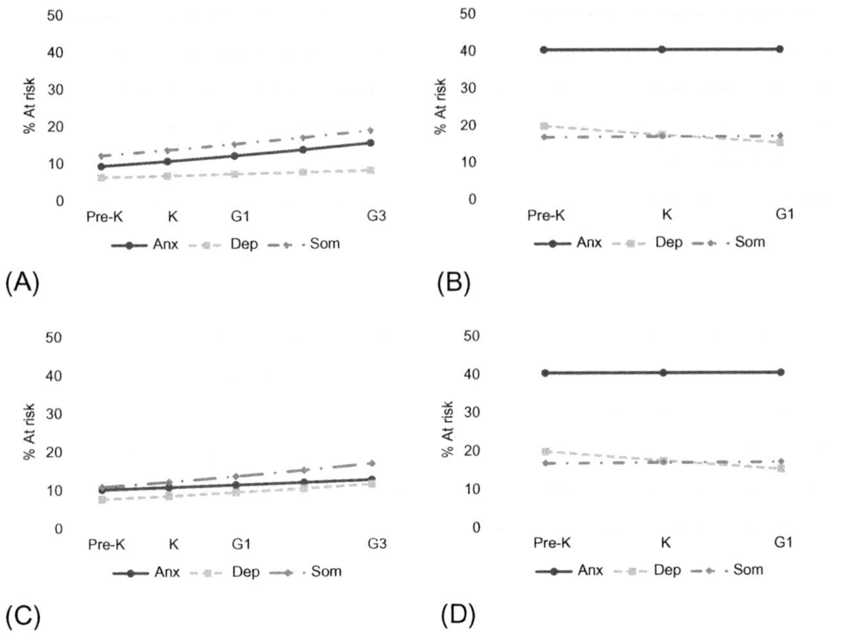

FIG. 2 (A) Teacher report of internalizing problems in girls, (B) mother report of internalizing problems in girls, (C) teacher report of internalizing problems in boys and (D) mother report of internalizing problems in boys.

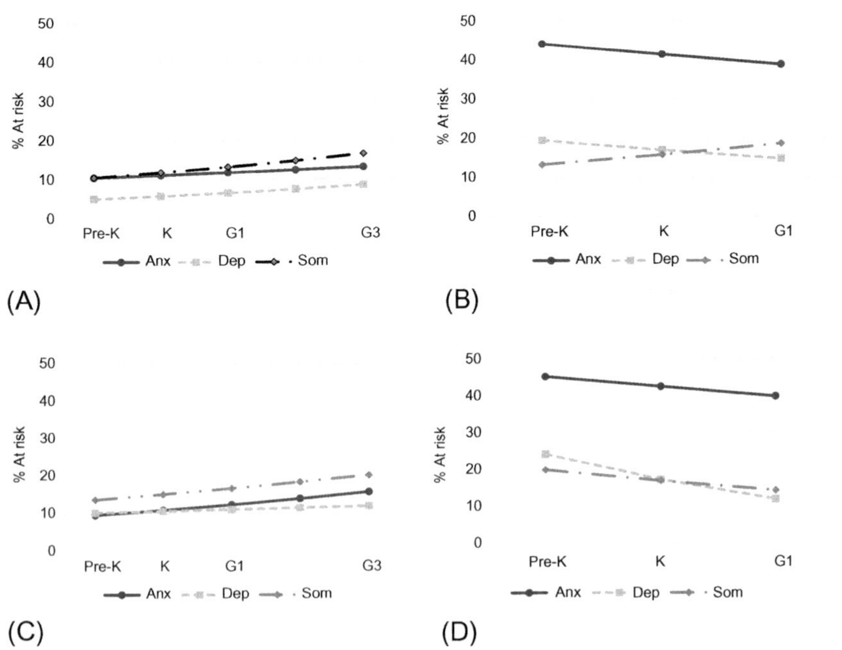

FIG. 3 (A) Teacher report of internalizing problems MA children, (B) mother report of internalizing problems MA children, (C) teacher report of internalizing problems DA children, and (D) mother report of internalizing problems DA children.

Predictors of internalizing behavior problem trajectories

Our second aim was to examine the home environment predictors of internalizing problems. We included each variable (family poverty status, socialization of *respeto*, socialization of independence, authoritarian parenting, authoritative parenting, social support from family and school) as a time-varying predictor (along with time-varying internalizing problems from pre-K to G1) as main effects in the model. We controlled for three potential confounding variables—ethnicity, child gender, and time enrolled in the study (pre-K or K) (Table 2).

As shown in Table 3, none of the home environment variables was significant in predicting teacher-rated anxiety, depression, and somatization problems. However, poverty status, socialization practices, parenting, and social support showed significant associations with mother-rated internalizing problems. Specifically, more socialization of independence, authoritarian practices, authoritative practices, and social support from family were all associated with greater anxiety in children. In addition, more authoritarian practices were associated with greater depressive symptoms. Finally, poverty status, more authoritarian practices, and socialization of *respeto* were associated with more somatization in children.

Next, we tested whether the associations between predictors and outcomes were consistent across time by adding predictor-by-time interaction terms in the model. We found no significant interactions, suggesting similar associations between predictors and internalizing problems at each timepoint (pre-K, K, and G1). Finally, because there were ethnic group differences on teacher- and mother-rated internalizing problem trajectories, we carried out a final set of analyses to test whether the associations between predictors and outcomes were consistent across MA and DA children by adding predictor-by-ethnicity interaction terms in the model. We found no significant interactions, suggesting similar associations for MA and DA children.

Discussion

Internalizing problems often have their onset in early childhood when an individual child and ecological factors combine to initiate a cascade toward mental health problems in adolescence (Shonkoff et al., 2012). In the Latinx population, anxiety and depression are highly prevalent among adolescents but understudied in childhood. To address this gap, the present study examined specific domains of internalizing problems over time with a large, community sample of young Latinx children. Our findings suggest alarming rates of anxiety, depression, and somatization problems starting when children enter school (i.e., at age 4 or 5).

Patterns of internalizing problems over time

According to mothers, who rated children in pre-K, K, and G1, approximately 40% of children were at risk for anxiety and 18% for somatization consistently

TABLE 2 Internalizing behavior problem trajectories predicted by time, ethnicity, and gender.

	Teacher rating (pre-K, K, G1, G3)			Mother rating (pre-K, K, G1)		
	Anxiety	Depression	Somatization	Anxiety	Depression	Somatization
	Estimate (SE)	Estimate (SE)	Estimate (SE)	Estimate (SE)	Estimate (SE)	Estimate (SE)
Continuous outcomes						
Intercept	46.98 (.40)***	46.51 (.35)***	47.89 (.46)***	57.71 (.52)***	48.85 (.50)***	49.22 (.50)***
Time	.10 (.20)	.30 (.18)	.53 (.19)**	−.17 (.37)	.24 (.37)	.17 (.36)
Binary outcomes ($T \geq 60$)						
Intercept	−2.19 (.12)***	−2.54 (.14)***	−2.01 (.13)***	−.21 (.09)*	−1.30 (.12)	−1.66 (.13)***
Time	.10 (.05)*	.09 (.06)	.13 (.05)*	−.11 (.07)	−.28 (.09)**	.02 (.09)
Binary outcomes ($T \geq 60$)						
Intercept	−2.20 (.15)	−2.98 (.18)***	−2.08 (.16)***	−.19 (.11)*	−1.34 (.15)***	−1.94 (.22)***
Time	.10 (.05)*	.09 (.06)	.13 (.05)*	.11 (.07)	−.28 (.09)**	.22 (.13)+
Ethnicity	.08 (.15)	.55 (.16)***	.28 (.13)*	.04 (.10)	−.05 (.14)	. 53 (.25)*
Gender	−.07 (.16)	.29 (.17)	−.13 (.12)	−.08 (.11)	.13 (.13)	.11 (.25)

Note: Time was coded as pre-K = 0, K = 1, G1 = 2, and G3 = 4. Models were based on 10 imputed data sets. In the last model that include ethnicity and gender, we also conducted analysis by including Ethnicity × Time and Gender × Time. The significant interaction effect is shown in Fig. 3 (see below).
*$P < .05$.
**$P < .01$.
***$P < .001$.

TABLE 3 Predictors of internalizing behavior problems over time.

	Teacher rating (pre-K, K, G1)			Parent rating (pre-K, K, G1)		
	Anxiety	Depression	Somatization	Anxiety	Depression	Somatization
	Estimate (SE)	Estimate (SE)	Estimate (SE)	Estimate (SE)	Estimate (SE)	Estimate (SE)
Main effects model						
Intercept	46.79 (.70)***	47.79 (.70)***	48.41 (.71)***	57.97 (.69)***	48.55 (.62)***	48.34 (.67)***
Poverty	−.81 (.60)	−.81 (.60)	−.73 (.67)	−.86 (.69)	.21 (.60)	1.36 (.61)*
Respeto	−.82 (.98)	−.82 (.98)	−.38 (1.28)	.30 (.97)	1.23 (.89)	1.57 (.76)*
Independence	.02 (1.26)	.02 (1.26)	.88 (1.27)	2.18 (1.09)*	.08 (1.24)	.92 (1.16)
Authoritarian practices	.58 (.81)	.58 (.81)	.61 (1.00)	3.48 (.67)***	6.42 (.82)***	3.39 (.75)***
Authoritative practices	.70 (.57)	.70 (.57)	−.26 (.59)	2.28 (.53)***	−1.14 (.85)	−.52 (.63)
Family support	−.20 (.33)	−.20 (.33)	−.45 (.32)	.73 (.29)*	−.43 (.40)	−.37 (.36)
School support	−.11 (.23)	−.11 (.23)	.38 (.25)	.17 (.25)	−.06 (.20)	.06 (.19)
Time	−.17 (.45)	−.17 (.45)	.55 (.41)	.04 (.38)	.33 (.37)	.08 (.38)
Interaction model						
Poverty × Time	.61 (.80)	1.13 (.66)	.73 (.81)	1.09 (.80)	1.14 (.79)	−.04 (.81)
Respeto × Time	−.49 (1.25)	−.62 (1.00)	.41 (1.48)	−.66 (1.13)	.02 (1.02)	.15 (.95)
Independence × Time	.38 (1.61)	.28 (1.28)	1.60 (1.56)	.93 (1.31)	1.94 (1.62)	.61 (1.33)

Continued

TABLE 3 Predictors of internalizing behavior problems over time—cont'd

	Teacher rating (pre-K, K, G1)			Parent rating (pre-K, K, G1)		
	Anxiety	Depression	Somatization	Anxiety	Depression	Somatization
	Estimate (SE)	Estimate (SE)	Estimate (SE)	Estimate (SE)	Estimate (SE)	Estimate (SE)
Authoritarian × Time	.01 (1.01)	−1.12 (.66)	.26 (1.18)	−.51 (.79)	−1.11 (.92)	1.28 (.80)
Authoritative × Time	−.60 (.77)	.20 (.64)	−.22 (.77)	−.12 (.69)	−.18 (.88)	.04 (.75)
Family support × Time	.13 (.48)	.19 (.32)	.18 (.39)	.36 (.38)	−.53 (.42)	−.32 (.41)
School support × Time	−.18 (.27)	−.21 (.20)	−.08 (.36)	−.19 (.28)	.23 (.24)	.42 (.26)

Note: Time was coded as pre-K = 0, K = 1, and G1 = 2. Models were based on 10 imputed data sets. Outcomes were based on standardized *T* scores (on continuous scale). The sample include 70% poor families (income to need ratio ≤1). Models controlled for ethnicity, gender, and time enrolled in the study (not shown). The continuous predictors were centered at the mean.
*$P<.05$.
**$P<.01$.
***$P<.001$.

over time. Ratings of depression decreased over time, such that by G1, 13% of children were classified at risk (compared to the baseline rate of 21%). Teacher ratings, which were provided in pre-K, K, G1, and G3, were lower. However, in contrast with mother ratings, anxiety and depression as observed by teachers increased over time (somatization remained stable). By G3, ratings identified 14% of children at risk for depression, 10% for anxiety, and 18% for somatization. That is, despite the relatively modest rates reported by teachers compared to mothers, *all* ratings (mother and teacher) at all time points and on all domains were higher than would be expected based on population norms (see Ghandour et al., 2019).

This pattern of findings builds on our initial results (over a 12-month period; Calzada et al., 2017) by documenting high and stable risk, especially for anxiety, through age 9. Past research on developmental trajectories has found that children who begin with high levels of internalizing problems tend to remain high; those who are low tend to remain low; and those who are moderate may be most susceptible to variation depending on stressors (Sterba et al., 2007). An important next step for LINCs will be to use person-centered approaches to distinguish between children who are high and stable from those whose symptomatology varies depending on changes in context.

In considering child gender, we found that boys and girls were at similar risk for internalizing problems on both mother and teacher reports. This finding is consistent with the broader literature in suggesting that gender disparities in anxiety and depression emerge in preadolescence, likely as a function of the interrelation of physiological and social factors (Côté, Tremblay, Nagin, Zoccolillo, & Vitaro, 2002; Zahn-Waxler et al., 2000). In considering child ethnicity, we found that DA and MA children had similar profiles of risk on anxiety but DA children had higher ratings of depression and somatization. In addition, mother ratings of somatization increased over time in MA children but decreased in DA children. Ethnic group differences have been documented in the literature, but primarily based on pan-ethnic categorizations; country of origin differences have been found, but primarily with adults (Alegria et al., 2007; Keyes et al., 2012). Still, it is not surprising that MA and DA children differ in some ways given their unique ecologies, even within New York City (Yoshikawa, 2011). Our own past work has consistently shown higher rates of internalizing and externalizing problems among DA children (Calzada et al., 2012, 2017). In follow-up analyses, we found racial differences (operationalized as researcher ratings of skin color) and specifically, that dark-skinned Afro-Latinx (i.e., DA, not MA) children were twice as likely to be rated as depressed by teachers (Calzada, Kim, & O'Gara, 2019). The race is a determinant of discrimination (Dixon & Telles, 2017) and discrimination increases the risk for Latinx depression (Zeiders, Umaña-Taylor, & Derlan, 2013), but these associations have seldom been studied before adolescence in racially diverse Latinx children.

Similarly, we highlight the increase in anti-Latinx, antiimmigrant policies and rhetoric since the 2016 presidential election as a source of stress and distress for parents and children (Barajas-Gonzalez, Ayón, & Torres, 2018). A recent study found that anxiety, sleep problems, and blood pressure increased significantly after the 2016 presidential election due to fear and worry about US immigration policy (Eskenazi et al., 2019). Evidence shows that antiimmigration policies have population-wide impacts (Roche, Vaquera, White, & Rivera, 2018), but legal vulnerability (i.e., undocumented or temporary status) has particularly negative consequences for parents and children (Barajas-Gonzalez et al., 2018). We did not assess the impact of immigration policies or the legal vulnerability in LINCs, but similar factors may have influenced the well-being of our sample (which took place from 2010 to 2017). Future research on the influence of racism and xenophobia on Latinx families is urgently needed.

Predictors of internalizing problems

The home-level predictors we examined were not significantly associated with teacher report of child anxiety, depression, or somatization. It may be that classroom factors, particularly teacher-student interactions, are more associated with internalizing problems as reported by teachers (Baker, Grant, & Morlock, 2008; Zatto & Hoglund, 2019). Starting in pre-K, teachers appear to hold more negative perceptions of Latinx and African-American students compared with White students (Gilliam, Maupin, Reyes, Accavitti, & Shic, 2016), with negative implications for teacher-student interactions (Okonofua & Eberhardt, 2015). Past literature has focused on externalizing behaviors, but given the high rates of internalizing problems observed in the present study, research on how teachers influence the emotional functioning of young Latinx children is equally important.

Several characteristics of the home environment predicted mother reports of child internalizing problems, consistent with our past work. As expected, authoritarian parenting emerged as the most robust risk factor (Calzada et al., 2012, 2017; Gil-Rivas et al., 2003), predicting anxiety, depression, and somatization. We also replicated findings showing that *respeto* and independence both exert direct influences on child internalizing problems (Calzada et al., 2017); *respeto* predicted somatization symptoms (even as it may make children more obedient) and independence predicted anxiety (even as it may make children more autonomous). Increasingly, scholars recognize the dynamic complexities of culture as shaped not only by traditional histories, values, and norms but also by current environmental influences (White, Nair, & Bradley, 2018). In the case of cultural values, the incongruence between Latinx and mainstream cultures may make the maintenance (e.g., of *respeto*) or adoption (e.g., of independence) of a given value challenging as parents and children balance the respective behavioral demands of home and outside settings. Without understanding these complexities, we emphasize that, in spite of our findings, cultural values may well be protective but also caution against assumptions that they are uniformly protective for all children in all domains of well-being.

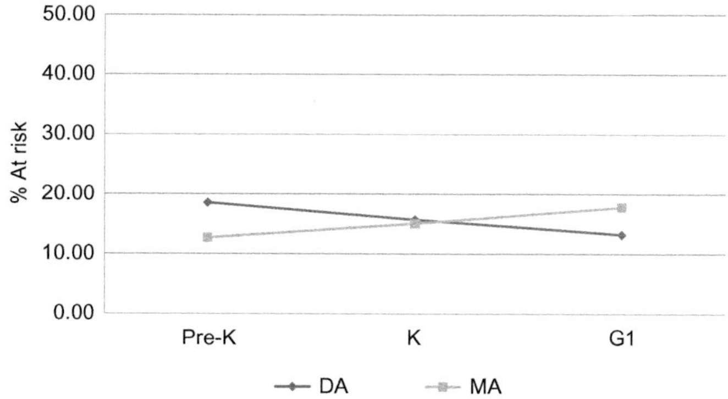

FIG. 4 Trajectories of mother-reported somatization problems by ethnicity.

Our findings also identified authoritative parenting and familial support as predictors of mother-rated anxiety. It may be that at least some aspects of authoritative parenting help to maintain anxious symptoms, similar to findings that solicitous parenting (high in proximity, positive affect, and positive control) at age 4 maintain social wariness in children through age 7 (Degnan, Henderson, Fox, & Rubin, 2008). Alternately or additionally, our findings may reflect child-evocative effects or the ways in which child characteristics, especially behavior problems, elicit certain parental responses (Bates, Schermerhorn, & Petersen, 2012; Hollenstein, Granic, Stoolmiller, & Snyder, 2004). The surprising association between familial support and anxiety may similarly reflect the ways in which the family system accommodates to the emotional needs of a child.

Finally, poverty status was related to more somatization problems (mother report), a finding that is consistent with research showing that poverty undermines child mental health (Mendoza et al., 2017) (Fig. 4). In fact, it is not clear why poverty was not a more robust risk factor for internalizing problems in the present study, but it may be that there was not enough variation in socioeconomic status (SES) in our sample (i.e., 70% of families were living in poverty) or because of changes in poverty status over the course of the study (Dawson & Williams, 2008). It will be important to address this methodological limitation in future studies by sampling Latinx families from diverse SES backgrounds.

Limitations and conclusions

There are a number of notable limitations to the present study. For example, our assessment of the home environment was quite narrow and neglected a number of other factors relevant to developmental psychopathology. For example, maternal depression has robust effects on children, especially on childhood internalizing problems and in early childhood (Goodman et al., 2011). Given the ongoing exposure to stressors related to immigration, acculturation, racism, and poverty faced by many Latinx parents, the risk for maternal depression is high and warrants more scholarly attention (Calzada & Sales, 2019). Factors outside the home, such as neighborhood context, have also been found to influence Latinx child mental health, both directly and indirectly through interactions with family-level processes (White, Zeiders, Gonzales, Tein, & Roosa, 2013). Future research should consider more comprehensive developmental models that capture these contextual influences.

Another limitation was our reliance on behavior ratings to measure childhood internalizing symptoms. Although behavior ratings, particularly from parents, have been shown to correlate to clinical assessments of psychopathology (Luby, 2013), they cannot be interpreted as evidence of psychopathology without an assessment of functional impairment (Canino & Alegria, 2009). On the other hand, research shows that even subclinical levels of depression may be as impairing as clinical depression in children (Avenevoli, Knight, Kessler, & Merikangas, 2008). Similarly, symptoms of anxiety and somatization, especially in childhood, have known clinical implications (Beesdo et al., 2009). Still, we recommend that future studies of Latinx child functioning include diagnostic instruments.

Nonetheless, the present study is significant in bringing attention to the issue of internalizing problems in young, Latinx children. Findings showed a concerning pattern of risk for anxiety, depression, and somatization symptoms from age 4 to 9 and implicate authoritarian parenting as a robust predictor of these problem behaviors. We encourage broader dissemination of supports for Latinx families and specifically of evidence-based and culturally informed parenting interventions during early childhood.

References

Alegria, M., Mulvaney-Day, N., Torres, M., Polo, A., Cao, Z., & Canino, G. (2007). Prevalence of psychiatric disorders across Latino subgroups in the United States. *American Journal of Public Health*, *97*, 68–75. https://doi.org/10.2105/AJPH.2006.087205.

Avenevoli, S., Knight, E., Kessler, R. C., & Merikangas, K. R. (2008). Epidemiology of depression in children and adolescents. In J. R. Z. Abela & B. L. Hankin (Eds.), *Handbook of depression in children and adolescents* (pp. 6–32). New York, NY: Guilford Press.

Baker, J. A., Grant, S., & Morlock, L. (2008). The teacher-student relationship as a developmental context for children with internalizing or externalizing behavior problems. *School Psychology Quarterly*, *23*(1), 3–15. https://doi.org/10.1037/1045-3830.23.1.3.

Bámaca-Colbert, M. Y., Umaña-Taylor, A. J., & Gayles, J. G. (2012). A developmental contextual model of depressive symptoms in Mexican-origin female adolescents. *Developmental Psychology*, *48*(2), 406. https://doi.org/10.1037/a0025666.

Barajas-Gonzalez, R. G., Ayón, C., & Torres, F. (2018). Applying a community violence framework to understand the impact of immigration enforcement threat on Latino children. *Social Policy Report*, *31*(3), 1–24. https://doi.org/10.1002/sop2.1.

Barajas-Gonzalez, R. G., & Brooks-Gunn, J. (2014). Income, neighborhood stressors, and harsh parenting: Test of moderation by ethnicity, age, and gender. *Journal of Family Psychology*, *28*(6), 855. https://doi.org/10.1037/a0038242.

Bates, J. E., Schermerhorn, A. C., & Petersen, I. T. (2012). Temperament and parenting in developmental perspective. In M. Zentner & R. L. Shiner (Eds.), *Handbook of temperament* (pp. 425–441). New York, NY: Guilford Press.

Baumrind, D. (1995). *Child maltreatment and optimal caregiving in social contexts.* Garland Publishing.

Bayer, J. K., Sanson, A. V., & Hemphill, S. A. (2006). Parent influences on early childhood internalizing difficulties. *Journal of Applied Developmental Psychology, 27*(6), 542–559. https://doi.org/10.1016/j.appdev.2006.08.002.

Beesdo, K., Knappe, S., & Pine, D. S. (2009). Anxiety and anxiety disorders in children and adolescents: Developmental issues and implications for DSM-V. *Psychiatric Clinics, 32*(3), 483–524. https://doi.org/10.1016/j.psc.2009.06.002.

Beidel, D. C., Christ, M. A. G., & Long, P. J. (1991). Somatic complaints in anxious children. *Journal of Abnormal Child Psychology, 19*(6), 659–670. https://doi.org/10.1007/BF00918905.

Bufferd, S. J., Dougherty, L. R., & Olino, T. M. (2017). Mapping the frequency and severity of depressive behaviors in preschool-aged children. *Child Psychiatry & Human Development, 48*(6), 934–943. https://doi.org/10.1007/s10578-017-0715-2.

Bufferd, S. J., Dyson, M. W., Hernandez, I. G., & Wakschlag, L. S. (2016). Explicating the "developmental" in preschool psychopathology. In D. Cicchetti (Ed.), *Developmental psychopathology* (pp. 152–186). New York, NY: Wiley. https://doi.org/10.1002/9781119125556.devpsy305.

Calzada, E. J., Barajas-Gonzalez, R. G., Huang, K. Y., & Brotman, L. (2017). Early childhood internalizing problems in Mexican-and Dominican-origin children: The role of cultural socialization and parenting practices. *Journal of Clinical Child & Adolescent Psychology, 46*(4), 551–562. https://doi.org/10.1080/15374416.2015.1041593.

Calzada, E. J., & Eyberg, S. M. (2002). Self-reported parenting practices in Dominican and Puerto Rican mothers of young children. *Journal of Clinical Child and Adolescent Psychology, 31*(3), 354–363.

Calzada, E. J., Fernandez, Y., & Cortes, D. E. (2010). Incorporating the cultural value of respeto into a framework of Latino parenting. *Cultural Diversity and Ethnic Minority Psychology, 16*(1), 77. https://doi.org/10.1037/a0016071.

Calzada, E. J., Huang, K. Y., Anicama, C., Fernandez, Y., & Brotman, L. M. (2012). Test of a cultural framework of parenting with Latino families of young children. *Cultural Diversity and Ethnic Minority Psychology, 18*(3), 285. https://doi.org/10.1037/a0028694.

Calzada, E. J., Kim, Y., & O'Gara, J. (2019). Skin color as a predictor of mental health in young Latinx children. *Social Science & Medicine, 238*, https://doi.org/10.1016/j.socscimed.2019.112467.

Calzada, E. J., & Sales, A. (2019). Depression among Mexican-origin mothers: Exploring the immigrant paradox. *Cultural Diversity and Ethnic Minority Psychology, 25*(2), 288–298. https://doi.org/10.1037/cdp0000214.

Calzada, E. J., Sales, A., & O'Gara, J. (2019). Maternal depression and acculturative stress impacts on Mexican-origin children through authoritarian parenting. *Journal of Applied Developmental Psychology, 63*, 65–75. https://doi.org/10.1016/j.appdev.2019.05.001.

Canino, G. (2004). Are somatic symptoms and related distress more prevalent in Hispanic/Latino youth? Some methodological considerations. *Journal of Clinical Child and Adolescent Psychology, 33*(2), 272–275. https://doi.org/10.1207/s15374424jccp3302_8.

Canino, G., & Alegria, M. (2009). Understanding psychopathology among the adult and child Latino population from the United States and Puerto Rico: An epidemiologic perspective. In F. A. Villarruel, G. Carlo, J. M. Contreras Grau, M. Azmitia, & N. J. Cabrera (Eds.), *Handbook of US Latino psychology: Developmental and community-based perspectives* (pp. 31–44). Thousand Oaks, CA: Sage.

Child Trends. (2018). *Racial and ethnic composition of the child population*. Retrieved from https://www.childtrends.org/indicators/racial-and-ethnic-composition-of-the-child-population.

Child Trends. (2019). *Children in poverty*. Retrieved from https://www.childtrends.org/?indicators=children-in-poverty.

Cicchetti, D., Rogosch, F. A., & Toth, S. L. (2000). The efficacy of toddler-parent psychotherapy for fostering cognitive development in offspring of depressed mothers. *Journal of Abnormal Child Psychology*, *28*(2), 135–148. https://doi.org/10.1023/A:1005118713814.

Coley, R. L., Kull, M. A., & Carrano, J. (2014). Parental endorsement of spanking and children's internalizing and externalizing problems in African American and Hispanic families. *Journal of Family Psychology*, *28*(1), 22–31. https://doi.org/10.1037/a0035272.

Côté, S., Tremblay, R. E., Nagin, D., Zoccolillo, M., & Vitaro, F. (2002). The development of impulsivity, fearfulness, and helpfulness during childhood: Patterns of consistency and change in the trajectories of boys and girls. *Journal of Child Psychology and Psychiatry*, *43*(5), 609–618. https://doi.org/10.1111/1469-7610.00050.

Dallaire, D. H., Pineda, A. Q., Cole, D. A., Ciesla, J. A., Jacquez, F., LaGrange, B., & Bruce, A. E. (2006). Relation of positive and negative parenting to children's depressive symptoms. *Journal of Clinical Child & Adolescent Psychology*, *35*(2), 313–322. https://doi.org/10.1207/s15374424jccp3502_15.

Dawson, B. A., & Williams, S. A. (2008). The impact of language status as an acculturative stressor on internalizing and externalizing behaviors among Latino/a children: A longitudinal analysis from school entry through third grade. *Journal of Youth and Adolescence*, *37*(4), 399–411. https://doi.org/10.1007/s10964-007-9233-z.

Degnan, K. A., Henderson, H. A., Fox, N. A., & Rubin, K. H. (2008). Predicting social wariness in middle childhood: The moderating roles of child care history, maternal personality and maternal behavior. *Social Development*, *17*(3), 471–487. https://doi.org/10.1111/j.1467-9507.2007.00437.x.

Dixon, A. R., & Telles, E. E. (2017). Skin color and colorism: Global research, concepts, and measurement. *Annual Review of Sociology*, *43*, 405–424. https://doi.org/10.1146/annurev-soc-060116-053315.

Dougherty, L. R., Tolep, M. R., Bufferd, S. J., Olino, T. M., Dyson, M., Traditi, J., … Klein, D. N. (2013). Preschool anxiety disorders: Comprehensive assessment of clinical, demographic, temperamental, familial, and life stress correlates. *Journal of Clinical Child & Adolescent Psychology*, *42*(5), 577–589. https://doi.org/10.1080/15374416.2012.759225.

Egger, H. L., & Angold, A. (2006). Common emotional and behavioral disorders in preschool children: Presentation, nosology, and epidemiology. *Journal of Child Psychology & Psychiatry*, *47*(3–4), 313–337. https://doi.org/10.1111/j.1469-7610.2006.01618.x.

Eminson, M., Benjamin, S., Shortall, A., Woods, T., & Faragher, B. (1996). Physical symptoms and illness attitudes in adolescents: An epidemiological study. *Journal of Child Psychology and Psychiatry*, *37*(5), 519–528. https://doi.org/10.1111/j.1469-7610.1996.tb01438.x.

Eskenazi, B., Fayeh, C. A., Kogut, K., Gunier, R., Torres, J., Gonzales, N., … Deardorff, J. (2019). Association of perceived immigration policy vulnerability with mental and physical health among US-born Latino adolescents in California. *JAMA Pediatrics*, *173*(8), 744–753. https://doi.org/10.1001/jamapediatrics.2019.1475.

Fanti, K. A., & Henrich, C. C. (2010). Trajectories of pure and co-occurring internalizing and externalizing problems from age 2 to age 12: Findings from the National Institute of Child Health and Human Development Study of Early Child Care. *Developmental Psychology*, *46*(5), 1159–1175. https://doi.org/10.1037/a0020659.

Ghandour, R. M., Sherman, L. J., Vladutiu, C. J., Ali, M. M., Lynch, S. E., Bitsko, R. H., & Blumberg, S. J. (2019). Prevalence and treatment of depression, anxiety, and conduct problems in U.S. children. *Journal of Pediatrics*, *206*, 256–267. E3 https://doi.org/10.1016/j.jpeds.2018.09.021.

Gilliam, W., Maupin, A., Reyes, C., Accavitti, M., & Shic, F. (2016). *Do early educators' implicit biases regarding sex and race relate to behavior expectations and recommendations of preschool expulsions and suspensions?*. Retrieved from http://ziglercenter.yale.edu/publications/Preschool%20Implicit%20Bias%20Policy%20Brief_final_9_26_276766_5379.pdf.

Gilliom, M., & Shaw, D. S. (2004). Codevelopment of externalizing and internalizing problems in early childhood. *Development and Psychopathology*, *16*(2), 313–333. https://doi.org/10.1017/S0954579404044530.

Gil-Rivas, V., Greenberger, E., Chen, C., & Montero y López-Lena, M. (2003). Understanding depressed mood in the context of a family oriented culture. *Adolescence*, *38*, 93–109.

Goodman, S. H., Rouse, M. H., Connell, A. M., Broth, M. R., Hall, C. M., & Heyward, D. (2011). Maternal depression and child psychopathology: A meta-analytic review. *Clinical Child and Family Psychology Review*, *14*, 1–27. https://doi.org/10.1007/s10567-010-0080-1.

Guarnaccia, P. J., Lewis-Fernández, R., & Marano, M. R. (2003). Toward a Puerto Rican popular nosology: Nervios and ataque de nervios. *Culture, Medicine and Pychiatry*, *27*(3), 339–366. https://doi.org/10.1023/A:1025303315932.

Hirshfeld-Becker, D. R., Masek, B., Henin, A., Blakely, L. R., Pollock-Wurman, R. A., McQuade, J., … Biederman, J. (2010). Cognitive behavioral therapy for 4-to 7-year-old children with anxiety disorders: A randomized clinical trial. *Journal of Consulting and Clinical Psychology*, *78*(4), 498. https://doi.org/10.1037/a0019055.

Hollenstein, T., Granic, I., Stoolmiller, M., & Snyder, J. (2004). Rigidity in parent–child interactions and the development of externalizing and internalizing behavior in early childhood. *Journal of Abnormal Child Psychology*, *32*(6), 595–607. https://doi.org/10.1023/B:JACP.0000047209.37650.41.

Kann, L., McManus, T., Harris, W. A., Shanklin, S., Flint, K., Queens, B., … Ethier, K. A. (2018). Youth Risk Behavior Surveillance—United States, 2017. *MMWR Surveillance Summaries*, *67*(8), 1–114. https://doi.org/10.15585/mmwr.ss6708a1.

Kessler, R. C. (2012). The costs of depression. *Psychiatric Clinics*, *35*(1), 1–14. https://doi.org/10.1016/j.psc.2011.11.005.

Keyes, K. M., Martins, S. S., Hatzenbuehler, M. L., Blanco, C., Bates, L. M., & Hasin, D. S. (2012). Mental health service utilization for psychiatric disorders among Latinos living in the United States: The role of ethnic subgroup, ethnic identity, and language/social preferences. *Social Psychiatry and Psychiatric Epidemiology*, *47*(3), 383–394. https://doi.org/10.1007/s00127-010-0323-y.

Kleylamp, M., & Tienda, M. (2004). Physical and mental health status of adolescent girls: A comparative ethnic perspective. *Research on Social Stratification and Mobility*, *22*, 149–185. https://doi.org/10.1016/S0276-5624(04)22006-6.

Lengua, L. J. (2006). Growth in temperament and parenting as predictors of adjustment during children's transition to adolescence. *Developmental Psychology*, *42*(5), 819–832. https://doi.org/10.1037/0012-1649.42.5.819.

Linver, M. R., Brooks-Gunn, J., & Kohen, D. E. (2002). Family processes as pathways from income to young children's development. *Developmental Psychology*, *38*(5), 719–734. https://doi.org/10.1037/0012-1649.38.5.719.

Lorenzo-Blanco, E. I., Meca, A., Unger, J. B., Romero, A., Szapocznik, J., Piña-Watson, B., … Soto, D. W. (2017). Longitudinal effects of Latino parent cultural stress, depressive symptoms, and family functioning on youth emotional well-being and health risk behaviors. *Family Process*, *56*(4), 981–996. https://doi.org/10.1111/famp.12258.

Luby, J. L. (2013). Treatment of anxiety and depression in the preschool period. *Journal of the American Academy of Child & Adolescent Psychiatry*, *52*(4), 346–358. https://doi.org/10.1016/j.jaac.2013.01.011.

Luby, J. L., Heffelfinger, A. K., Mrakotsky, C., Brown, K. M., Hessler, M. J., Wallis, J. M., & Spitznagel, E. L. (2003). The clinical picture of depression in preschool children. *Journal of the American Academy of Child & Adolescent Psychiatry*, *42*(3), 340–348. https://doi.org/10.1097/00004583-200303000-00015.

Mak, W. W., & Zane, N. W. (2004). The phenomenon of somatization among community Chinese Americans. *Social Psychiatry and Psychiatric Epidemiology*, *39*(12), 967–974. https://doi.org/10.1007/s00127-004-0827-4.

McLeod, B. D., Weisz, J. R., & Wood, J. J. (2007). Examining the association between parenting and childhood depression: A meta-analysis. *Clinical Psychology Review*, *27*(8), 986–1003. https://doi.org/10.1016/j.cpr.2007.03.001.

McLeod, B. D., Wood, J. J., & Weisz, J. R. (2007). Examining the association between parenting and childhood anxiety: A meta-analysis. *Clinical Psychology Review*, *27*(2), 155–172. https://doi.org/10.1016/j.cpr.2006.09.002.

Mendoza, M. M., Dmitrieva, J., Perreira, K. M., Hurwich-Reiss, E., & Watamura, S. E. (2017). The effects of economic and sociocultural stressors on the well-being of children of Latino immigrants living in poverty. *Cultural Diversity and Ethnic Minority Psychology*, *23*(1), 15. https://doi.org/10.1037/cdp0000111.

Nair, R. L., White, R. M. B., Roosa, M., & Zeiders, K. (2013). Cultural stressors and mental health symptoms among Mexican Americans: A prospective study examining the impact of the family and neighborhood context. *Journal of Youth and Adolescence*, *42*(10), 1611–1623. https://doi.org/10.1007/s10964-012-9834-z.

Okonofua, J. A., & Eberhardt, J. L. (2015). Two strikes: Race and the disciplining of young students. *Psychological Science*, *26*, 617–624. https://doi.org/10.1177/0956797615570365.

Parker, G., Cheah, Y. C., & Roy, K. (2001). Do the Chinese somatize depression? A cross cultural study. *Social Psychiatry and Psychiatric Epidemiology*, *36*(6), 287–293. https://doi.org/10.1007/s001270170046.

Pina, A. A., & Silverman, W. K. (2004). Clinical phenomenology, somatic symptoms, and distress in Hispanic/Latino and European American youths with anxiety disorders. *Journal of Clinical Child and Adolescent Psychology*, *33*(2), 227–236. https://doi.org/10.1207/s15374424jccp3302_3.

Polo, A. J., & Lopez, S. R. (2009). Culture, context, and the internalizing distress of Mexican American youth. *Journal of Clinical Child & Adolescent Psychology*, *38*(2), 273–285. https://doi.org/10.1080/15374410802698370.

Potochnick, S. R., & Perreira, K. M. (2010). Depression and anxiety among first-generation immigrant Latino youth: Key correlates and implications for future research. *Journal of Nervous and Mental Disease*, *198*(7), 470–477.

Reynolds, C. R., & Kamphaus, R. W. (2004). *BASC: Behavioral assessment system for children*. Circle Pines, MN: AGS Publishing.

Roberts, R. E., Roberts, C. R., & Chen, Y. R. (1997). Ethnocultural differences in prevalence of adolescent depression. *American Journal of Community Psychology*, *25*(1), 95–110. https://doi.org/10.1023/A:1024649925737.

Robinson, C. C., Mandleco, B., Olsen, S. F., & Hart, C. H. (1995). Authoritative, authoritarian, and permissive parenting practices: Development of a new measure. *Psychological Reports*, *77*(3), 819–830. https://doi.org/10.2466/pr0.1995.77.3.819.

Roche, K. M., Lambert, S. F., White, R. M., Calzada, E. J., Little, T. D., Kuperminc, G. P., & Schulenberg, J. E. (2019). Autonomy-related parenting processes and adolescent adjustment in Latinx immigrant families. *Journal of Youth and Adolescence*, *48*(6), 1161–1174. https://doi.org/10.1007/s10964-019-01010-5.

Roche, K. M., Vaquera, E., White, R., & Rivera, M. I. (2018). Impacts of immigration actions and news and the psychological distress of U.S. Latino parents raising adolescents. *Journal of Adolescent Health*, *62*(5), 525–531. https://doi.org/10.1016/j.jadohealth.2018.01.004.

Shanahan, L., Zucker, N., Copeland, W. E., Bondy, C. L., Egger, H. L., & Costello, E. J. (2015). Childhood somatic complaints predict generalized anxiety and depressive disorders during young adulthood in a community sample. *Psychological Medicine*, *45*(8), 1721–1730. https://doi.org/10.1017/S0033291714002840.

Shelby, G. D., Shirkey, K. C., Sherman, A. L., Beck, J. E., Haman, K., Shears, A. R., … Walker, L. S. (2013). Functional abdominal pain in childhood and long-term vulnerability to anxiety disorders. *Pediatrics*, *132*(3), 475–482. https://doi.org/10.1542/peds.2012-2191.

Shonkoff, J. P., Garner, A. S., Siegel, B. S., Dobbins, M. I., Earls, M. F., McGuinn, L., … Committee on Early Childhood, Adoption, and Dependent Care. (2012). The lifelong effects of early childhood adversity and toxic stress. *Pediatrics*, *129*(1), e232–e246. https://doi.org/10.1542/peds.2011-2663.

Sterba, S., Prinstein, M., & Cox, M. (2007). Trajectories of internalizing problems across childhood: Heterogeneity, external validity, and gender differences. *Development and Psychopathology*, *19*, 345–366. https://doi.org/10.1017/S0954579407070174.

Varela, R. E., Sanchez-Sosa, J. J., Biggs, B. K., & Luis, T. M. (2008). Anxiety symptoms and fears in Hispanic and European American children: Cross-cultural measurement equivalence. *Journal of Psychopathology and Behavioral Assessment*, *30*(2), 132–145. https://doi.org/10.1007/s10862-007-9056-y.

Whalen, D. J., Dixon-Gordon, K., Belden, A. C., Barch, D., & Luby, J. L. (2015). Correlates and consequences of suicidal cognitions and behaviors in children ages 3 to 7 years. *Journal of the American Academy of Child & Adolescent Psychiatry*, *54*(11), 926–937. https://doi.org/10.1016/j.jaac.2015.08.009.

White, R. M. B., Nair, R. L., & Bradley, R. H. (2018). Theorizing the benefits and costs of adaptive cultures for development. *American Psychologist*, *73*(6), 727–739. https://doi.org/10.1037/amp0000237.

White, R. M., Roosa, M. W., Weaver, S. R., & Nair, R. L. (2009). Cultural and contextual influences on parenting in Mexican American families. *Journal of Marriage and Family*, *71*, 1–26. https://doi.org/10.1111/j.1741-3737.2008.00580.x.

White, R. M. B., Roosa, M. W., & Zeiders, K. H. (2012). Neighborhood and family intersections: Prospective implications for Mexican American adolescents' mental health. *Journal of Family Psychology*, *26*(5), 793–804. https://doi.org/10.1037/a0029426.

White, R. M. B., Zeiders, K. H., Gonzales, N. A., Tein, J., & Roosa, M. W. (2013). Cultural values, U.S. neighborhood danger, and Mexican American parents' parenting. *Journal of Family Psychology*, *27*, 265–275. https://doi.org/10.1037/a0032888.

World Health Organization. (2017). *Depression and other common mental disorders: Global health estimates*. Retrieved from https://apps.who.int/iris/bitstream/handle/10665/254610/WHO-MSD-MER-2017.2-eng.pdf.

Yildirim, E. D., & Roopnarine, J. L. (2015). The mediating role of maternal warmth in the associations between harsh parental practices and externalizing and internalizing behaviors in Hispanic American, African American, and European American families. *Cultural Diversity and Ethnic Minority Psychology*, *21*(3), 430. https://doi.org/10.1037/a0038210.

Yoshikawa, H. (2011). *Immigrants raising citizens: Undocumented parents and their young children*. New York, NY: Russell Sage.

Zahn-Waxler, C., Klimes-Dougan, B., & Slattery, M. J. (2000). Internalizing problems of childhood and adolescence: Prospects, pitfalls, and progress in understanding the development of anxiety and depression. *Development and Psychopathology*, *12*(3), 443–466. https://doi.org/10.1017/S0954579400003102.

Zatto, B., & Hoglund, W. (2019). Children's internalizing problems and teacher-child relationship quality across preschool. *Early Childhood Research Quarterly*, *49*, 28–39. https://doi.org/10.1016/j.ecresq.2019.05.007.

Zeiders, K. H., Umaña-Taylor, A. J., & Derlan, C. L. (2013). Trajectories of depressive symptoms and self-esteem in Latino youths: Examining the role of gender and perceived discrimination. *Developmental Psychology*, *49*(5), 951–963. https://doi.org/10.1037/a0028866.

Zeiders, K. H., Umaña-Taylor, A. J., Jahromi, L. B., Updegraff, K. A., & White, R. M. B. (2016). Discrimination and acculturation stress: A longitudinal study of children's well-being from prenatal development to 5 years of age. *Journal of Development and Behavioral Pediatrics*, *37*, 557–564. https://doi.org/10.1097/DBP.0000000000000321.

Zimet, G. D., Dahlem, N. W., Zimet, S. G., & Farley, G. K. (1988). The multidimensional scale of perceived social support. *Journal of Personality Assessment*, *52*(1), 30–41.

Further reading

Zeiders, K. H., Updegraff, K., Umaña-Taylor, A. J., Wheeler, L. A., Perez-Brena, N. J., & Rodriquez, S. A. (2013). Mexican-origin youths' trajectories of depressive symptoms: The role of familism values. *Journal of Adolescent Health*, *53*, 648–654. https://doi.org/10.1016/j.jadohealth.2013.06.008.

Chapter 13

Risk and protective factors for insomnia among Asian, Black, and Latinx adult immigrants in the United States: A socioecological analysis

Luciana Giorgio Cosenzo, Sarah Valentina Diaz, Melanie Morris and Carmela Alcántara
School of Social Work, Columbia University, New York, NY, United States

Introduction

Insomnia, a psychiatric disorder characterized by difficulty initiating sleep, maintaining sleep or waking up too early, accompanied by sleepiness the next day and clinical impairment, is one of the most prevalent sleep-wake disorders in the United States (US) affecting 14.7%–23.6% of adults (American Psychiatric Association, 2013; Roth et al., 2011). People with insomnia have an increased risk of mental and physical health conditions such as depression, anxiety, cardiovascular and cardiometabolic diseases, and mortality (Hale & Rivero-Fuentes, 2011; Javaheri & Redline, 2017; Laugsand, Strand, Platou, Vatten, & Janszky, 2014; Ozminkowski, Wang, & Walsh, 2007; Sarsour, Kalsekar, Swindle, Foley, & Walsh, 2011).

In the past decade, the age-adjusted prevalence of insomnia has increased from 17.4% to 18.8% in the general US population (Ford, Cunningham, Giles, & Croft, 2015). Among racial/ethnic minority adult populations, the prevalence of insomnia has also significantly increased by 2%–3% from 2002 to 2012, most notably among African Americans (from 9.4% to 12%) and Latinxs (from 8.8% to 10.9%) (Ford et al., 2015). While a sizeable proportion of the racial/ethnic minority US population is composed of immigrants, including 66.4% who identify as Asian, 9.44% who identify as non-Latino Black, and 34.36% who identify as Latinx (United States Census Bureau Population Division, n.d.), the prevalence of insomnia and its associated risk and protective factors remain

Mental and Behavioral Health of Immigrants in the United States
https://doi.org/10.1016/B978-0-12-816117-3.00013-0

understudied among racial/ethnic minority immigrants. This is problematic because the US immigrant population is aging (Radford & Noe-Bustamante, 2019). For example, current estimates indicate that 13.4% of the US population is made up of immigrants, of which 39.2% are between 25 and 44 years old, followed by 33% who are between 45 and 64 years old, and 14.8% who are older than 65 (Radford & Noe-Bustamante, 2019). Additionally, although the immigrant health paradox posits that immigrants have better health than US-born Whites and their US-born counterparts despite typically occupying positions of low socioeconomic status (Alcántara, Estevez, & Alegría, 2017), it is unclear whether these patterns are observed for insomnia. Importantly for mental health conditions, an immigrant health advantage is not always observed, and this may differ by specific country of origin and type of mental health condition. For example, among Latinx populations, Cuban and Puerto Rican migrants only exhibited an immigrant health advantage for substance use disorders and not depression or anxiety disorders (Alegria, Canino, Stinson, & Grant, 2006).

Notably, most of the widely utilized psychosocial models of the pathogenesis of insomnia explain insomnia as stemming from a combination of predisposing, precipitating, and perpetuating factors, which may be biological, psychological, behavioral, or social factors (Borbély, 1982; Spielman, Caruso, & Glovinsky, 1987). Most of these models focus almost exclusively on individual-level risk factors associated with insomnia while ignoring the influence of contextual factors on sleep, even though there is well-established evidence that contextual factors shape individual health (Marmot, Allen, Bell, Bloomer, & Goldblatt, 2012). Contextual factors can include social level factors such as sociocultural stressors or macro-level factors such as neighborhood quality. Numerous studies with racial/ethnic minority communities have established links between contextual level factors and insomnia, however, migration-related factors remain understudied (Mezick et al., 2008; Nam et al., 2018; Robbins et al., 2019).

Integrating Bronfenbrenner's classic socioecological framework (Bronfenbrenner & Morris, 2007) that emphasizes persons within their environments, as well as the National Institute of Minority Health and Health Disparities (NIMHD) research framework (Alvidrez, Castille, Laude-Sharp, Rosario, & Tabor, 2019) which emphasizes the influence of the social determinants of health across socioecological levels, we illustrate how migration-related contextual factors may affect insomnia and poor sleep quality directly and indirectly through behavioral, psychological, and cognitive factors (Fig. 1). For example, among immigrants, low English language proficiency could increase stress particularly for immigrants living in English dominant neighborhoods, which may, in turn, increase the risk for insomnia and poor sleep quality. Additionally, migration-related factors, such as acculturation stress, a type of psychological distress in response to the process of adapting and integrating to a new culture, can directly impact risk for insomnia through its effects on biological and cognitive pathways, such as hyperarousal and rumination. This, in turn, would negatively affect sleep. Also included in the conceptual model are

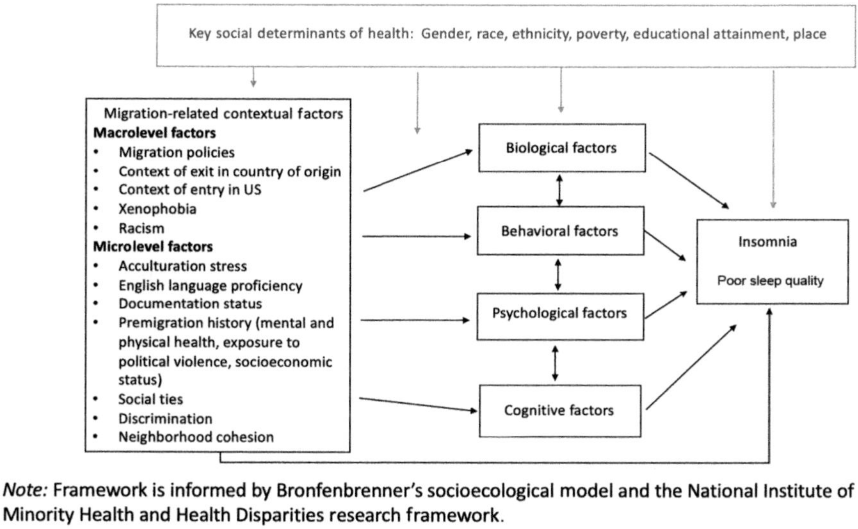

FIG. 1 Conceptual framework for the relationship between migration-related contextual factors and insomnia/poor sleep quality.

key social determinants of health (e.g., race, ethnicity, gender, socioeconomic status, place) that intersect with migration-related contextual factors and associated biological, psychological, cognitive, and behavioral mechanisms that affect risk for insomnia or poor sleep quality. Although a thorough discussion of these factors is beyond the scope of this chapter, previous research has demonstrated differential health outcomes at the intersections of these social determinants including socioeconomic status, race, and immigration status (Viruell-Fuentes, Miranda, & Abdulrahim, 2012).

Using a socioecological framework, we conducted a systematic review of the literature on insomnia and sleep quality among racial/ethnic minority immigrants living in the United States to (a) describe the sociodemographic characteristics of articles focused on immigrants and insomnia and related sleep quality, (b) describe the prevalence of insomnia and poor sleep quality among immigrants, and (c) summarize the state of the science on risk and protective factors of insomnia in Asian, Black, and Latinx immigrant samples, as well as combined US-born and immigrant racial/ethnic minority samples. Lastly, we discuss the implications for future research and clinical practice.

Methods

We searched the electronic databases PubMed, PsychINFO, CINAHL, and EBSCO for English-language or Spanish-language research articles published in peer-reviewed journals examining sleep outcomes in immigrant populations from inception until August 14, 2019. Search terms included variations of migrant identifications (e.g., immigrant, foreign-born, etc.), varying terms associated with insomnia and sleep quality (e.g., sleep disturbance, sleep disorder, etc.), searches with and without an age group identifier (i.e., adult), and variations of *United States*.

Article selection for inclusion in the systematic review was conducted through a two-step process. First, authors LGC, SVD, and MM conducted an initial title and abstract review of articles identified in the searches described above. To increase reliability, the authors reviewed 40 articles as a group to clarify inclusion and exclusion criteria. Studies were included into the next review process if they met the following inclusion criteria: included racial/ethnic minority populations and/or immigrant populations, assessed sleep quality-related outcomes, and focused on adults over the age of 18. Systematic reviews, meta-analyses, conference abstracts, dissertations, and case studies were not included in the second review.

In the second step of the review process, LGC, SVD, and MM conducted a full-text assessment to determine eligibility for inclusion in the final analysis. Two authors reviewed each article and determined its eligibility, noting reasons for exclusion. All discrepancies were discussed in the pairs. If the pairs did not reach consensus, a larger discussion with all study authors was held until a final decision was made. Studies were excluded if they: (1) were not conducted in the US mainland, Puerto Rico, or US territories, (2) were not in English or Spanish, (3) did not include immigrant populations in the sample or did not include factors associated with acculturation or migration-related processes in the analysis (e.g., nativity status, duration in the United States). Articles were additionally excluded for wrong study design and wrong sleep outcome.

Once the final set of articles was determined, the authors extracted relevant data from each article using a data extraction form. The authors extracted six articles in pairs until reaching above 70% internal reliability. The data extraction form included article information (title, author, and publication date), sample sociodemographic characteristics (average age, percentage race/ethnicity, percent female, percent or average years of education, income, and unemployment status), predictors, outcomes, and main findings. Individual-level factors were categorized into sociodemographic factors (e.g., gender), mental health conditions, migration-related factors (e.g., nativity status), and health behaviors and conditions. Importantly, acculturation, the active process of adopting and adapting to a new culture (Schwartz, Unger, Zamboanga, & Szapocznik, 2010), and acculturation stress, the psychological distress associated with the process of acculturation (Cervantes, Padilla, & Salgado de Snyder, 1991), were also included in migration-related factors. Social level factors were placed in two categories: social relationships (e.g., social support) or sociocultural stress (e.g., discrimination). Macro-level factors included those referring to housing, neighborhood, occupational, and health-care access factors. If articles included combined US-born and immigrant adults, we described moderation analyses by nativity status where appropriate. Below, we summarize the major findings by Asian, Black, Latinx, and multiethnic samples; multiethnic samples refer to articles that included three or more racial/ethnic groups in their analysis.

Results

In total, 482 unique records were identified and evaluated for initial inclusion in the title and abstract screening (Fig. 2). Of the 482 articles, 183 were reviewed in the full-text screening process. Of those, 153 did not meet eligibility criteria due to wrong participant population ($n=80$), wrong outcomes ($n=35$), wrong setting ($n=21$), and wrong study design ($n=17$). Only 30 articles met eligibility criteria and were included in the synthesis review.

Study characteristics

Study characteristics are summarized in Table 1. The range in sample size was 32–33,865. Most participants were female (60.51%), and immigrants (66.01%). On average, 39.48% received less than a high school education and 32.16% were unemployed. The average age of participants was 49.64 (SD=16.41). Only 11 (35.48%) articles exclusively sampled immigrants. Of these, 18.18% described the prevalence of insomnia and poor sleep quality in Asian immigrants. The remaining 81.82% articles examined the association of risk and protective factors with insomnia or poor sleep quality in immigrant samples. Of these, most (54.56%) articles exclusively sampled Latinx immigrants, followed by Asians immigrants (27.27%), and 0% Black immigrants. Combined US-born and immigrant samples were included in 19 articles examining the associations between acculturation or other migration-related factors and insomnia or sleep quality.

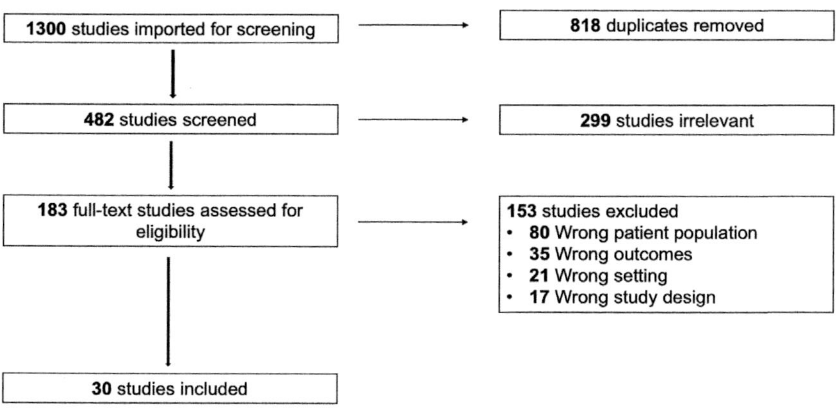

FIG. 2 PRISMA flow diagram.

TABLE 1 Sociodemographic characteristics of articles including Asian, Black, and Latinx immigrants in combined (US-born and immigrant) and immigrant only samples.

Article	Total *N*	% Immigrant	% Female	% White	% Latinx	% Black/AA	% Asian
Asian immigrants in combined (US-born and immigrant) and immigrant only samples							
Hirooka, Takedai, and D'Amico (2012)	93	100	59.1	NR	NR	NR	100
Hsu (2001)	80	100	NR	NR	NR	NR	100
Riley, Nazareno, and Malish (2016)	32	100	78	NR	NR	NR	NR
Sok (2008)	52	100	59.62	NR	NR	NR	100
Young, Xiong, Finn, and Young (2013)	747	100	38	NR	NR	NR	100
Black immigrants in combined (US-born and immigrant) and immigrant only samples							
Consedine, Magai, Cohen, and Gillespie (2002)	1118	54.38	62	39.99	NR	60.02	NR
Jean-Louis et al. (2001)	1118	54	62	40	NR	60	NR
Jean-Louis et al. (2008)	1394	67	100	22.45	11.84	43.54	NR
Latinx immigrants in combined (US-born and immigrant) and immigrant only samples							
Alcántara, Patel, et al. (2017)	5313	78.04	54.85	NA	100	NA	NA
Alcántara et al. (2019)	1192	72.3	NR	NR	100	NR	NR
D'Anna-Hernandez, Garcia, Coussons-Read, Laudenslager, & Ross (2016)	60	NR	100	NR	100	NR	NR

Age (M or %)	Country of origin	Education (% or M)	Yearly household income (% or M)	Unemployed
37.3(5.5)	Japan	NR	NR	54.8%
76.13	China	28.8% <High school	NR	NR
51	Philippines	NR	NR	NR
71.83	Korea	11.5% <High school	49.9% ≤$20,000	67.3%
40(13)	Vietnam	NR	NR	NR
73.8(5.9)	Jamaica, Trinidad, Barbados, Ukraine, Russia, Poland, and other Eastern European countries	40.04% <High school	$18.45K[a]	NR
74	Caribbean, mostly Eastern Europe, US	49% <High school	$18.5K[a]	NR
59.42	US, English-speaking Caribbean Islands, Haiti, Dominican Republic Eastern Europe	11.98 years	$31.52K[a]	NR
43.54% ≥45	Central American, Cuban, Dominican, Mexican, Puerto Rican, South American, More than one	32.53% <High school	71.44% <$30,000	NA
NR	NR	29.3% <High school	47.7% ≤$20,000	53.6%
96.7% <40	Mexico and US	55% <High school	88.3% ≤$30,000	35%

Continued

TABLE 1 Sociodemographic characteristics of articles including Asian, Black, and Latinx immigrants in combined (US-born and immigrant) and immigrant only samples—cont'd

Article	Total *N*	% Immigrant	% Female	% White	% Latinx	% Black/AA	% Asian
Garcini et al. (2018)	1332	29.65	56.8	NR	100	NR	NR
Green et al. (2010)	419	NR	100	33.89	66.11	NR	NR
Grzywacz et al. (2011)	122	100	10.7	NR	100	NR	NR
Latinx immigrants in combined (US-born and Immigrant) and immigrant only samples							
Heilemann et al. (2012)	312	53	10	NR	100	NR	NR
Kelly (2010)	33	100	100	NR	100	NR	NR
Manber et al. (2013)	1289	39.80	100	NR	100	NR	NR
Martinez-Miller et al. (2019)	2929	GEN1[b]: 50.1; GEN2[b]: 24.6, GEN1-parents[b]: 49.3, GEN2-offspring[b]: 25.5	62.73	NR	100	NR	NR
Riley et al. (2008)	911	74	71	NR	NR	NR	NR
Sandberg et al. (2012)	300	100	15(5)	NR	100	NR	NR
Sandberg et al. (2014)	371	100	0	NR	100	NR	NR
Sandberg et al. (2016)	147	100	0	NR	100	NR	NR
Seicean and Seicean (2010)	1806	100	47.23	NR	100	NR	NR
Seicean, Neuhauser, Strohl, and Redline (2011)	5160	12	58.24	NR	20.19	NR	NR

Age (M or %)	Country of origin	Education (% or M)	Yearly household income (% or M)	Unemployed
46(14.9)	Primarily Mexico	10.7(3.5)	NR	38.5%
46.3	Central America, South America, Puerto Rico, Dominican Republic, Cuba	53.5% >High school	NR	NR
41% ≥40	NR	50.8% 0–6 years; 40.2% 7–9; 9% 10+	NR	0%
28 (5.6)	Mexican descent	39.5% <High school	91% ≤$2900	54%
39.7	NR	NR	NR	NR
26.5 (6.7)	NR	48.9% <High school	90% ≤$30,000	73.8%
61.85	Mexico, Central America, South America	52.55% <High school	NR	4.95%
NR	NR	NR	NR	NR
32% ≥40	NR	53.7% 0–6 years; 46.3% 7 or more years	NR	0%
≥40 26.7%	NR	NR	NR	0%
39.18 (7.5)	Mexico	91.84% <High school	NR	0%
40.98	Mexico or other Latin American country	56.98% <High school	35.43%[c]	NR
40.97	Mexico and US	36.5% <High school	2.47[d]	NR

Continued

TABLE 1 Sociodemographic characteristics of articles including Asian, Black, and Latinx immigrants in combined (US-born and immigrant) and immigrant only samples—cont'd

Article	Total *N*	% Immigrant	% Female	% White	% Latinx	% Black/AA	% Asian
Latinx immigrants in combined (US-born and immigrant) and immigrant only samples							
Simonelli et al. (2017)	2156	83.12	64.75	NR	100	NR	NR
Multiethnic immigrants in combined (US-born and immigrant) and immigrant only samples							
Chen, Redline, Shields, Williams, and Williams (2014)	3330	21.38	47.48	47.84	19.07	21.38	NR
Cunningham, Ford, Chapman, Liu, and Croft (2015)	33,865	18.91	55.74	59.86	16.94	14.74	6.07
Grandner et al. (2013)	5,587	Born in Mexico: 4.14 Born in Other Country: 9.7	48.05	72.81	12.15	10.29	4.75
Hale, Troxel, Kravitz, Hall, and Matthews (2014)	1180	34.75	100	41.1	28.20	NR	Chinese: 32.8 Japanese 39.0
Slopen and Williams (2014)	2983	14.08	52.9	42	26	32	NR

Notes: This table includes articles with immigrant samples exclusively and US-born and immigrant combined samples.
[a] *Average household income $K.*
[b] *This sample included GEN1: older adults from the Sacramento Area Latino Study on Aging (SALSA), GEN2: middle-aged ad… from Niños Lifestyle and Diabetes Study (NLDS), GEN1-parents: Matched parents from SALSA with offspring from NLDS, and GEN2-offspring: Matched offspring with parents from SALSA.*
[c] *This refers to family income below or at the US poverty level.*
[d] *Measured using poverty income ratio.*

Age (M or %)	Country of origin	Education (% or M)	Yearly household income (% or M)	Unemployed
47 (11.6)	Central America, Cuba, Dominican Republic, Mexico, Puerto Rico, South America	NR	49.4% <$20,000	41.80%
≥40 76.29%	NR	26.79% <High school	22.73%[d] Low Income	NR
> 65 78.82%	NR	15.88% <High school	NR	NR
46.54	Mexico and other countries	32.68% <High school	13.52% <$20,000	NR
45.8(2.7)	China, Japan, Latin America	25.4% <High school	NR	19.7%
42.3 (0.4)	NR	23.5% <High school	36.8% ≤$30,000	38.9%

Prevalence

Asian immigrants

There were no population-based articles that provided estimates on the prevalence of insomnia exclusively among Asian immigrants. However, in a large national sample of 1180 middle-aged women, Hale et al. (2014) found that overall 25.4% of Chinese, Japanese, and Latinx immigrants experienced at least one insomnia symptom. Results from a regional study with a convenience sample of 52 Korean American immigrant older adults living in Pittsburgh indicate that 82.60% reported having interrupted sleep and 17.80% met criteria for clinically significant insomnia (Sok, 2008). Results from a regional study with a convenience sample of 95 Japanese immigrants living in Pittsburgh found that 21.6% of Japanese men and 27.3% of Japanese women reported not sleeping well (Hirooka et al., 2012).

Black immigrants

While there were no population-based articles that provided estimates on the prevalence of insomnia among Black immigrants, two community-based studies with sizeable samples of Black immigrants provided data on the distribution of sleep quality. In a large study of adults living in Brooklyn, New York, Jean-Louis et al. (2001) found that among 435 Caribbean immigrants, 16% reported difficulty initiating sleep, 6% had difficulty maintaining sleep, and 13% experienced early morning awakenings. In a related study also conducted in Brooklyn, New York with a random sample of 1440 African American and African Caribbean women, 9% of English-speaking Caribbean women, 19% of Haitian women, and 35% of Dominican women reported difficulty initiating sleep (Jean-Louis et al., 2008). Difficulty maintaining sleep was reported by 32% of English-speaking Caribbean women, 26% of Haitian women, and 62% of Dominican women. Lastly, 15% of English-speaking Caribbean women, 20% of Haitian women, and 54% of Dominican women reported early morning awakening. Although it is unclear whether all of the women in the study by Jean-Louis et al. (2008) were immigrants, this is the only article that provided estimates on the distribution of cardinal insomnia symptoms by ethnicity in a large sample of Black adults.

Latinx immigrants

There were two population-based articles that used data from the National Health and Nutrition Examination Survey (NHANES) to generate estimates on the prevalence of insomnia among Latinx immigrants. Seicean and Seicean (2010) found that in a sample of 1806 Mexican and Latinx immigrants, 12.08% of men and 22.14% of women reported mild/moderate insomnia (insomnia symptoms 6–15 times per month) and 4.30% of men and 9.42% of women reported severe insomnia (insomnia symptoms more than 15 times per month).

Similarly, in a related study using NHANES data of US-born Mexican and immigrant Mexican adults, Seicean et al. (2011) found that 11.8% and 21.3% of immigrant Mexican men and women reported mild/moderate insomnia, respectively, and 4.2% of immigrant men and 7.17% of immigrant women reported severe insomnia (Seicean et al., 2011).

In combined samples of US-born and immigrant Latinx adults, the prevalence of insomnia varied from 14.9% to 29.83% in population-based samples (Alcántara et al., 2019; Alcántara, Patel, et al., 2017). In a state-level sample of menopausal women living in New Jersey, 66.1% of Puerto Rican women, 26.4% of Cuban women, 51.7% of Central American women, and 45.3% of South American women reported trouble sleeping due to difficulty initiating or maintaining sleep, early morning awakenings, and overall poor sleep quality (Green et al., 2010). Although Green et al. (2010) did not specify if women included in the sample were immigrants, this is the only article reporting differences by country of origin in a Latinx sample.

Risk and protective factors of insomnia and poor sleep quality in immigrant adults

Table 2 summarizes the major findings for the risk and protective factors of insomnia among racial/ethnic minority immigrants categorized by socioecological levels of analysis. Among the subset of 11 articles focused on immigrants, five articles sampled Asian immigrants exclusively and six sampled Latinx immigrants exclusively. None exclusively sampled Black immigrants. Of these 11 articles, two did not provide analyses of risk and/or protective factors of insomnia, and therefore, are not discussed below. The nine articles described included at least one individual-level factor, including acculturation and migration-related factors in their analyses. Macro-level factors were the next most commonly examined factors ($n=5$), and finally social level factors ($n=1$).

Asian immigrants

Sociodemographic factors

In a convenience sample of 32 Filipino live-in caregivers in Los Angeles, women reported significantly lower sleep quality and restfulness than men (Riley et al., 2016). In contrast, results from a population-based sample of 747 Hmong immigrants living in Wisconsin indicated that being male was significantly associated with increased odds of difficulty sleeping and restless sleep when compared to being female (Young et al., 2013). The relationship between age and insomnia symptoms was not statistically significant among convenience samples of Hmong immigrants or Chinese immigrant older adults living in Seattle (Hsu, 2001; Young et al., 2013).

TABLE 2 Risk and protective factors for insomnia and poor sleep quality among Asian, Black, and Latinx US immigrant adults.

Article	Study location	Country of origin	Duration in US	Outcomes	Major findings
Asian immigrants					
Hsu (2001)	Seattle, Washington	China	25% 5–19 years; 27.5%11–15 years; 13.8%16–20 years; 13.8% 21–25 years; 16.2%> 25 years	Sleep quality[a]	**Statistically significant risk factors**: Increasing depression symptom severity and increasing number of medical conditions were significantly and positively correlated with worsening sleep quality in Chinese immigrants (r=0.478, P<.001; r=0.221, P=.049)
					Not statistically significant: Age, napping, exercise, church attendance, and the length of residence in the US were not statistically associated with sleep quality
Riley et al. (2016)	Los Angeles, California	Philippines	NR	Sleep quality	**Statistically significant risk factors**: Women rated their sleep quality and restfulness significantly lower than men (2.9 vs. 3.8, P=.019, 2.8 vs. 3.8, P=.021). Filipino immigrants reported significantly lower sleep quality and feeling less restfulness on workdays than nonworkdays (3.2 vs. 3.8, 3.1 vs. 3.8, P<.05). They also reported significantly more days with trouble sleeping and or waking on mixed work and nonworkdays when compared to full workdays (2.9 vs. 3.8, 2.8 vs. 3.8, P<.05)
					Not statistically significant: Though not significantly different, those hired through homecare agencies reported lower sleep quality scores than those hired directly by patients or guardians
Young et al. (2013)	Wisconsin	Vietnam	15 (6) years	Insomnia	**Statistically significant risk factors**: Being male was associated with increased odds of having difficulty getting to sleep and restless sleep in Vietnamese immigrants (OR=1.67, 1.58, P<.0001). Experiencing dab tsog[b] and having chronic pain were associated with increased odds of having difficulty getting to sleep and having restless sleep (OR=1.86, 1.49, P<.001; OR=2.72, 3.31, P<.001). Having stressful experiences in the Vietnam War were associated with increased in odds of having restless sleep (OR=1.91, P<.001)
					Not statistically significant: Age, knowing instances of SUNDS[c] among relatives or friends and acculturation proxies (practicing Shamanism, adhering to a Hmong diet and number of years living in United States), diabetes, heart problems, hypertension, and average number living in household were not statistically associated with insomnia symptoms

Black immigrants					
					No articles examining risk and protective factors in exclusively Black immigrant samples
Latinx immigrants					
Grzywacz et al. (2011)	North Carolina	NR	NR	Daytime sleepiness[d]	**Statistically significant risk factors**: Increasing depressive symptom severity was associated with increasing daytime sleepiness ($\beta=0.20$, SE=0.05, $P<.001$) in Latinx farmworkers
					Not statistically significant: Gender, a history of depressive symptoms, and having a H-2A visa were not statistically associated with daytime sleepiness
Kelly (2010)	Urban area in New England	NR	NR	Sleep difficulty	**Statistically significant risk factors**: Having a PTSD diagnosis, an MDD diagnosis, and co-morbid PTSD and MDD were also positively associated with increasing sleep difficulty ($r=0.476$, 0.86, 0.391, $P<.001$) in Latinx sample of immigrant women. Increasing PTDS symptoms severity and increasing MDD symptoms severity were both associated with increasing sleeping difficulty ($r=0.751$, 0.568, $P<.01$). Childhood sexual assault was positively correlated with increasing sleeping difficulty ($r=0.349$, $P<.05$). Worsening health-related quality of life outcomes were positively correlated with increasing sleeping difficulty (physical health appraisal: $r=0.433$, mental health appraisal: $r=0.521$, days physical health not good: $r=0.483$, days mental health not good: $r=0.411$, impaired daily activity: $r=0.400$, all at $P<.01$). Documentation status was positively associated with increasing sleeping difficulty ($r=0.428$, $P<.05$)
					Not statistically significant: Severity of psychological abuse, physical abuse, sexual abuse, adult sexual assault, and adult sexual assault in the past year were not statistically correlated with sleeping difficulty in Latinx immigrant women

Continued

TABLE 2 Risk and protective factors for insomnia and poor sleep quality among Asian, Black, and Latinx US immigrant adults—cont'd

Article	Study location	Country of origin	Duration in US	Outcomes	Major findings
Latinx immigrants					
Sandberg et al. (2012)	North Carolina	NR	13.7% ≤ 1 year in US agriculture; 47% 2–7 years in US agriculture; 39.3% ≥ 8 + years in US agriculture	Daytime Sleepines[d]	**Statistically significant risk factors**: In bivariate analyses, those who were 40 years of age or older reported elevated daytime sleepiness significantly more frequently than their younger counterparts (56.3% vs. 18–24: 3.1%, 25–29: 15.6%, 30–39: 25%, $P=.01$) in a Latinx male farmworkers. Increasing depressive symptom severity was positively correlated with increasing daytime sleepiness ($r=0.27$, $P<.001$). Those who had 8 or more years in US agriculture (i.e., number of seasons spent in cyclical migration due to farm work) reported elevated daytime sleepiness significantly more frequently (62.5%) than those with 1 year or less (6.3%) or 2–7 years (31.3%) in agriculture ($P=.01$)
					Statistically significant protective factors: Increasing musculoskeletal pain severity was negatively correlated with daytime sleepiness ($r=-0.15$, $P<.01$)
					Not statistically significant: There was no statistically significant differences in elevated daytime sleepiness by educational attainment, gender, or language spoken (English vs. Indigenous)
Sandberg et al. (2014)	North Carolina	NR	NR	Sleep quality[e]	**Statistically significant risk factors**: Elevated anxiety was associated with 0.96 decreased odds of good sleep quality in a sample of 371 Latinx immigrant men (OR = 0.96, 95% CI: 0.93–0.99)
					Statistically significant protective factors: Few depressive symptoms and no or low pain were associated with increased odds of good sleep quality when compared to elevated depressive symptoms and elevated pain (OR = 3.19, 95% CI: 1.39–7.32; OR = 3.41, 95% CI: 1.76–6.61). Having air conditioning in housing unit was associated with increase in odds of having good sleep quality (OR = 2.43, 95% CI: 1.33–4.43)
					Not statistically significant: Educational attainment, age, marital status, reporting good health, alcohol consumption, smoking status, the number of people in the housing unit, and the quality of the sleep room were not statistically associated with good sleep quality

Latinx immigrants					
Sandberg et al. (2016)	North Carolina	Mexico	NR	Sleep quality[a]	**Statistically significant risk factors**: Those with elevated depressive symptoms were significantly more likely to report poor sleep quality than good sleep quality (44.44% vs. 55.56%, $P<.001$) in Mexican immigrant men. Those with few depressive symptoms were more likely to report good sleep quality than poor sleep quality (85.51% vs. 14.49%, $P<.001$)
					Not statistically significant: There was no statistically significant associations between working more than 40 hours a week, working when the heat index reached 91, workplace safety, workplace flexibility, workplace vulnerability, lifetime pesticide exposure, age, problem drinking, smoking status, caffeine intake, obesity, chronic conditions, educational attainment, or anxiety, and sleep quality. Working more than 40 hours a week and having a high lifetime pesticide exposure were marginally associated with poor sleep quality ($P<.10$)
Seicean and Seicean (2010)	National sample	Mexico and other Latin American Countries	Proportion of lifetime in migration: 39% Mexican born Males; 46% non-Mexico born Males; 42%, Mexico-born females; 45% non-Mexico born Females	Insomnia	**Statistically significant risk factors**: Having elevated depressive symptoms was associated with increased odds of having severe insomnia among Latin American immigrants (OR = 7.80, 95% CI: 3.50–19.50). Reporting fair or poor overall general health was associated with increased odds of severe insomnia among Latin American immigrants (OR = 2.90, 95% CI: 1.50–5.70)
					Statistically significant protective factors: Being a Mexico-born immigrant was associated with decreased odds of severe insomnia than being an immigrant from another Latin American country (OR = 0.40, 95% CI: 0.20–0.70)
					Not statistically significant: Educational attainment, age, gender, poverty income ratio, living without a partner, the proportion of lifetime in immigration, being an adult at the time of emigration, speaking mostly English or only English language at home, not having health insurance, were not statistically associated with severe insomnia among immigrants from a Latin American country of origin other than Mexico

Notes: This table includes only articles with exclusively sampled Asian and Latinx immigrants and tested the relationship between risk and protective factors of insomnia and sleep quality across socioecological levels. There were no articles on risk and protective factors that exclusively sampled Black immigrants. There were two additional articles that exclusively sampled immigrants, but these did not assess risk and protective factors. The remaining 19 articles included combined US-born and immigrant samples and are not described qualitatively in the Results.

[a] *Measured with Pittsburgh Sleep Quality Index.*

[b] *Dab tsog is a culturally specific indicator of distress in Hmong culture.*

[c] *SUNDS refers to Sudden Unexplained Nocturnal Death Syndrome.*

[d] *Measured with Epworth Sleepiness Scale.*

[e] *Measured with Sleep Timing and Sleep Quality Screening Questionnaire.*

Mental health conditions

Hsu (2001) found that depressive symptoms severity was significantly and positively correlated with worsening sleep quality among Chinese older adults. In a sample of Hmong immigrants, Sudden Unexplained Nocturnal Death Syndrome (SUNDS), sudden death during sleep prevalent in South East Asian communities, was not statistically associated with difficulty falling asleep or restless sleep (Young et al., 2013). However, knowledge and experience of dab tsog, a culturally specific indicator of distress, and having any traumatic experience (e.g., being in the army, being exposed to chemical warfare, losing family or relatives, etc.) in the Vietnam War were associated with increased odds of restless sleep in this sample (Young et al., 2013). In one of the few studies to test protective factors for insomnia, frequency of church attendance was not significantly associated with sleep quality among Chinese immigrant older adults (Hsu, 2001).

Acculturation and migration-related factors

Duration in the United States, measured by the number of years since immigration, was not significantly associated with insomnia symptoms or poor sleep quality among Chinese immigrant older adults and Hmong immigrants (Hsu, 2001; Young et al., 2013). Cultural practices such as practicing Shamanism, a prominent religion in Hmong culture, and adhering to a Hmong diet, both utilized as acculturation proxies, were not significantly related to insomnia symptoms among Hmong immigrants (Young et al., 2013).

Other acculturation factors were also tested in combined US-born and immigrant samples of Asian adults. In a national sample of middle-aged US-born and immigrant Japanese, Chinese, and Latinx women, being US-born was not statistically associated with sleep complaints but being more acculturated, defined as speaking English more often than another language, was associated with a 1.09 increase in odds (95% CI: 1.01–1.17) of reporting sleep complaints among Japanese women (Hale et al., 2014). In contrast, among Chinese women being US-born was associated with 2.41 increased odds of reporting sleep complaints (95% CI: 1.03–5.61) and being more acculturated was not associated with sleep complaints.

Health behaviors and health conditions

Among Chinese immigrant older adults, the number of naps, a potential risk factor, and regular exercise, a potential protective factor, were not significantly associated with poor sleep quality (Hsu, 2001). Young et al. (2013) found that chronic pain was associated with increased odds of experiencing difficulty falling asleep and restless sleep, respectively, but diabetes, heart problems, and hypertension were not significantly associated with these insomnia symptoms among Hmong adults (Young et al., 2013).

Macro-level factors

Young et al. (2013) found that the number of people living in a household was not significantly associated with difficulty falling asleep or restless sleep among

Hmong immigrants. Filipino live-in caregivers rated their sleep quality and restfulness significantly lower on workdays than on nonworkdays (Riley et al., 2016). These caregivers also reported having trouble sleeping and waking significantly more frequently on days when they worked part of the time or did not work at all (trouble sleeping: 51% vs. 71%, 72%; trouble waking: 65% vs. 88%, 80%, $P < .05$) (Riley et al., 2016). Caregivers hired by home care agencies reported lower sleep quality than those hired by patients or guardians directly although these differences were not statistically significant (Riley et al., 2016).

Summary of findings for Asian immigrants

While gender was inconsistently associated with insomnia and poor sleep quality across Asian immigrant samples from Vietnam, China, Japan, and the Philippines, age was not associated with insomnia. Depression, experiencing trauma, and pain were associated with worsening sleep quality. Although in immigrant samples duration in the United States and acculturation were not significantly associated with insomnia, in a combined immigrant and US-born sample acculturation and nativity status were associated with sleep complaints. The only macro-level factor associated with poor sleep quality was the work schedule of Filipino live-in caregivers.

Black immigrants

Acculturation and migration-related factors

Although none of the articles sampled Black immigrants exclusively, three articles examined risk and protective factors among US-born and immigrant Black adults. In a sample of 1118 older African American, African Caribbean, European American, and Eastern European adults, identifying as a African Caribbean, meaning being an immigrant from a English-speaking Caribbean country including Jamaica, Trinidad, and Barbados, was significantly and negatively associated with sleep disturbances when compared to US-born European Americans (Consedine et al., 2002). In a similar study, Jean-Louis et al. (2001) found that those who identified as African Caribbean, meaning being born or having parents who were born in a Caribbean country, reported fewer sleep complaints than US-born African Americans, though this difference was not statistically tested. In a sample of 1140 menopausal women, Jean-Louis et al. (2008) found that Dominican women (35%) had a significantly higher prevalence of difficulty sleeping than Haitian women (19%) and significantly higher prevalence of difficulty maintaining sleep (62%), and early morning awakening (54%) than Haitian (26%; 20%) and English-Speaking Caribbean women (32%; 15%).

Mental health conditions

Consedine et al. (2002) found that immigrant status significantly modified the association between negative affect (anger, sadness, fear, and shame) and sleep disturbances and the relationship between emotion inhibition and sleep disturbances in a sample of African American, African Caribbean, European American, and Eastern European adults. In particular, the adverse effect of negative affect and emotion inhibition on sleep disturbances was reduced for African Caribbean immigrants compared to US-born European Americans (Consedine et al., 2002).

Summary of findings for Black immigrants

Three articles included Black immigrants from Jamaica, Trinidad, Barbados, Haiti, the Dominican Republic, and other English-speaking Caribbean countries in their samples. Identifying as an African Caribbean immigrant vs. identifying as European American was associated with lower sleep complaints and a more attenuated association between negative affect and emotion inhibition and sleep disturbances.

Latinx immigrants

Sociodemographic factors

Educational attainment was not statistically associated with daytime sleepiness, sleep quality, or insomnia among samples of Latinx farmworkers and an aggregate Latinx immigrant sample (Sandberg et al., 2012, 2016; Seicean & Seicean, 2010). Socioeconomic status, measured by the poverty income ratio, was also not significantly associated with severe insomnia (Seicean & Seicean, 2010). Similarly, age when measured continuously was not significantly related to sleep quality or severe insomnia among Mexican male farmworkers (Sandberg et al., 2016). However, when age was tested as a categorical variable in a sample of Latinx male and female farmworkers, participants aged 40 or older reported elevated daytime sleepiness significantly more frequently than their younger counterparts in unadjusted bivariate analyses (Sandberg et al., 2012). In a nationally representative sample of Latinx immigrants, univariate analyses found that a 5-year increase in age was significantly associated with 1.20 increased odds of severe insomnia (95% CI: 1.10–1.20), but this relationship was no longer statistically significant when adjusting for other sociodemographic characteristics, health insurance, and health characteristics (Seicean & Seicean, 2010).

The findings on the association of gender with insomnia, and/or sleep quality were consistently not statistically significant in samples of Mexican and Latinx farmworkers and in a nationally representative sample of Latinx immigrants (Grzywacz et al., 2011; Sandberg et al., 2012; Seicean & Seicean, 2010).

Marital status was not significantly associated with sleep quality among a sample of 371 male Spanish-speaking Latinx farmworkers in North Carolina (Sandberg et al., 2014). Relatedly, not living with a partner was not significantly associated with severe insomnia in a national sample of Latinx immigrants (Seicean & Seicean, 2010).

Mental health conditions

Depression

Having a diagnosis of major depressive disorder (MDD) and MDD symptom severity were positively correlated with worsening sleep difficulty among Latina immigrant women who experienced intimate partner violence (IPV) (Kelly, 2010). Elevated depressive symptoms were also associated with poor sleep quality among four separate samples of Mexican and Latinx farmworkers (Grzywacz et al., 2011; Sandberg et al., 2012, 2016, 2014). In a nationally representative sample of Latinx immigrants, having elevated depressive symptoms were also associated with 7.80 increased odds of severe insomnia (95% CI: 3.50–17.50) (Seicean & Seicean, 2010).

Anxiety

While higher levels of anxiety were significantly associated with 0.96 decreased odds of good sleep quality (95% CI: 0.93–0.99) when controlling for housing quality, health quality, health behaviors, and sociodemographic characteristics among Spanish-speaking male Latino farmworkers (Sandberg et al., 2014), in a similar study conducted by Sandberg et al. (2016), there was no statistically significant relationship between anxiety and sleep quality among Mexican male farmworkers in North Carolina. Among Latina women who experienced IPV, PTSD symptoms and worsening mental health status were positively correlated with sleep difficulty (Kelly, 2010). Kelly (2010) also found that experiencing childhood sexual assault was significantly and positively correlated with sleep difficulty, while other types of trauma were not significantly associated with sleep difficulty.

Acculturation and migration-related factors

Documentation status

In a small sample of 33 immigrant Latina women, being undocumented was positively correlated with increasing sleep difficulty at statistically significant levels (Kelly, 2010). Among Latinx immigrant farmworkers, those who did not possess an H-2A visa, a temporary visa specifically granted for agricultural work, had elevated daytime sleepiness when compared to those who had an H-2A visa, though this difference was not statistically significant (Grzywacz et al., 2011).

Language use

Findings on the association of language use with insomnia symptoms/poor sleep quality are mixed. For example, neither speaking English nor an Indigenous language were statistically associated with daytime sleepiness in Latinx immigrant farmworkers in North Carolina (Sandberg et al., 2012). However, in a study sampling 1289 pregnant Latina women, completing study measures in English was associated with 2.61 increased odds (95% CI: 1.80–3.79) of having clinically significant insomnia compared to those who completed the measures in Spanish (Manber et al., 2013). Similarly, in a national sample of 1118 menopausal Latina women, speaking more English than Spanish was associated with increased odds of sleep complaints (Hale et al., 2014). In contrast, in a sample of 911 Latinx adults in South Florida, speaking Spanish more often than English was associated with a significant increase in sleep difficulty (Riley et al., 2008). Yet another study in national sample of 1042 US-born and immigrant Mexican adults, speaking Spanish and English equally in comparison to speaking only Spanish was associated with increased odds of insomnia in unadjusted models (Seicean et al., 2011), but after further adjustment for sociodemographic and psychosocial factors, the association was no longer statistically significant.

Duration in United States

Among Latinx farmworkers, those who had spent 8 or more years in US agriculture (i.e., number of seasons spent in cyclical migration due to farm work), were more likely to report elevated daytime sleepiness than those who had spent fewer years in seasonal agricultural work in bivariate analyses (Sandberg et al., 2012). Relatedly, in a national sample of Latinx immigrants, Seicean and Seicean (2010) found that proportion lifetime in immigration, estimated by dividing the duration in the United States by the participant's age at the time of data collection, was not significantly associated with severe insomnia. Being an adult at the time of immigration, was also not significantly associated with severe insomnia (Seicean & Seicean, 2010).

Country of origin

In a national sample of Mexican and Other Latinx immigrants, being a Mexico-born immigrant compared to being born in another Latin American country was associated with a 60% decrease in odds of severe insomnia adjusting for sociodemographic factors, health conditions, and health-care access (Seicean & Seicean, 2010).

Nativity status

Results from combined samples testing differences in insomnia or poor sleep quality by nativity status (whether US-born or immigrant) found that being an immigrant was inconsistently associated with sleep quality. In a national sample of menopausal Latina women, being an immigrant was not statistically associated with sleep complaints (Hale et al., 2014). However, convenience and population-based study both found that being an immigrant was associated with less sleep difficulty when compared to being US-born (Riley et al., 2008; Seicean et al., 2011). More specifically, in a community sample of US-born and immigrant adults in Sacramento, California, being a third-generation immigrant or greater was associated with a 40% decrease in prevalence of restless sleep when compared to the first-generation immigrant, while second-generation immigrants did not have a significantly different prevalence of restless sleep than first-generation immigrants (Martinez-Miller et al., 2019).

Acculturation

Although acculturation was not tested in immigrant only studies, there was evidence of the importance of this sociocultural factor for insomnia and sleep quality among combined US-born and immigrant Latinx adult samples. In a convenience sample of 60 Mexican-American pregnant women, higher levels of US acculturation was associated with feeling less refreshed upon awakening (D'Anna-Hernandez et al., 2016). Similarly, in a sample of 911 Latinx adults in South Florida, identifying more with US culture, an indicator of acculturation, was associated with increased sleep difficulty (Riley et al., 2008). In one of the first studies to examine the relationship between intergenerational acculturation and sleep in a Latinx sample using parent-offspring matched subsamples from the longitudinal studies Sacramento Area Latino Study on Aging and Niños Lifestyle and Diabetes Study, Martinez-Miller et al. (2019) found that intergenerational US acculturation, operationalized as the match or discrepancy in the level of US acculturation between parents and children across their lifetime, was not significantly associated with prevalence of restless sleep among the adult children (Martinez-Miller et al., 2019).

Acculturation stress

The only studies examining the relationship between acculturation stress and insomnia were conducted in combined population-based samples of US-born and immigrant Latinx adults. Alcántara et al. (2019) and Alcántara, Patel, et al. (2017) found that increasing acculturation stress was significantly associated with increasing insomnia symptom severity when adjusting for sociodemographic, health, other psychosocial stressors, and mental health conditions. This association was no longer statistically significant with a final adjustment for depressive symptoms. Importantly, nativity status (US-born vs. immigrants) did not modify the association of acculturation stress and insomnia (Alcántara et al., 2019).

Health behaviors and health conditions

In both a nationally representative sample of Latinx immigrants and samples of Mexican and Latinx farmworkers in North Carolina, alcohol consumption, smoking cigarettes, and caffeine intake were not significantly associated with severe insomnia or sleep quality (Sandberg et al., 2016, 2014; Seicean & Seicean, 2010).

Among Latina immigrant women who experienced IPV, measures indicating poor health status (e.g., perceived poor physical health, number of days with poor health, daily activity impairment) were positively correlated with increasing sleep difficulty (Kelly, 2010). Similarly, in a national sample of Latinx immigrants, fair to poor overall general health was associated with increased odds of severe insomnia (Seicean & Seicean, 2010). On the other hand, good to excellent health was not significantly associated with sleep quality among male Latinx farmworkers (Sandberg et al., 2016). More specific measures of physical health such as obesity, central obesity, and chronic conditions were not significantly associated with severe insomnia among Latinx immigrants or among male Latino farmworkers (Sandberg et al., 2014; Seicean & Seicean, 2010). Increasing musculoskeletal pain severity had a weak but statistically significant negative correlation with daytime sleepiness among Latinx male and female farmworkers in North Carolina (Sandberg et al., 2012). In a similar sample of male Latinx farmworkers, no or low pain was associated with increased odds of reporting good sleep quality when compared to elevated pain (Sandberg et al., 2014).

Sociocultural stress and social relationships

Sandberg et al. (2016) tested the effects of social support from employers and sleep quality among Mexican male farmworkers and found that it was not statistically related to sleep quality. Other sociocultural stressors were tested in combined US-born and immigrant Latinx adult samples. Alcántara et al. (2019) and Alcántara, Patel, et al. (2017) found that both ethnic discrimination and chronic stress burden were significantly associated with increasing insomnia symptom severity, nativity status did not moderate these associations (Alcántara et al., 2019). Similarly, in mediation analyses, perceived racial/ethnic discrimination was directly and indirectly associated with sleep disturbances through psychological distress and this relationship was comparable between US-born and immigrant Latinx adults (Garcini et al., 2018). In a convenience sample of White, Black, US-born Latinx, and immigrant Latinx adults living in Chicago, there were no significant differences in the number of sleep difficulties reported between immigrant Latinx adults and US-born Whites in models adjusting for racial and nonracial discrimination experiences (Slopen & Williams, 2014).

Macro-level factors

Housing

Sandberg et al. (2014) found that the availability of air conditioning in the home was statistically associated with 2.43 increased odds of good sleep quality (95% CI: 1.33–4.43) when controlling for sociodemographic characteristics, health conditions, and other housing quality measures. Other housing-related features (i.e., number of people in the housing unit and the quality of the room used for sleeping) were not statistically associated with sleep quality (Sandberg et al., 2014).

Occupational environment

Among a sample of male Latino farmworkers, the effects of lifetime pesticide exposure and working when the heat index reaches 91°F were not statistically associated with poor sleep quality (Sandberg et al., 2016). Among Mexican immigrant male farmworkers, occupational factors (i.e., workplace safety and flexibility) were also not significantly associated with sleep quality (Sandberg et al., 2016). However, working more than 40 hours a week was marginally associated with sleep quality in unadjusted models (Sandberg et al., 2016).

Neighborhood

In a combined US-born and immigrant Latinx population-based sample, insomnia was 4.4% points higher in neighborhoods perceived as noisy when compared to those not perceived as noisy in models adjusted for sociodemographic factors, sleep apnea severity, and depressive symptoms (Simonelli et al., 2017). In contrast, perceived neighborhood violence and safety were not significantly associated with insomnia symptoms (Simonelli et al., 2017). Importantly, nativity status did not moderate the relationship between neighborhood noise and insomnia (Simonelli et al., 2017).

Health-care access

In a nationally representative sample of Mexican and other Latinx US immigrants, health insurance status was not significantly associated with insomnia (Seicean et al., 2011).

Summary of findings for Latinx immigrants

Educational attainment, socioeconomic status, gender, and marital status were not significantly associated with insomnia across Latinx samples from Mexico and other Latin American countries. Increasing age was inconsistently associated with insomnia symptoms. Depression, PTSD, pain, and physical health were consistently associated with poor sleep quality while the findings of anxiety and sleep quality were mixed. Several migration-related and macro-level factors (i.e., acculturation and acculturation stress, discrimination, neighborhood noise levels, etc.) were associated with poor sleep outcomes, though not all analyses found statistically significant associations.

Multiethnic immigrant samples

Sociodemographic factors

Although immigrant specific outcomes were not reported, Cunningham et al. (2015) found that the relationship between educational attainment and insomnia was moderated by race/ethnicity. Among Latinx adults, an increase in educational attainment was associated with an increase in odds of insomnia when adjusting for nativity status, but this relationship was not observed among Asian, Black, or other races/ethnicities.

Acculturation and migration-related factors

Two studies using national samples of multiethnic US-born and immigrant adults including one study sampling Black/African American, Mexican American, Latinx, and Asian adults, and the other sampling Latina, Chinese, Japanese, and White menopausal women found that being an immigrant was associated with decreased odds of reporting insomnia symptoms (Grandner et al., 2013; Hale et al., 2014). A third study, using a national sample of 3330 African American, Latinx, White, and other racial/ethnic US adults, found no significant differences between US-born and immigrant adults in the relationship between allostatic load, measured through nine biomarkers of cardiovascular, inflammatory, and metabolic system functioning, and insomnia in stratified analyses by nativity status (Chen et al., 2014).

Hale et al. (2014) also tested the relationship between acculturation and insomnia symptoms in a sample of Latina, Chinese, and Japanese US-born and immigrant women, and found that among all immigrants greater acculturation to US culture was associated with 1.05 increased odds of reporting sleep complaints in models adjusting for nativity status, sociodemographic characteristics, health behaviors, BMI, depressive symptoms, use of folk and sleep medicines (95% CI: 1.01–1.09) (Hale et al., 2014).

Summary of finding for multiethnic immigrant samples

In multiethnic national samples of immigrant and US-born Chinese, Japanese, Black, Mexican, and Latinx adults, immigrant status was associated with lower sleep complaints when compared to US-born status. Acculturation was associated with increased odds of reporting sleep complaints among a sample of Latina, Chinese, and Japanese women.

Discussion

In the United States, about 30% of people experience insomnia in their lifetime, yet the risk and protective factors associated with this sleep-wake disorder are understudied, especially among racial/ethnic immigrant minorities (Ford et al., 2015). Using a socioecological framework, our aims in this systematic review were to describe the sociodemographic characteristics of peer-reviewed published articles on insomnia and sleep quality in Asian, Black, and Latinx immigrants in the United States, describe the prevalence of insomnia and poor sleep quality in these populations and summarize the state of the science on the risk and protective factors of insomnia and poor sleep quality for these racial/ethnic immigrant groups. Of 482 eligible articles, 6.22% met inclusion criteria, and 1.87% included racial/ethnic minority immigrant only samples. The main findings of this review and implications for future research and clinical practice are discussed below.

Our first aim was to describe the sociodemographic characteristics of included articles. Of the articles that included immigrant only samples, 16.7% focused on Asian immigrants, 20% focused on Latinx immigrants, and 0% focused on Black immigrants. These relative percentages do not correspond to the demographic composition of the immigrant population in the United States. For example, Latinx immigrants compose 45.1% of the immigrant population, followed by Asian immigrants at 26.5%, and Black immigrants at 8.9%, and yet the immigration focused scholarship on insomnia and sleep quality did not surpass 20% for Asian and Latinx immigrants, and was 0% for Black immigrants (United States Census Bureau Population Division, n.d.). This represents a significant gap because the Black immigrant US population, particularly those originating from African countries, has grown exponentially in the past decade (United States Census Bureau Population Division, n.d.; Hamilton & Hummer, 2011). Further, disaggregation by country of origin was not the norm for included articles; though there were some exceptions for articles that included Asian immigrants from Japan, China, and Vietnam, Black Caribbean immigrants from English-speaking Caribbean countries, Haiti, and the Dominican Republic (Jean-Louis et al., 2008), and Latinx immigrants from Mexico. The inattention to country of origin differences in research on immigrant sleep health is problematic because of the vast heterogeneity within the immigrant population in the United States, as well as the consistent research showing important health differences by country of origin, and cohort of arrival (Alcántara, Patel, et al., 2017; Hamilton & Hummer, 2011). For example, the top five sending countries for Black immigrants in the United States include Jamaica, Haiti, Nigeria, Ethiopia, and Trinidad & Tobago (Anderson & Lopez, 2018), which represent different cultures and living conditions that may affect health. Future research should prioritize the exploration of the country of origin differences within each of the major immigrant groups in relation to insomnia. Further, there is an urgent need for research on risk and protective factors in Black immigrants from the diaspora, with an emphasis on understanding country of origin differences.

Our second aim was to describe the population prevalence of insomnia and poor sleep quality for Asian, Black, and Latinx US immigrants. Only 10% of included articles were of representative regional samples in the United States, and 23.33% were of nationally representative samples. As such, our review indicates that the national prevalence of insomnia among racial/ethnic minority immigrants is largely unknown, particularly for Asian and Black immigrants. From the best available evidence based on convenience samples, the prevalence of insomnia or insomnia symptoms ranges from 17% to 27% among Asian immigrants (Hirooka et al., 2012; Sok, 2008), and 6%–54% for African Caribbean immigrants or Black immigrants depending on the symptom (Jean-Louis et al., 2008, 2001). Population-based data indicate that the prevalence of insomnia among Latinx immigrants is 21.12% (Seicean & Seicean, 2010). Importantly, none of the articles on insomnia in Latinx immigrants examined differences by self-identified race (Black vs. White), and at times ethnicity was conflated with race [as in the case of Dominicans who were identified as Black immigrants by study investigators in the absence of a self-assessment of race (Jean-Louis et al., 2008)]. Future research should use population-based studies with valid and reliable insomnia measures to estimate the prevalence of insomnia in racial/ethnic immigrant communities, particularly for Asian and Black immigrants, and by country of origin. Moreover, future research on the intersections of race and Latinx ethnicity and its effect on sleep is warranted given the mounting evidence that self-identified Black race vs. White race among Latinxs is associated with worse health (Cuevas, Dawson, & Williams, 2016).

Our third aim was to conduct a socioecological analysis of the risk and protective factors associated with insomnia and poor sleep quality in Asian, Black, and Latinx immigrants. Traditional sociodemographic factors such as female gender, older age, and low educational attainment were not consistently associated with increased insomnia risk. For example, while one study with Asian immigrants found that women had worse sleep quality than men (Riley et al., 2016), which is consistent with gender findings in studies of the general population (Theorell-Haglöw et al., 2018), the remaining studies found either increased odds for insomnia among Asian immigrant men vs. Asian immigrant women (Young et al., 2013), or no statistically significant gender differences in insomnia or sleep quality in Latinx immigrants (Grzywacz et al., 2011;Sandberg et al., 2012; Seicean & Seicean, 2010). Similarly, contrary to prior research indicating that increased age and lower socioeconomic status are risk factors for insomnia (Gellis et al., 2005; Green, Espie, & Benzeval, 2014; Ohayon, 2002), the majority of articles found no statistically significant associations between age and insomnia or poor sleep quality, and educational attainment and insomnia in Latinx adults (Hsu, 2001; Sandberg et al., 2012, 2014; Seicean & Seicean, 2010; Young et al., 2013). Of note, other work has found significant differences in sleep outcomes when examining the interaction of socioeconomic status indicators with race, ethnicity, and other racial/ethnic minority-related factors (Alcántara et al., 2019; Cunningham, Wheaton, Ford, & Croft, 2016; Jackson et al., 2014), yet these interactions were not tested in articles of immigrant only samples. As such, future research should examine how social identities such as race, socioeconomic status, age, and gender intersect with immigrant status as a means to uncover unique predisposing, precipitating, and perpetuating factors of insomnia among racial/ethnic minority immigrants, information that could be incorporated into behavioral treatments for insomnia.

Among mental health conditions and psychosocial factors, depression was the most studied and consistently associated with increased risk of insomnia across immigrant groups (Grzywacz et al., 2011; Hsu, 2001; Kelly, 2010; Sandberg et al., 2012, 2016, 2014; Seicean & Seicean, 2010), which is consistent with prior research with US-born Whites (Alvaro, Roberts, & Harris, 2013). Additionally, while traumatic experiences were identified as a risk factor for insomnia in Asian immigrants (Young et al., 2013), no articles examined premigration traumatic experiences, though one article with Asian immigrants examined cultural concepts of distress that included trauma (Young et al., 2013). This is important because premigration exposure to political violence and trauma is broadly associated with underutilization of mental health care and poor health (Del Gaizo, Elhai, & Weaver, 2011; Fortuna, Porche, & Alegria, 2008). Future research on premigration traumatic experiences and cultural concepts of distress may elucidate important precipitating factors of insomnia and inform the development and enhancement of insomnia treatments in immigrant populations that are not otherwise specified in prevailing treatment models (Borbély, 1982; Spielman et al., 1987). Importantly, only one article sampling Black immigrants examined emotion regulation strategies (Consedine et al., 2002), even though emotion regulation has been associated with insomnia (Carney, Harris, Falco, & Edinger, 2013; Palmer & Alfano, 2017). Relatedly, only 3.33% of articles examined coping strategies as protective factors for insomnia (Hsu, 2001). Research on coping strategies in immigrants could help identify strength-based treatments for insomnia that capitalize on protective coping strategies that are consonant with the specific country of origin cultural strengths and values.

Acculturation and migration-related factors were inconsistently associated with insomnia and sleep quality across racial/ethnic minority immigrants. Duration in the United States was significantly associated with insomnia symptoms in one Latinx immigrant sample (Sandberg et al., 2012) but not in a population-based Latinx immigrant sample or in Asian immigrant samples (Hsu, 2001; Seicean & Seicean, 2010). Language proficiency was not significantly associated with insomnia or sleep quality among Latinx immigrants (Sandberg et al., 2012; Seicean & Seicean, 2010), though speaking English was associated with an increased risk of insomnia in combined US-born and immigrant Latinx samples (Hale et al., 2014; Manber et al., 2013; Riley et al., 2008). US-born status vs. immigrant status and other Latin American born status vs. Mexico-born status were significantly associated with poor sleep in Black and Latinx immigrants (Consedine et al., 2002; Seicean & Seicean, 2010). Importantly, acculturation stress was only examined in two articles with combined US-born and immigrant Latinx samples (Alcántara et al., 2019; Alcántara, Patel, et al., 2017), with only one article testing moderation by nativity status (Alcántara et al., 2019). By and large, most studies of acculturation and migration-related factors did not use validated measures of acculturation processes or strategies, or sociocultural stressors. This scientific gap presents an opportunity to improve mental health care for racial/ethnic minority immigrants by assessing and addressing culturally relevant stressors in insomnia interventions. Indeed, a systematic review of randomized controlled trials (RCTs) of cultural adaptations of psychological interventions for sleep-wake disorders (Alcántara et al., n.d.), found that none of the RCTs focused on immigrant populations.

Of note, racial/ethnic discrimination, an important psychosocial and sociocultural stressor was not examined in any of the immigrant only articles.

Although racial/ethnic discrimination has been associated with poor sleep health outcomes among racial/ethnic minorities (Slopen, Lewis, & Williams, 2016), this type of sociocultural stress was only examined in Latinx immigrant samples (Alcántara et al., 2019; Alcántara, Patel, et al., 2017; Garcini et al., 2018; Slopen & Williams, 2014). Considering US-born and immigrant racial/ethnic minorities experience racial/ethnic discrimination at high rates in the United States (Lee, Perez, Boykin, & Mendoza-Denton, 2019), greater understanding of how racial/ethnic discrimination affects insomnia, especially among racial/ethnic minority immigrants who may face antiimmigrant discrimination in addition to racial/ethnic discrimination is necessary for the delivery of high quality culturally sensitive behavioral health care.

Macro-level factors were examined in 16.67% of Asian and Latinx immigrant only articles. Housing conditions and work environments were inconsistently associated with insomnia symptoms and poor sleep health, though one study found a significant relationship between the availability of air conditioning and sleep quality among farmworkers in North Carolina (Sandberg et al., 2014). Access to health care, measured through the availability of health insurance, and employment characteristics were the only structural factors examined among Asian and Latinx immigrants. Because environmental and neighborhood factors influence sleep health (Johnson, Billings, & Hale, 2018), future research should identify macro-level intervention targets that can be addressed to improve sleep health at community and populations levels. Future research should also examine the impact of other macro-level factors such as immigration policies, context of exit, and reception, which may also have a direct and indirect effect on sleep.

Overall, there was no clear pattern of similarities and differences in risk and protective factors of insomnia or poor sleep quality across immigrant groups, with the exception of depression, which was a consistent risk factor of insomnia for Asian and Latinx immigrants. Of three articles sampling multiethnic immigrant adults, only one article compared risk factors for sleep complaints across Chinese, Japanese, and Latinx middle-aged women (Hale et al., 2014). Acculturation, operationalized as speaking English more frequently than other languages, was a common risk factor for sleep complaints among Japanese and Latinx immigrant women but not among Chinese women while being US-born vs. being an immigrant was associated with increased sleep complaints among Chinese women but not Japanese or Latinx women (Hale et al., 2014). Although the behavioral, psychological, and cognitive mechanisms of insomnia and poor sleep quality are not expected to differ across immigrant groups, what may differ across racial/ethnic immigrant groups is the exposure to key migration-related contextual factors. Race and ethnicity may interact with key migration-related contextual factors such as premigration socioeconomic status, English language proficiency, and migration policies at the time of arrival to differently shape risk of insomnia and poor sleep quality across racial/ethnic immigrant groups. For example, the risk of insomnia for Black immigrants with high-socioeconomic status backgrounds who migrate from an English-speaking country may be different or similar from the risk of insomnia for White Latinx immigrants with low socioeconomic status backgrounds who migrate from a Spanish-speaking country based on differential exposure to stress resulting from racism, language barriers, and financial strain, all risk factors for insomnia. Future research should examine the similarities and differences of risk and protective factor of insomnia across immigrant groups, with special attention to differences in exposure to migration-related contextual factors and stress.

This systematic review has several limitations. Articles included in this review measured insomnia and sleep quality outcomes differently, therefore, a proper evaluation of study quality and risk of bias could not be completed. Comparisons across studies and across immigrant groups of risk and protective factors were also limited by the heterogeneity of insomnia and sleep quality measures. Other limitations of this review included limited generalizability of findings because most articles included convenience samples. We also did not assess risk and protective factors for non-Latinx White immigrants because we limited our review to the top three racial/ethnic minority immigrant groups in the United States. Lastly, as with other systematic reviews, there is a risk that relevant articles may not have been included in the initial search, although several databases were searched to decrease risk.

Conclusion

Insomnia is prevalent in the United States and associated with high public health and societal costs in the US-born adult population. Yet, the risk and protective factors of insomnia and poor sleep quality among racial/ethnic immigrants in the United States are understudied. We used a socioecological framework to conduct a systematic review to describe the state of science on the prevalence as well as the risk and protective factors of insomnia among Asian, Black, and Latinx immigrant groups, the three largest immigrant groups in the United States. Of the articles that included immigrant only samples, 16.7% focused on Asian immigrants, 20% focused on Latinx immigrants, and 0% focused on Black immigrants. More research is needed to understand the prevalence, risk, and protective factors of insomnia across socioecological levels, particularly among Black immigrants who were disproportionality underrepresented in the articles that met inclusion criteria in this review. The racial/ethnic minority immigrant population constitutes an important proportion of the US population (Radford & Noe-Bustamante, 2019), therefore, in order to advance the health of the nation, it is essential to identify the risk and protective factors of insomnia. The application of a socioecological perspective to prevailing treatment models for insomnia may lead to more accurate assessment of predisposing, precipitating, and perpetuating factors at the individual, social, and macro levels, which may lead to better treatment and treatment outcomes, particularly for marginalized racial/ethnic minority immigrant communities who may face stressors that may not be recognized in traditional psychosocial models of insomnia.

References

Alcántara, C., Estevez, C. D., & Alegría, M. (2017). Latino and Asian immigrant adult health. In S. J. Schwartz & J. Unger (Eds.), *The Oxford Handbook of Acculturation and Health*. New York, NY: Oxford University Press.

Alcántara, C., Gallo, L. C., Wen, J., Dudley, K. A., Wallace, D. M., Mossavar-Rahmani, Y., et al. (2019). Employment status and the association of sociocultural stress with sleep in the Hispanic Community Health Study/Study of Latinos (HCHS/SOL). *Sleep*, *42*(4). https://doi.org/10.1093/sleep/zsz002.

Alcántara, C., Giorgio Cosenzo, L., McCullough, E., Vogt, T., Falzon, A. L., & Perez Ibarra, I. (n.d.). Cultural adaptation of psychological interventions for prevalent sleep-wake disorders in the United States: A systematic review (in preparation).

Alcántara, C., Patel, S. R., Carnethon, M., Castaneda, S., Isasi, C. R., Davis, S., et al. (2017). Stress and sleep: Results from the Hispanic Community Health Study/Study of Latinos Sociocultural Ancillary Study. *SSM—Population Health*, *3*, 713–721. https://doi.org/10.1016/j.ssmph.2017.08.004.

Alegria, M., Canino, G., Stinson, F. S., & Grant, B. F. (2006). Nativity and DSM-IV psychiatric disorders among Puerto Ricans, Cuban Americans, and non-Latino Whites in the United States: Results from the National Epidemiologic Survey on alcohol and related conditions. *The Journal of Clinical Psychiatry*, *67*(1), 56–65. https://doi.org/10.4088/jcp.v67n0109.

Alvaro, P. K., Roberts, R. M., & Harris, J. K. (2013). A systematic review assessing bidirectionality between sleep disturbances, anxiety, and depression. *Sleep*, *36*(7), 1059–1068. https://doi.org/10.5665/sleep.2810.

Alvidrez, J., Castille, D., Laude-Sharp, M., Rosario, A., & Tabor, D. (2019). The National Institute on Minority Health and Health Disparities Research Framework. *American Journal of Public Health*, *109*(S1), S16–S20.

American Psychiatric Association. (2013). Sleep-wake disorders. In *Diagnostic and statistical manual of mental disorders*. American Psychiatric Association. https://doi.org/10.1176/appi.books.9780890425596.dsm12.

Anderson, M., & Lopez, G. (2018). *Key facts about black immigrants in the U.S.* Retrieved from Pew Research Center website: https://www.pewresearch.org/fact-tank/2018/01/24/key-facts-about-black-immigrants-in-the-u-s/.

Borbély, A. A. (1982). A two process model of sleep regulation. *Human Neurobiology*, *1*(3), 195–204.

Bronfenbrenner, U., & Morris, P. A. (2007). The bioecological model of human development. In *Handbook of child psychology*. https://doi.org/10.1002/9780470147658.chpsy0114.

Carney, C. E., Harris, A. L., Falco, A., & Edinger, J. D. (2013). The relation between insomnia symptoms, mood, and rumination about insomnia symptoms. *Journal of Clinical Sleep Medicine*, *9*(6), 567–575. https://doi.org/10.5664/jcsm.2752.

Cervantes, R. C., Padilla, A. M., & Salgado de Snyder, N. (1991). The Hispanic Stress Inventory: A culturally relevant approach to psychosocial assessment. *Psychological Assessment: A Journal of Consulting and Clinical Psychology*, *3*(3), 438–447. https://doi.org/10.1037/1040-3590.3.3.438.

Chen, X., Redline, S., Shields, A. E., Williams, D. R., & Williams, M. A. (2014). Associations of allostatic load with sleep apnea, insomnia, short sleep duration, and other sleep disturbances: Findings from the National Health and Nutrition Examination Survey 2005 to 2008. *Annals of Epidemiology*, *24*(8), 612–619. https://doi.org/10.1016/j.annepidem.2014.05.014.

Consedine, N. S., Magai, C., Cohen, C. I., & Gillespie, M. (2002). Ethnic variation in the impact of negative affect and emotion inhibition on the health of older adults. *The Journals of Gerontology. Series B, Psychological Sciences and Social Sciences*, *57*(5), P396–P408. https://doi.org/10.1093/geronb/57.5.p396.

Cuevas, A. G., Dawson, B. A., & Williams, D. R. (2016). Race and Skin Color in Latino Health: An Analytic Review. *American Journal of Public Health*, *106*(12), 2131–2136. https://doi.org/10.2105/AJPH.2016.303452.

Cunningham, T. J., Ford, E. S., Chapman, D. P., Liu, Y., & Croft, J. B. (2015). Independent and joint associations of race/ethnicity and educational attainment with sleep-related symptoms in a population-based US sample. *Preventive Medicine*, *77*, 99–105. https://doi.org/10.1016/j.ypmed.2015.05.008.

Cunningham, T. J., Wheaton, A. G., Ford, E. S., & Croft, J. B. (2016). Racial/ethnic disparities in self-reported short sleep duration among US-born and foreign-born adults. *Ethnicity & Health*, *21*(6), 628–638. https://doi.org/10.1080/13557858.2016.1179724.

D'Anna-Hernandez, K. L., Garcia, E., Coussons-Read, M., Laudenslager, M. L., & Ross, R. G. (2016). Sleep moderates and mediates the relationship between acculturation and depressive symptoms in pregnant Mexican-American women. *Maternal and Child Health Journal*, *20*(2), 422–433. https://doi.org/10.1007/s10995-015-1840-9.

Del Gaizo, A. L., Elhai, J. D., & Weaver, T. L. (2011). Posttraumatic stress disorder, poor physical health and substance use behaviors in a national trauma-exposed sample. *Psychiatry Research*, *188*(3), 390–395. https://doi.org/10.1016/j.psychres.2011.03.016.

Ford, E. S., Cunningham, T. J., Giles, W. H., & Croft, J. B. (2015). Trends in insomnia and excessive daytime sleepiness among US adults from 2002 to 2012. *Sleep Medicine*, *16*(3), 372–378. https://doi.org/10.1016/j.sleep.2014.12.008.

Fortuna, L. R., Porche, M. V., & Alegria, M. (2008). Political violence, psychosocial trauma, and the context of mental health services use among immigrant Latinos in the United States. *Ethnicity & Health*, *13*(5), 435–463. https://doi.org/10.1080/13557850701837286.

Garcini, L. M., Chirinos, D. A., Murdock, K. W., Seiler, A., LeRoy, A. S., Peek, K., et al. (2018). Pathways linking racial/ethnic discrimination and sleep among U.S.-born and foreign-born Latinxs. *Journal of Behavioral Medicine*, *41*(3), 364–373. https://doi.org/10.1007/s10865-017-9907-2.

Gellis, L. A., Lichstein, K. L., Scarinci, I. C., Durrence, H. H., Taylor, D. J., Bush, A. J., et al. (2005). Socioeconomic status and insomnia. *Journal of Abnormal Psychology*, *114*(1), 111–118. https://doi.org/10.1037/0021-843X.114.1.111.

Grandner, M. A., Petrov, M. E. R., Rattanaumpawan, P., Jackson, N., Platt, A., & Patel, N. P. (2013). Sleep symptoms, race/ethnicity, and socioeconomic position. *Journal of Clinical Sleep Medicine*, *9*(9), 897–905. 905A-905D https://doi.org/10.5664/jcsm.2990.

Green, M. J., Espie, C. A., & Benzeval, M. (2014). Social class and gender patterning of insomnia symptoms and psychiatric distress: A 20-year prospective cohort study. *BMC Psychiatry*, *14*(1), 152. https://doi.org/10.1186/1471-244X-14-152.

Green, R., Polotsky, A. J., Wildman, R. P., McGinn, A. P., Lin, J., Derby, C., et al. (2010). Menopausal symptoms within a Hispanic cohort: SWAN, the Study of Women's Health Across the Nation. *Climacteric: The Journal of the International Menopause Society*, *13*(4), 376–384. https://doi.org/10.3109/13697130903528272.

Grzywacz, J. G., Chatterjee, A. B., Quandt, S. A., Talton, J. W., Chen, H., Weir, M., et al. (2011). Depressive symptoms and sleepiness among Latino farmworkers in eastern North Carolina. *Journal of Agromedicine*, *16*(4), 251–260. https://doi.org/10.1080/1059924X.2011.605722.

Hale, L., & Rivero-Fuentes, E. (2011). Negative acculturation in sleep duration among Mexican immigrants and Mexican Americans. *Journal of Immigrant and Minority Health*, *13*(2), 402–407. https://doi.org/10.1007/s10903-009-9284-1.

Hale, L., Troxel, W. M., Kravitz, H. M., Hall, M. H., & Matthews, K. A. (2014). Acculturation and sleep among a multiethnic sample of women: The study of Women's Health Across the Nation (SWAN). *Sleep*, *37*(2), 309–317. https://doi.org/10.5665/sleep.3404.

Hamilton, T. G., & Hummer, R. A. (2011). Immigration and the health of U.S. black adults: Does country of origin matter? *Social Science & Medicine (1982)*, *73*(10), 1551–1560. https://doi.org/10.1016/j.socscimed.2011.07.026.

Heilemann, M. V., Choudhury, M. V., Kury, S. M., & Lee, K. A. (2012). Factors associated with sleep disturbance in women of Mexican descent. *Journal of Advanced Nursing (John Wiley & Sons, Inc)*, *68*(10), 2256–2266. https://doi.org/10.1111/j.1365-2648.2011.05918.x. cin20.

Hirooka, N., Takedai, T., & D'Amico, F. (2012). Lifestyle characteristics assessment of Japanese in Pittsburgh, USA. *Journal of Community Health*, *37*(2), 480–486. https://doi.org/10.1007/s10900-011-9467-2.

Hsu, H. C. (2001). Relationships between quality of sleep and its related factors among elderly Chinese immigrants in the Seattle area. *The Journal of Nursing Research*, *9*(5), 179–190.

Jackson, C. L., Hu, F. B., Redline, S., Williams, D. R., Mattei, J., & Kawachi, I. (2014). Racial/ethnic disparities in short sleep duration by occupation: The contribution of immigrant status. *Social Science & Medicine*, *118*, 71–79. https://doi.org/10.1016/j.socscimed.2014.07.059.

Javaheri, S., & Redline, S. (2017). Insomnia and risk of cardiovascular disease. *Chest*, *152*(2), 435–444. https://doi.org/10.1016/j.chest.2017.01.026.

Jean-Louis, G., Magai, C., Casimir, G. J., Zizi, F., Moise, F., McKenzie, D., et al. (2008). Insomnia symptoms in a multiethnic sample of American women. *Journal of Women's Health (2002)*, *17*(1), 15–25. https://doi.org/10.1089/jwh.2006.0310.

Jean-Louis, G., Magai, C. M., Cohen, C. I., Zizi, F., von Gizycki, H., DiPalma, J., et al. (2001). Ethnic differences in self-reported sleep problems in older adults. *Sleep*, *24*(8), 926–933. https://doi.org/10.1093/sleep/24.8.926.

Johnson, D. A., Billings, M. E., & Hale, L. (2018). Environmental determinants of insufficient sleep and sleep disorders: Implications for population health. *Current Epidemiology Reports*, *5*(2), 61–69. https://doi.org/10.1007/s40471-018-0139-y.

Kelly, U. (2010). Intimate partner violence, physical health, posttraumatic stress disorder, depression, and quality of life in latinas. *The Western Journal of Emergency Medicine*, *11*(3), 247–251.

Laugsand, L. E., Strand, L. B., Platou, C., Vatten, L. J., & Janszky, I. (2014). Insomnia and the risk of incident heart failure: A population study. *European Heart Journal*, *35*(21), 1382–1393. https://doi.org/10.1093/eurheartj/eht019.

Lee, R. T., Perez, A. D., Boykin, C. M., & Mendoza-Denton, R. (2019). On the prevalence of racial discrimination in the United States. *PLoS One*, *14*(1), e0210698. https://doi.org/10.1371/journal.pone.0210698.

Manber, R., Steidtmann, D., Chambers, A. S., Ganger, W., Horwitz, S., & Connelly, C. D. (2013). Factors associated with clinically significant insomnia among pregnant low-income Latinas. *Journal of Women's Health (2002)*, *22*(8), 694–701. https://doi.org/10.1089/jwh.2012.4039.

Marmot, M., Allen, J., Bell, R., Bloomer, E., & Goldblatt, P. (2012). WHO European review of social determinants of health and the health divide. *Lancet*, *380*(9846), 1011–1029 [NLM].

Martinez-Miller, E. E., Prather, A. A., Robinson, W. R., Avery, C. L., Yang, Y. C., Haan, M. N., et al. (2019). US acculturation and poor sleep among an intergenerational cohort of adult Latinos in Sacramento, California. *Sleep*, *42*(3). https://doi.org/10.1093/sleep/zsy246.

Mezick, E. J., Matthews, K. A., Hall, M., Strollo, P. J. J., Buysse, D. J., Kamarck, T. W., et al. (2008). Influence of race and socioeconomic status on sleep: Pittsburgh SleepSCORE project. *Psychosomatic Medicine*, *70*(4), 410–416. https://doi.org/10.1097/PSY.0b013e31816fdf21.

Nam, S., Whittemore, R., Jung, S., Latkin, C., Kershaw, T., & Redeker, N. S. (2018). Physical neighborhood and social environment, beliefs about sleep, sleep hygiene behaviors, and sleep quality among African Americans. *Sleep Health*, *4*(3), 258–264. https://doi.org/10.1016/j.sleh.2018.03.002.

Ohayon, M. M. (2002). Epidemiology of insomnia: What we know and what we still need to learn. *Sleep Medicine Reviews*, *6*(2), 97–111. https://doi.org/10.1053/smrv.2002.0186.

Ozminkowski, R. J., Wang, S., & Walsh, J. K. (2007). The direct and indirect costs of untreated insomnia in adults in the United States. *Sleep*, *30*(3), 263–273.

Palmer, C. A., & Alfano, C. A. (2017). Sleep and emotion regulation: An organizing, integrative review. *Sleep Medicine Reviews*, *31*, 6–16. https://doi.org/10.1016/j.smrv.2015.12.006.

Radford, J., & Noe-Bustamante, L. (2019). *Immigrants in America: Key charts and facts*. Retrieved from Pew Research Center website https://www.pewresearch.org/hispanic/2019/06/03/facts-on-u-s-immigrants/.

Riley, J. L., 3rd, Gibson, E., Zsembik, B. A., Duncan, R. P., Gilbert, G. H., & Heft, M. W. (2008). Acculturation and orofacial pain among Hispanic adults. *The Journal of Pain: Official Journal of the American Pain Society*, *9*(8), 750–758. https://doi.org/10.1016/j.jpain.2008.03.007.

Riley, K., Nazareno, J., & Malish, S. (2016). 24-hour care: Work and sleep conditions of migrant Filipino live-in caregivers in Los Angeles. *American Journal of Industrial Medicine*, *59*(12), 1120–1129. https://doi.org/10.1002/ajim.22647.

Robbins, R., Jean-Louis, G., Gallagher, R. A., Hale, L., Branas, C. C., Gooneratne, N., et al. (2019). Examining social capital in relation to sleep duration, insomnia, and daytime sleepiness. *Sleep Medicine*, *60*, 165–172. https://doi.org/10.1016/j.sleep.2019.03.019.

Roth, T., Coulouvrat, C., Hajak, G., Lakoma, M. D., Sampson, N. A., Shahly, V., et al. (2011). Prevalence and perceived health associated with insomnia based on DSM-IV-TR; International Statistical Classification of Diseases and Related Health Problems, Tenth Revision; and Research Diagnostic Criteria/International Classification of Sleep Disorders, Second Edition Criteria: Results from the America Insomnia Survey. *Biological Psychiatry*, *69*(6), 592–600. https://doi.org/10.1016/j.biopsych.2010.10.023.

Sandberg, J. C., Grzywacz, J. G., Talton, J. W., Quandt, S. A., Chen, H., Chatterjee, A. B., et al. (2012). A cross-sectional exploration of excessive daytime sleepiness, depression, and musculoskeletal pain among migrant farmworkers. *Journal of Agromedicine*, *17*(1), 70–80. https://doi.org/10.1080/1059924X.2012.626750.

Sandberg, J. C., Nguyen, H. T., Quandt, S. A., Chen, H., Summers, P., Walker, F. O., et al. (2016). Sleep quality among Latino farmworkers in North Carolina: Examination of the job control-demand-support model. *Journal of Immigrant and Minority Health*, *18*(3), 532–541. https://doi.org/10.1007/s10903-015-0248-3.

Sandberg, J. C., Talton, J. W., Quandt, S. A., Chen, H., Weir, M., Doumani, W. R., et al. (2014). Association between housing quality and individual health characteristics on sleep quality among Latino farmworkers. *Journal of Immigrant and Minority Health*, *16*(2), 265–272. https://doi.org/10.1007/s10903-012-9746-8.

Sarsour, K., Kalsekar, A., Swindle, R., Foley, K., & Walsh, J. K. (2011). The association between insomnia severity and healthcare and productivity costs in a health plan sample. *Sleep*, *34*(4), 443–450.

Schwartz, S. J., Unger, J. B., Zamboanga, B. L., & Szapocznik, J. (2010). Rethinking the concept of acculturation: Implications for theory and research. *The American Psychologist*, *65*(4), 237–251. https://doi.org/10.1037/a0019330.

Seicean, S., Neuhauser, D., Strohl, K., & Redline, S. (2011). An exploration of differences in sleep characteristics between Mexico-born US immigrants and other Americans to address the Hispanic paradox. *Sleep*, *34*(8), 1021–1031. https://doi.org/10.5665/SLEEP.1154.

Seicean, S., & Seicean, A. (2010). Insomnia in adult Latino immigrants in the United States. *Hispanic Health Care International*, *8*(4), 227–234. https://doi.org/10.1891/1540-4153.8.4.227.

Simonelli, G., Dudley, K. A., Weng, J., Gallo, L. C., Perreira, K., Shah, N. A., et al. (2017). Neighborhood factors as predictors of poor sleep in the Sueno Ancillary Study of the Hispanic Community Health Study/Study of Latinos. *Sleep*, *40*(1). https://doi.org/10.1093/sleep/zsw025.

Slopen, N., Lewis, T. T., & Williams, D. R. (2016). Discrimination and sleep: A systematic review. *Sleep Medicine*, *18*, 88–95. https://doi.org/10.1016/j.sleep.2015.01.012.

Slopen, N., & Williams, D. R. (2014). Discrimination, other psychosocial stressors, and self-reported sleep duration and difficulties. *Sleep*, *37*(1), 147–156. https://doi.org/10.5665/sleep.3326.

Sok, S. R. (2008). Sleep patterns and insomnia management in Korean-American older adult immigrants. *Journal of Clinical Nursing*, *17*(1), 135–143. https://doi.org/10.1111/j.1365-2702.2006.01869.x.

Spielman, A. J., Caruso, L. S., & Glovinsky, P. B. (1987). A behavioral perspective on insomnia treatment. *Psychiatric Clinics*, *10*(4), 541–553.

Theorell-Haglöw, J., Miller, C. B., Bartlett, D. J., Yee, B. J., Openshaw, H. D., & Grunstein, R. R. (2018). Gender differences in obstructive sleep apnoea, insomnia and restless legs syndrome in adults—What do we know? A clinical update. *Sleep Medicine Reviews*, *38*, 28–38. https://doi.org/10.1016/j.smrv.2017.03.003.

United States Census Bureau Population Division. (n.d.). Selected characteristics of the Native and Foreign-born populations: 2013–2017 American Community Survey 5-Year estimates. Retrieved 30 September 2019, from https://factfinder.census.gov/faces/tableservices/jsf/pages/productview.xhtml?src=CF.

Viruell-Fuentes, E. A., Miranda, P. Y., & Abdulrahim, S. (2012). More than culture: Structural racism, intersectionality theory, and immigrant health. *Social Science & Medicine*, *75*(12), 2099–2106. https://doi.org/10.1016/j.socscimed.2011.12.037.

Young, E., Xiong, S., Finn, L., & Young, T. (2013). Unique sleep disorders profile of a population-based sample of 747 Hmong immigrants in Wisconsin. *Social Science & Medicine (1982)*, *79*, 57–65. https://doi.org/10.1016/j.socscimed.2012.06.009.

Index

Note: Page numbers followed by *f* indicate figures and *t* indicate tables.

B

J

L

M

N

O

P

R

S

9780128161173